Case Studies in Cardiomyopathy

Case Studies in Cardiomyopathy

Editor: Orlando Gray

AMERICAN
MEDICAL PUBLISHERS
www.americanmedicalpublishers.com

AMERICAN
MEDICAL PUBLISHERS
www.americanmedicalpublishers.com

Cataloging-in-Publication Data

Case studies in cardiomyopathy / edited by Orlando Gray.
p. cm.
Includes bibliographical references and index.
ISBN 979-8-88740-594-0
1. Myocardium--Diseases. 2. Heart--Diseases. 3. Cardiology. I. Gray, Orlando.
RC685.M9 C37 2023
616.124--dc23

American Medical Publishers,
41 Flatbush Avenue,
1st Floor, New York,
NY 11217, USA

ISBN 979-8-88740-594-0 (Hardback)

Contents

Preface

Cardiomyopathy refers to a group of diseases that affect the heart muscles. Such diseases impair the ability of the heart to pump blood efficiently. In some cases, the heart rhythm may also be disrupted. Hypertrophic cardiomyopathy, restrictive cardiomyopathy, dilated cardiomyopathy, transthyretin amyloid cardiomyopathy (ATTR-CM), and arrhythmogenic right ventricular dysplasia (ARVD) are the most common types of cardiomyopathies. In the early stages of development of cardiomyopathy, there may be no symptoms or signs of cardiomyopathy. However, as the disease progresses, symptoms and signs start to show up. Common symptoms include bloating of the abdomen due to fluid buildup, exhaustion, breathlessness during activity or at rest, and coughing while lying down. Tests like electrocardiogram (EKG/ECG), ambulatory monitoring, myocardial biopsy, and exercise stress test are used to diagnose cardiomyopathy. The treatment of cardiomyopathies may include either or a combination of lifestyle modifications, surgery, and medications. These treatments can alleviate symptoms, reduce difficulties, and ensure that the disease does not progress. This book presents case studies on cardiomyopathies in the most comprehensible and easy-to-understand language. A number of latest researches have been included to keep the readers up-to-date with the global concepts in this medical condition.

This book unites the global concepts and researches in an organized manner for a comprehensive understanding of the subject. It is a ripe text for all researchers, students, scientists or anyone else who is interested in acquiring a better knowledge of this dynamic field.

I extend my sincere thanks to the contributors for such eloquent research chapters. Finally, I thank my family for being a source of support and help.

Editor

1

Severe Hyponatremia-Induced Stress Cardiomyopathy

Irushna Perera,[1] Sanjeewa Rajapakse,[1] and Shamila T. De Silva[1,2]

[1]*Colombo North Teaching Hospital, Ragama, Sri Lanka*
[2]*Faculty of Medicine, University of Kelaniya, Sri Lanka*

Correspondence should be addressed to Irushna Perera; irushna.p@gmail.com
Academic Editor: Kathleen Ngu

Takotsubo or stress cardiomyopathy is a non ischemic disease affecting the myocardium, which presents with typical features of myocardial ischemia. Although the presentation with acute central chest pain and shortness of breath mimics acute myocardial ischemia, there is an absence of actual disruption of cardiac blood supply via the coronaries due to acute plaque rupture or vascular spasm. The underlying pathophysiology of this clinical entity remains largely unclear, but a definite association with physical or emotional stress has been well established, hence the term "stress cardiomyopathy." The list of potential triggers continues to grow as the disorder is increasingly detected by clinicians and cardiologists, with better clinical insight and improved availability of cardiac investigations. We report a patient with Takotsubo cardiomyopathy associated with severe hyponatremia.

1. Introduction

Takotsubo cardiomyopathy is a potentially reversible disorder affecting the myocardium. It is characterized by transient apical ballooning of the left ventricle, evident on transthoracic echocardiography. Typically, the disease is seen in postmenopausal women, who present with central tightening chest pain and shortness of breath, with electrocardiographic changes which mimic coronary artery disease and a mild elevation of cardiac enzymes [1]. The condition is usually benign and has a self-limiting course, with recovery within days to weeks following removal of the emotional or physical trigger. Rarely, the syndrome may be complicated by lethal ventricular arrhythmias or ventricular rupture [2].

2. Case Report

A 73-year-old woman was admitted to the Emergency Department with vomiting, diarrhea, and confusion for two days. She had been generally unwell during the preceding two weeks, with poor oral intake. She had also developed a few presyncopal episodes during this time, but she had not lost consciousness. She denied chest pain or fever. She was on treatment for hypertension with verapamil, losartan, and spironolactone, along with atorvastatin for elevated lipids.

On admission, she was unwell, with a heart rate of 100 beats/minute, blood pressure of 140/90 mmHg, peripheral oxygen saturation of 97% breathing ambient air, and respiratory rate of 25 breaths/minute. She did not appear dehydrated. Electrocardiogram revealed ST segment elevations in leads I, II, aVF, and V3 to V6. A cardiac biomarker assay revealed a Troponin I of 0.343 ng/ml (upper limit of reference 0.04 ng/ml). She was initiated on treatment for an acute coronary event, with loading doses of oral aspirin, clopidogrel, atorvastatin, and subcutaneous low molecular weight heparin. Echocardiography revealed apical ballooning of the left ventricle (Figure 1) with mild left ventricular systolic dysfunction, suggestive of stress cardiomyopathy. However, treatment of a presumed acute coronary event was continued.

She was severely hyponatremic, with serum sodium of 104 mmol/L. Serum potassium was 3.7 mmol/L, and serum chloride was 72 mmol/L. As the patient was symptomatic,

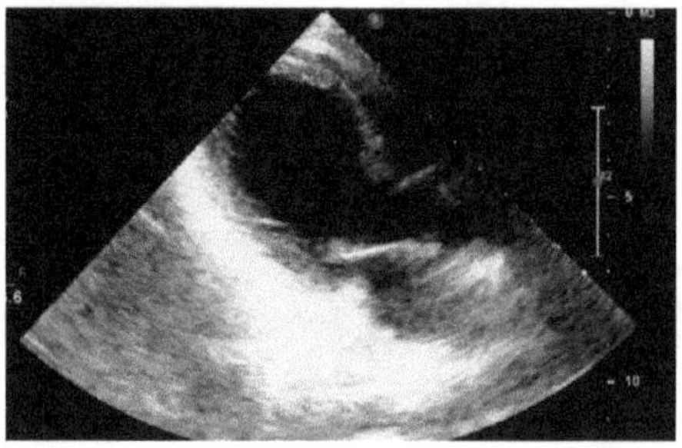

FIGURE 1: Echocardiogram long axis view revealed apical ballooning of the LV.

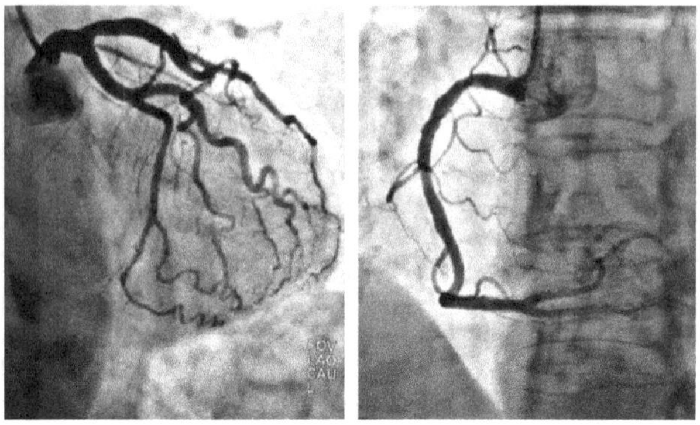

FIGURE 2: Coronary angiogram revealed normal coronary arteries.

serum sodium was corrected slowly, with 3% saline infusions over a few days. Concurrently, all medications liable to cause sodium depletion were withheld.

The day after admission, the patient developed a transient drop in blood pressure, which was managed with inotrope support for 18 hours, following which her hemodynamic status remained stable.

With the slow correction of serum sodium and treatment of a presumed acute coronary event, the patient's general condition improved, but she continued to have a residual amount of confusion. A psychiatry consultation was requested, and a diagnosis of a mixed anxiety, and depressive disorder was made. However, no drug treatment was given for her psychiatric illness, since the consulting psychiatrist felt counseling alone would be sufficient treatment.

A coronary angiogram was performed which failed to reveal any obstruction to the coronary blood flow (Figure 2), and a subsequent echocardiogram revealed a completely recovered myocardium with a left ventricular ejection fraction of 60% (Figure 3). These finding make stress cardiomyopathy the most likely diagnosis, possibly triggered by severe hyponatremia.

Investigations to identify the cause of hyponatremia revealed a serum osmolality of 234 mOsm/L, a urinary osmolality of 597 mOsm/L, and a urinary sodium excretion of 145 mmol/L. There was no evidence of renal or hepatic derangement, and thyroid functions were normal, making the syndrome of inappropriate ADH secretion (SIADH) a possible cause for hyponatremia. However, as the patient was on long-term angiotensin converting enzyme inhibitors and spironolactone for hypertension, a complex interplay of mechanisms could possibly have resulted in severe hyponatremia. Over the next six months at follow-up visits, the patient remained well, with normal serum sodium levels.

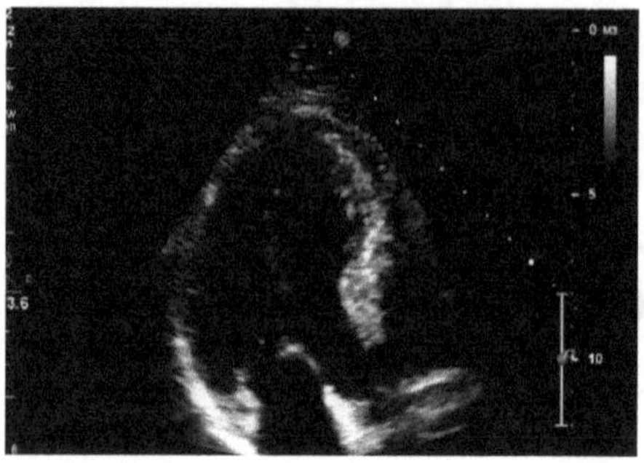

FIGURE 3: Subsequent echocardiogram revealing a completely recovered myocardium.

3. Discussion

Takotsubo cardiomyopathy is a syndrome characterized by transient, regional, systolic dysfunction of the left ventricle, mimicking regional wall motion abnormalities seen in coronary artery disease, but with absence of angiographic evidence of coronary artery obstruction [3]. The entity is also known as the apical ballooning syndrome due to its characteristic appearance on echocardiography and left ventriculography. Takotsubo in Japanese means "a fishing pot for trapping octopus," similar in shape to the left ventricle in patients with this condition [4]. Usually, the regional wall motion abnormality extends beyond the territory perfused by a single coronary artery [5].

The pathophysiology of Takotsubo cardiomyopathy remains poorly understood, even though numerous theories on its pathogenesis have been proposed. One of the postulated mechanisms is a surge of catecholamines in the circulation resulting in a stunned myocardium, microvascular dysfunction, and spasm of coronary arteries [1]. The proposed role of a catecholamine surge in the development of Takotsubo cardiomyopathy has been observed where cardiomyopathy has developed with infusions of noradrenaline and dopamine, initiated for causes other than cardiogenic shock [6, 7]. Limited data is available on possible triggers, even though the list keeps growing with increasing recognition of the disorder. Commonly, the onset follows intense emotional or physical stress. However, a few cases of Takotsubo cardiomyopathy associated with endocrine abnormalities and electrolyte disturbances have been described, where hyponatremia-associated Takotsubo cardiomyopathy has been reported [8–10].

Hyponatremia is a common electrolyte disorder, encountered especially among elderly patients, in whom finding the etiology of hyponatremia remains challenging as most often it tends to be multifactorial [7]. However, prescription drugs for various comorbidities, especially in the elderly, is the usual culprit, as was observed in our patient as well. The drugs with established potential to cause hyponatremia are diuretics, antidepressants, antipsychotics, and anticonvulsants, resulting in a significant number of Takotsubo cardiomyopathy cases being detected in patients on treatment for hypertension or heart failure and among those in psychiatry wards [8]. Development of Takotsubo cardiomyopathy, secondary to hyponatremia resulting from prescribed drugs, is well recognized. As with the well-known sequelae of hyponatremia, the rapidity with which the electrolyte disturbance develops is likely to be a deciding factor in the occurrence of Takotsubo cardiomyopathy, as chronic, persistent hyponatremia is a less likely trigger [9]. The mechanism of transient cardiac dysfunction in the setting of hyponatremia, whatever the etiology may be, remains unclear, but this association has been previously observed [10–13]. The possible mechanisms proposed are central nervous system dysfunction secondary to hyponatremia, which results in myocardial injury due to raised catecholamine levels, interference of myocardial contractility by low sodium concentration due to disruption of myocyte sodium and calcium exchange, and swelling of cardiac myocytes due to the resultant hypotonicity [9].

The case presented demonstrates the possible association of hyponatremia with stress cardiomyopathy, where the patient made a complete recovery from the cardiac disorder with correction of the electrolyte disturbance. As the detection rate of Takotsubo cardiomyopathy increases with increasing availability of sophisticated cardiac investigations, its possible triggers need to be kept in mind to guide clinicians towards an early and accurate diagnosis.

Consent

Written informed consent was obtained from the patient for publication of this case report.

Acknowledgments

We gratefully acknowledge the assistance given to us to collect clinical data by Drs. T N K Gamage and U. Illangasekera.

References

[1] Y. J. Akashi, D. S. Goldstein, G. Barbaro, and T. Ueyama, "Takotsubo Cardiomyopathy," *Circulation*, vol. 118, no. 25, pp. 2754-2762, 2008.

[2] K. M. Lampropoulos, D. Kotsas, and T. A. Iliopoulos, "Apical ballooning syndrome: a case report," *BMC Research Notes*, vol. 5, no. 1, 2012.

[3] K. A. Bybee, T. Kara, A. Prasad et al., "Systematic review: transient left ventricular apical ballooning: a syndrome that mimics ST-segment elevation myocardial infarction," *Annals of Internal Medicine*, vol. 141, no. 11, pp. 858–865, 2004.

[4] S. S. Virani, A. N. Khan, C. E. Mendoza, A. C. Ferreira, and E. de Marchena, "Takotsubo cardiomyopathy, or broken-heart syndrome," *Texas Heart Institute Journal*, vol. 34, no. 1, pp. 76–79, 2007.

[5] S. Y-Hassan and P. Tornvall, "Epidemiology, pathogenesis, and management of takotsubo syndrome," *Clinical Autonomic Research*, vol. 28, no. 1, pp. 53–65, 2018.

[6] A. Vieira, B. Batista, and T. Tribolet de Abreu, "Iatrogenic Takotsubo cardiomyopathy secondary to norepinephrine by continuous infusion for shock," *European Journal of Case Reports in Internal Medicine*, vol. 5, no. 7, p. 1, 2018.

[7] S. Hajsadeghi, "Dobutamine-induced takotsubo cardiomyopathy: a systematic review of the literature and case report," *The Anatolian Journal of Cardiology*, vol. 19, no. 6, pp. 412–416, 2018.

[8] M. Nakamura and T. Nagamine, "Severe lamotrigine-induced hyponatremia associated with Takotsubo cardiomyopathy," *Innov Clin Neurosci*, vol. 16, no. 7-08, pp. 32–34, 2019.

[9] E. Ç. Şimşek, "Unusual combined cause of Takotsubo cardiomiyopathy: hyponatremia and seizure," *Northern Clinics of Istanbul*, vol. 6, no. 3, pp. 304–307, 2018.

[10] S. Gupta, P. Goyal, S. Idrees, S. Aggarwal, D. Bajaj, and J. Mattana, "Association of endocrine conditions with Takotsubo cardiomyopathy: a comprehensive review," *Journal of the American Heart Association*, vol. 7, no. 19, article e009003, 2018.

[11] W. Elikowski, M. Małek-Elikowska, W. Greberska, M. Słomczyński, J. Marchlewska, and L. Korol, "Takotsubo syndrome in a patient with adrenal insufficiency, severe hyponatremia and coexistent coronary artery disease," *Pol Merkur Lekarski*, vol. 46, no. 274, pp. 182–186, 2019.

[12] F. Andreozzi, G. Cominetti, R. Karmali, and P. Kamgang, "Electrolyte disorders as triggers for Takotsubo cardiomyopathy," *European Journal of Case Reports in Internal Medicine*, vol. 5, no. LATEST ONLINE, p. 1, 2018, eCollection 2018.

[13] R. W. Schrier and S. Bansal, "Diagnosis and management of hyponatremia in acute illness," *Current Opinion in Critical Care*, vol. 14, no. 6, pp. 627–634, 2008.

2

A Case of Postpartum Takotsubo (Stress) Cardiomyopathy

Fadi Kandah,[1] Tanya Deol,[1] Pooja Dhruva,[1] Zachary Chandler,[1] Thaer Musa,[2] and Gladys Velarde[2]

[1]*Internal Medicine, UF Health Jacksonville, Dept. of Medicine, 655 W 8th Street, Jacksonville, FL 32209-6595, USA*
[2]*Cardiology, UF Health Jacksonville, Dept. of Cardiology, 655 W 8th Street, Jacksonville, FL 32209-6595, USA*

Correspondence should be addressed to Fadi Kandah; fadi.kandah@jax.ufl.edu

Academic Editor: Antonio de Padua Mansur

Takotsubo (stress) cardiomyopathy (TCM) is usually triggered by psychological and/or physical stress. Most often, it is seen in postmenopausal women. Cases of TCM related to pregnancy are rare. We present a unique case of a 35-year-old, two-day postpartum female who was diagnosed with TCM.

1. Introduction

Despite being described in the 1990s, TCM remains poorly understood. While known to be triggered by acute stressors, the exact mechanism is largely unknown. Numerous etiologies have been proposed, including excess catecholamine release during stress, hormones, microvascular ischemia, or spasms [1]. The syndrome mimics an acute coronary syndrome (ACS) presentation with angina-type chest pain, ischemic EKG changes, and elevated cardiac biomarkers. One of the hallmarks of the syndrome is findings on echocardiography which can show severe left ventricular dysfunction with regional dysfunction, most commonly a hypokinetic apex or apical ballooning. EKG abnormalities are very common, including ST elevations and diffuse T wave inversions and prolonged QTc with ST depressions being less common [1, 2]. Additionally, cardiac biomarkers can be elevated, although more modestly elevated compared to ST-elevated myocardial infarctions (STEMI) [2].

2. History of Presentation

A 35-year-old African-American woman (gravida 7, para 5) presented for evaluation of sudden onset substernal chest pain, diaphoresis, and dyspnea on exertion. Two days prior to presentation, she had a spontaneous vaginal delivery of a singleton healthy baby at term. Both her pregnancy and delivery were uncomplicated. At presentation, she had a temperature of 98.7°F, blood pressure of 140/87 mmHg, heart rate of 70 beats per minute, respiratory rate of 20 breaths per minute, and oxygen saturation of 97% on room air. Cardiopulmonary examination revealed no accessory muscle use, clear lungs to auscultation bilaterally, a regular rhythm, no cardiac murmurs or rub, and an S3 gallop without jugular venous distension. There was trace peripheral edema, and she had mild suprapubic tenderness with an otherwise unrevealing exam.

3. Past Medical History

The patient had a history of Roux-en-Y gastric bypass surgery (four years prior due to morbid obesity) and iron-deficiency anemia due to menorrhagia on oral iron supplementation. She did experience preeclampsia with a prior pregnancy without sequelae. She was a nonsmoker, consumed alcohol socially, and denied any illicit substance use.

4. Investigations

Initial chest radiographs and comprehensive metabolic panel were unremarkable. Only abnormality on complete blood count was hemoglobin level of 7.1 g/dL; patient's baseline hemoglobin was 8 g/dL. Chest computed tomography ruled out pulmonary embolism. The initial high-sensitivity troponin T (TnT) was 99 ng/L and 408 ng/L (reference range: 0-14 ng/L) an hour following. The initial electrocardiogram (EKG)

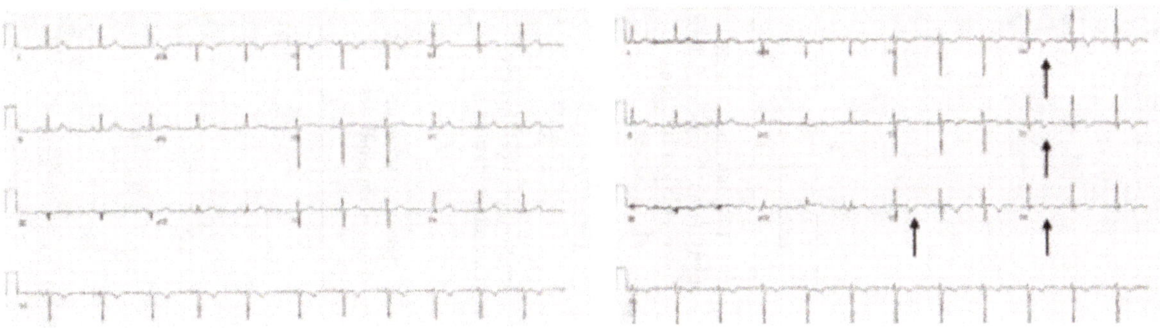

(a) (b)

Figure 1: (a) EKG on admission and (b) EKG two hours later showing dynamic T wave changes in leads V3-V6 (demonstrated by the arrows).

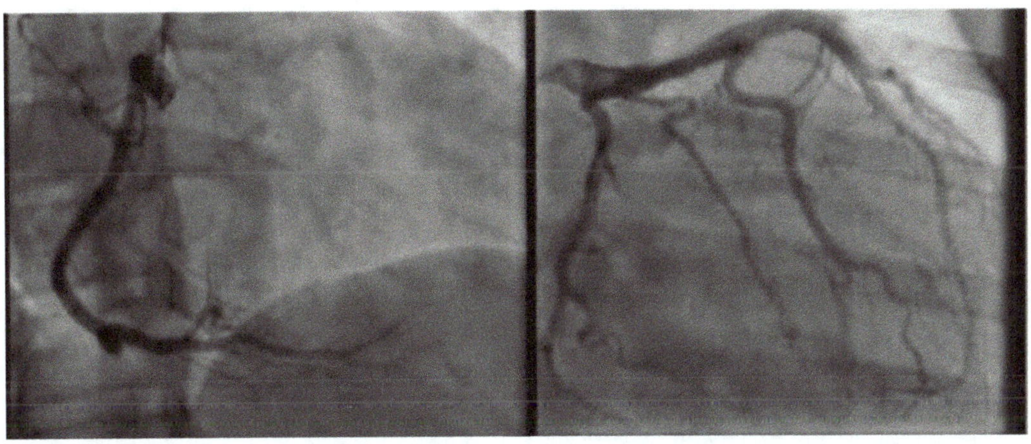

Figure 2: Left heart catheterization demonstrating angiographically normal coronary arteries.

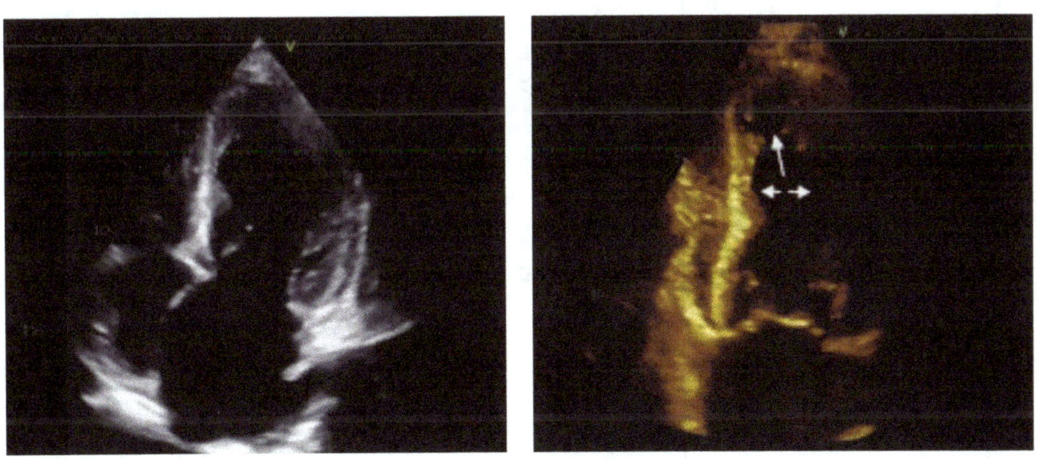

(a) (b)

Figure 3: Transthoracic echocardiogram four-chamber view (diastolic image on (a), systolic image on (b)) demonstrating classic pattern of apical akinesis and hypercontractility of midbasal segments of the LV (arrows on (b) emphasizing this specific pattern of wall motion abnormalities seen in Takotsubo's).

showed normal sinus rhythm without acute ischemic findings. EKG performed two hours later showed 0.5 mm ST elevation in leads II and aVF and dynamic T wave inversions in leads III, V3-V6 (Figure 1). The constellation of findings were initially most concerning for spontaneous coronary artery dissection (SCAD).

5. Differential Diagnosis

The differential diagnosis in this case included pulmonary emboli, spontaneous coronary artery dissection (SCAD), coronary artery spasm, ischemic obstructive coronary artery disease, peripartum cardiomyopathy, or TCM.

Table 1: Cardiac complications during pregnancy—distinctive features.

Condition	Timing	Cardiac biomarkers	LV dysfunction	LHC findings	Risk factors	Course recurrence/ prognosis	Treatment
TKSCM[1]	Antepartum, intrapartum, and/or immediate postpartum period	+	Present	Normal	Psychosocial stressors, comorbid psychological disorders	Recovery in 4-8 weeks; rare recurrence	Supportive care or guideline-directed medical therapy (GDMT) for heart failure with reduced ejection fraction
PPCM[3]	One month prepartum-5 months postpartum	+/−	Present	Normal	Advanced maternal age, preeclampsia, multiparity, twin gestations, black race	Recovery in 3-6 months; high recurrence rate	GDMT for heart failure with reduced EF
SCAD[10]	Third trimester-early postpartum	+	Absent	Radiolucent lumens	Black race, advanced maternal age, chronic hypertension, and preeclampsia	Variable prognosis; may recur	May require PCI, medical therapy, cardiac rehabilitation
Pre/ eclampsia[11]	Third trimester-decades later	+/−	Present or absent	Normal or coronary artery disease (increased risk later in life)	Advanced maternal age, black race, obesity, smoking, hypertension	Leads to increased risk for CAD, heart failure, stroke	Preventative measures, screening, and treatment of comorbidities

6. Management

She was initiated on aspirin and heparin infusion and taken urgently for left heart catheterization (LHC). This revealed no evidence of significant coronary artery disease, coronary dissection, spasm, or myocardial bridging (Figure 2).

Transthoracic echocardiogram (TTE) (Figure 3) was performed and revealed a preserved ejection fraction, left ventricular apical hypokinesis, a mildly enlarged right ventricle with normal systolic function, and no significant valvular pathologies. Based on these findings, the patient was diagnosed with TCM. The patient was observed for 36 hours with no recurrence of chest pain. The patient was initiated on goal-directed medical therapy and discharged from the hospital in stable condition. There were plans for close outpatient cardiology follow-up and repeat TTE in 2 months but was subsequently lost to follow-up.

7. Discussion

TCM is characterized by left ventricular systolic dysfunction, in the absence of obstructive coronary artery disease. Currently, about two percent of all patients undergoing emergency coronary angiography for suspected ACS have TCM [1]. About 90% of patients with TCM are postmenopausal women [1]. However, TCM in pregnancy or peripartum state is extremely rare. In general, acute cardiac complications during pregnancy or in the peripartum periods are difficult to differentiate at times. The two most common are ischemic heart disease and peripartum cardiomyopathy [3]. Peripartum cardiomyopathy occurs in 1 per 3,000 births and typically presents in the last month of pregnancy or in the first five months postpartum [1, 3]. As opposed to TCM, which presents more similarly to ACS, patients with peripartum cardiomyopathy present with signs and symptoms of congestive heart failure. TCM also differs in that it can develop shortly after delivery as opposed to peripartum cardiomyopathy that can take months to develop or manifest clinically. TCM can also present in the postpartum period with coexisting conditions associated with a heightened sympathetic response. Acute intracranial disease processes and injuries have been shown to be possible triggers for TCM. For example, a clinical case demonstrated a patient who initially presented with unrelenting headaches in the postpartum period with reversible cerebral vasoconstriction who developed chest pain and was diagnosed with TCM [4]. Furthermore, another rare trigger for postpartum TCM that has been cited is pheochromocytoma. Peripartum pheochromocytoma is difficult to diagnose as the symptoms can often mimic preeclampsia [5]. Establishing the trigger for TCM postpartum is vital so that management can be altered to focus on the underlying etiology.

Peripartum cardiomyopathy is more widely understood, and risk factors include older age, black race, preeclampsia, multiparity, and twin gestations [3]. Our patient had many of the risk factors usually associated with peripartum cardiomyopathy, including multiparity, twin gestations, and a previous pregnancy complicated by preeclampsia. Differentiating between the two syndromes is very important as they require different management and follow-up. For example, beta-adrenergic inotropic agents can be used in peripartum cardiomyopathy, while it is contraindicated in TCM [6]. Additionally, left ventricular function tends to recover fully and recovers more rapidly in TCM as compared to peripartum cardiomyopathy [5, 6]. See Table 1 for key differences between possible cardiac complications during pregnancy and the peripartum period.

The nomenclature and diagnostic criteria behind TCM continue to evolve. Initially, TCM was defined by Mayo's diagnostic criteria which was established in 2004 [7]. This includes hypokinesis of the left ventricular mid segment, with or without apical involvement, absence of coronary disease on angiography, new EKG or troponin abnormalities, and the absence of myocarditis or pheochromocytoma [7, 8]. Our patient fulfilled all these criteria which established the diagnosis. More recent research continues to further expand the diagnostic basis behind TCM and have separated it into "primary" and "secondary." In primary TCM, the initial stressor may not be clear, and the patient's cardiac symptoms are the main reason for seeking medical care. Secondary TCM requires the patient to be already hospitalized, whether for surgical, psychiatric, or obstetric reasons [9]. As in our patient, the inciting stressful trigger is presumed to be her pregnancy, which imposes both emotional and physical stressors. This is a valuable distinction as TCM should be included in the differential diagnosis of other pregnancy-related complications, such as peripartum cardiomyopathy, spontaneous coronary artery dissection (SCAD), and eclampsia.

8. Conclusions

In conclusion, although it is rare, TCM can present during pregnancy. Recognition of this condition and early diagnosis are important as it can rarely lead to cardiac rupture and death. It is also vital to distinguish this condition from the widely understood and more common cardiac complication seen in pregnancy—peripartum cardiomyopathy. Once diagnosed, management of hospitalized patients with TCM consists of close monitoring of hemodynamics inpatient for 1-2 days, as in our patient. All patients should have close cardiology follow-up with serial echocardiograms to monitor for improvement in LV function. Supportive care with goal-directed medical therapies for LV dysfunction and heart failure if present should be instituted in patients with TCM. Most patients will recover normal cardiac function within 4-8 weeks [7]. Unfortunately, our patient was lost to clinical follow-up and a repeat echocardiography was not done. However, although recurrence in premenopausal women is very rare, all patients should be counseled of the potential risks in further pregnancies.

Abbreviations

TCM: Takotsubo cardiomyopathy
SCAD: Spontaneous coronary artery dissection
TnT: Troponin T
LHC: Left heart catheterization

STEMI: ST-elevated myocardial infarction
ACS: Acute coronary syndrome.

Additional Points

Learning Objectives. (i) To have a high index of suspicion for TCM in the peripartum period in women presenting with symptoms resembling an acute coronary syndrome. (ii) To recognize key differences (risk factors, imaging findings, and prognosis) in cardiac complications in pregnancy and peripartum period.

Authors' Contributions

All authors have read, edited, and approved the submission of this manuscript.

References

[1] F. Pelliccia, J. C. Kaski, F. Crea, and P. G. Camici, "Pathophysiology of takotsubo syndrome," *Circulation*, vol. 135, no. 24, pp. 2426–2441, 2017.

[2] A. Prasad, A. Lerman, and C. S. Rihal, "Apical ballooning syndrome (Tako-Tsubo or stress cardiomyopathy): a mimic of acute myocardial infarction," *American Heart Journal*, vol. 155, no. 3, pp. 408–417, 2008.

[3] Y. Yaqub, L. A. Jenkins, K. M. Nugent, and W. Chokesuwattanaskul, "Postpartum depression and apical ballooning syndrome (takotsubo syndrome)," *Journal of Obstetrics and Gynaecology Canada*, vol. 31, no. 8, pp. 736–739, 2009.

[4] E. Enderton and M. Cardwell, "Postpartum takotsubo cardiomyopathy with reversible cerebral vasoconstriction syndrome: a case report," *Case Reports in Perinatal Medicine*, vol. 2, no. 1-2, pp. 21–24, 2013.

[5] M. Itagane, J. Nakazato, and M. Kinjo, "Postpartum pheochromocytoma-induced takotsubo syndrome," *BMJ Case Reports*, vol. 14, no. 3, article e240098, 2021.

[6] R. Citro, M. Bellino, F. Minichino, D. di Vece, D. Ferraioli, and R. Petta, "Subsequent safe pregnancy with cesarean delivery in a patient with a history of peripartum takotsubo syndrome complicated by cardiogenic shock," *Journal of Cardiovascular Echography*, vol. 27, no. 3, pp. 114–117, 2017.

[7] F. M. Oindi, E. Sequeira, H. R. Sequeira, and S. K. Mutiso, "Takotsubo cardiomyopathy in pregnancy: a case report and literature review," *BMC Pregnancy and Childbirth*, vol. 19, no. 1, p. 89, 2019.

[8] C. Templin, J. R. Ghadri, J. Diekmann et al., "Clinical features and outcomes of Takotsubo (stress) cardiomyopathy," *The New England Journal of Medicine*, vol. 373, no. 10, pp. 929–938, 2015.

[9] A. R. Lyon, E. Bossone, B. Schneider et al., "Current state of knowledge on Takotsubo syndrome: a position statement from the Taskforce on Takotsubo Syndrome of the Heart Failure Association of the European Society of Cardiology," *European Journal of Heart Failure*, vol. 18, no. 1, pp. 8–27, 2016.

[10] M. Garcia-Guimarães, T. Bastante, P. Antuña et al., "Spontaneous coronary artery dissection: mechanisms, diagnosis and management," *European Cardiology Review*, vol. 15, pp. 1–8, 2020.

[11] B. Thilaganathan and E. Kalafat, "Cardiovascular system in preeclampsia and beyond," *Hypertension*, vol. 73, no. 3, pp. 522–531, 2019.

3

A Rare Case of Sudden Death in a Patient with Takotsubo Cardiomyopathy Secondary to Cardiac Rupture

Tarun Dalia[1] **Bashar S. Amr,**[2] **Ankit Agrawal**[3] **Archana Gautam,**[4] **Venkata Rakesh Sethapati,**[5] **and Jared Kvapil**[2]

[1]*Internal Medicine, University of Kansas Medical Center, Kansas City, KS 66160, USA*
[2]*Department of Cardiovascular Medicine, University of Kansas Medical Center, Kansas City, KS 66160, USA*
[3]*Internal Medicine Residency Program, Rutgers Robert Wood Johnson Medical School-Saint Peter's University Hospital, New Brunswick, NJ 08901, USA*
[4]*Montgomery Internal Medicine Residency Program, University of Alabama, Montgomery, Alabama 36116, USA*
[5]*Department of Pathology & Laboratory Medicine, University of Kansas Medical Center, Kansas City, KS 66160, USA*

Correspondence should be addressed to Tarun Dalia; tdalia2@kumc.edu
Academic Editor: Antonio de Padua Mansur

Takotsubo cardiomyopathy (TCM), also known as broken heart syndrome or stress-induced cardiomyopathy, is a rare condition with an estimated incidence of 0.02% of all hospitalizations in United States and 2% of all acute coronary syndrome presentations. TCM predominately presents as a transient wall motion abnormality of the left ventricular apex due to emotional or physical stress. Cardiac rupture in the setting of TCM is an extremely rare phenomenon with limited published case reports. We present a case of a 75-year-old female who had cardiac rupture secondary to TCM and performed a literature review using Ovid MEDLINE for published cases showing this association. After the literature review, we found 20 cases showing this association, which are listed in a tabular fashion.

1. Introduction

Takotsubo cardiomyopathy (TCM), also known as stress-induced cardiomyopathy, was first described in Japan in 1990 [1]. It mimics acute coronary syndrome and is characterized by transient systolic and diastolic dysfunction of the left ventricle, wall motion abnormalities, and elevated cardiac biomarkers and is frequently preceded by emotional or physical stress [2]. Ballooning of the left ventricular apex with a finding of patent coronary arteries is typically present on left ventriculography and cardiac catheterization, respectively. It is diagnosed in 0.02% of all nationwide hospitalization and predominantly involves elderly females [3]. The inpatient mortality rate in patients with TCM is 4.5% [3]. There has been a gradual increase in the incidence of TCM with the realization that this entity is not as benign as it was thought to be. As per recent TCM registry, on long-term follow-up, rate of major adverse cardiac and cerebrovascular events was 9.9% per patient-year and death was 5.6% per patient-year [4]. While TCM is usually reversible, it may present with rare complications including systemic embolism, life-threatening ventricular arrhythmias, cardiogenic shock, and cardiac rupture leading to cardiac arrest [5]. We present an exceptional rare case of TCM leading to left ventricular wall rupture. To the best of our knowledge, only 20 cases have been reported so far showing this very rare outcome.

2. Case Presentation

A 75-year-old female with past medical history of coronary artery disease, hypertension, hyperlipidemia, paroxysmal atrial fibrillation, systemic lupus erythematosus, and deep venous thrombosis was transferred from an outside hospital for the management of non-ST segment elevation myocardial infarction (NSTEMI). The patient presented to the local emergency department with substernal chest pain radiating

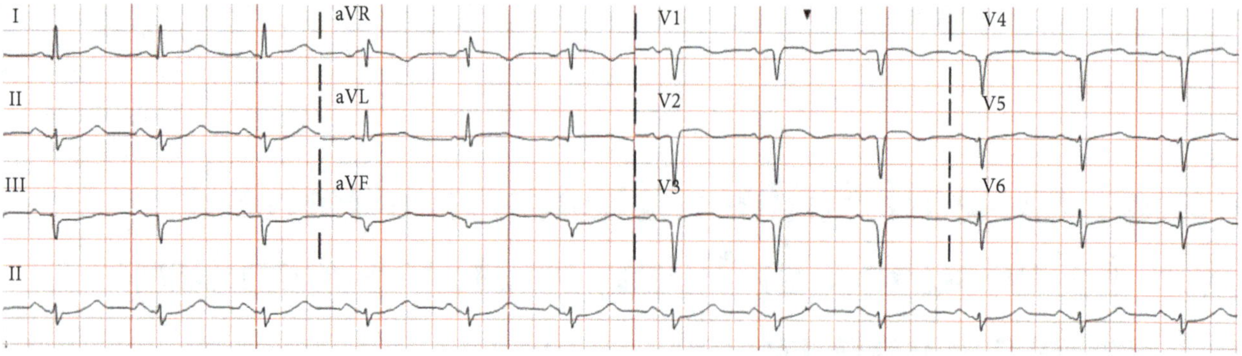

Figure 1: Electrocardiogram showing sinus rhythm at 74 beats/min, left axis deviation, Q waves in V1 to V3, 1 mm ST segment elevation of V2-V3, and poor R wave progression.

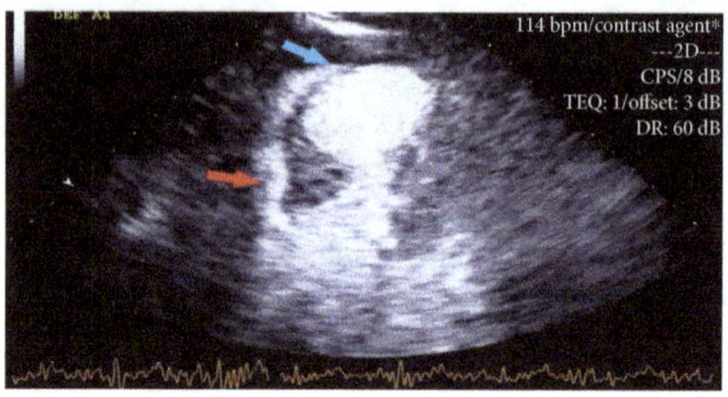

Figure 2: Transthoracic echo showing severely reduced ejection fraction of 30-35%, severe hypokinesis of mid to apical segment with more involvement of the mid anteroseptum, and anterior wall (blue arrow) with basal hyperkinesia and basal asymmetric hypertrophy of the septum (red arrow).

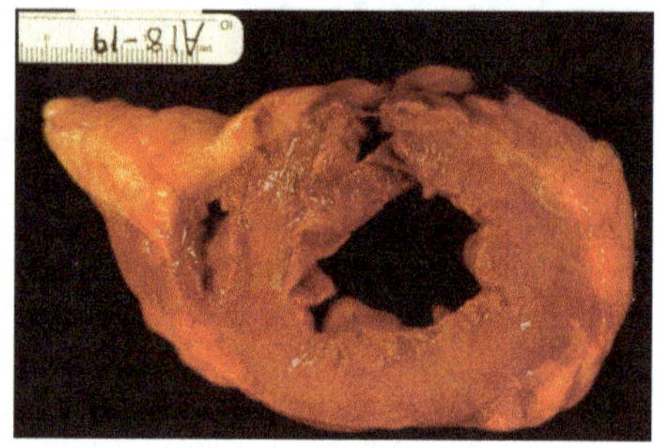

Figure 3: Gross pathology. A cut section of the left ventricle showing an anteriorly located, transmural slit-like rupture (1 cm × 0.8 cm) of the ventricular wall.

to the left jaw and arm and was found to have an elevated troponin (0.26 ng/ml). She was appropriately given aspirin, heparin, and nitroglycerine and was transferred to our medical centre for further care. On presentation, she was alert and oriented, her blood pressure was 200/100 mmHg, nontachycardic, nontachypneic, and sating at 97-98% on 2 litres per minute of oxygen. Pertinent physical exam findings include bibasilar crackles, no murmurs/rubs, normal heart sounds, and no pedal edema. Pertinent laboratory values include haemoglobin (14.2 gm/dl), platelet count (191 k/μl), white count (14.4 k/μl), INR (1.1), creatinine (0.66 mg/dl), and AST (87 μ/l). Electrocardiogram (ECG) on presentation showed sinus rhythm at 74 beats/min, left axis deviation, Q waves in V1 to V3, 1 mm ST segment elevation of V2-V3 (present in prior ECG), and poor R wave progression (Figure 1). A resting 2D Doppler echocardiogram was performed on admission which showed severely reduced ejection fraction of 30-35%, severe hypokinesis of mid to apical segment with more involvement of the mid anteroseptum, and anterior wall with basal hyperkinesia and basal asymmetric hypertrophy of the septum (Figure 2).

The decision was made to undergo urgent cardiac catheterization as her chest pain continued to worsen while on nitroglycerine drip, and the troponin on arrival to our facility was elevated (6.80 ng/ml). While in the elevator, en route to the cardiac catheterization laboratory, the patient became unresponsive. Resuscitation was immediately started, labs at the time of code blue were significant for acute drop in haemoglobin from 14.2 to 6.2, hypokalaemia of 2.5 mmol/l, and arterial blood gas showed metabolic acidosis (pH of 7.27, pCO2 of 34, pO2 of 28, bicarbonate of 15.2 mmol/l). The catheterization team was unable to establish arterial access hence coronary catheterization was not performed. Unfortunately, despite after aggressive resuscitative efforts for 50 minutes, the patient died.

Autopsy was performed and revealed 1000 ml of blood in chest wall cavity. Gross pathology revealed a slit-like rupture of 1 cm × 0.8 cm, transmural and located anteriorly 1.5 cm inferior to the base of the heart. The pericardial surface was smooth and tan red in colour (Figure 3). Microscopically, this area had coagulative necrosis, hypereosinophilic appearance of myocytes with abundant ghost cells (cells without nuclei), and cells with pyknotic nuclei. The neutrophilic infiltrate, haemorrhage, and contraction band necrosis can also be visualised (Figure 4). Sacha et al. reported similar rupture site changes indicative of new acute infarct and transmyocardial necrosis leading to rupture in TCM patient [6]. There was epicardial haemorrhage (3.5 cm in length) adjacent to the left anterior descending artery proximal to the site of rupture. Sections in this area revealed area of infarction with early signs of mottling grossly. Interestingly, this area lacked neutrophils suggesting an area of infarction of less than 10 hours. We speculated that this difference in timeline could be due to

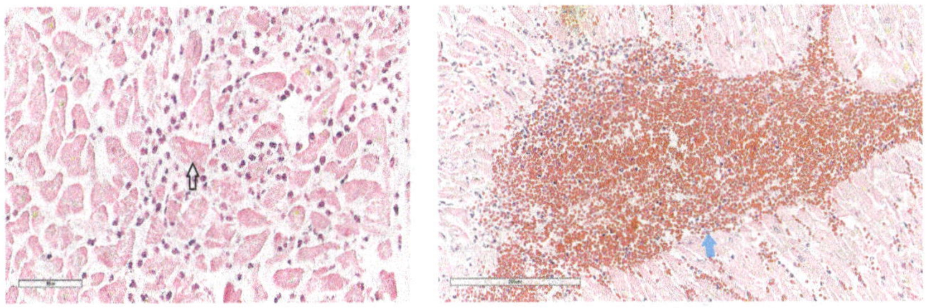

(a) (b)

FIGURE 4: (a) Microscopic pathology. Acute myocardial infarction, H&E, 400x. Note: neutrophilic infiltration of the myocardium, with contraction bands (arrow). (b) Myocardium, H&E, 400x, showing intraventricular haemorrhage (blue arrow).

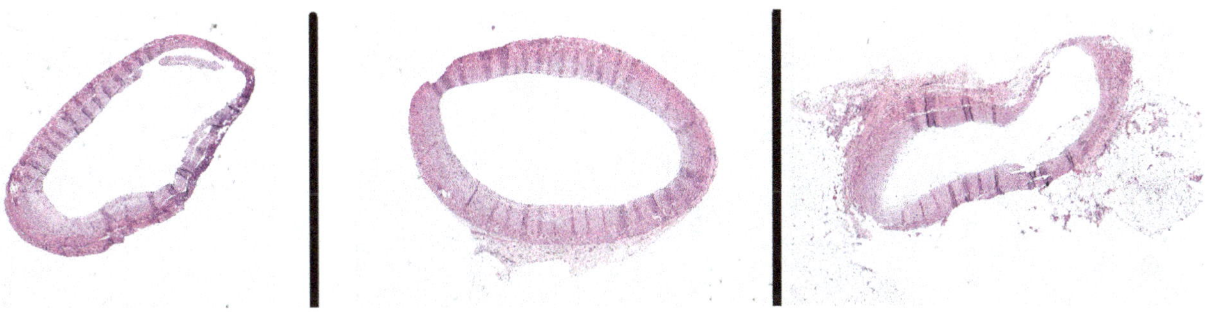

FIGURE 5: Cut sections of coronary arteries showing patent arteries with minimal atherosclerosis.

the discordance of myocardial contraction seen between the apex and base which is often seen in TCM. Most importantly, her major coronary arteries were patent with minimal atherosclerosis and without evidence of organizing thrombus (Figure 5), supporting the histopathological criteria for the diagnosis of TCM.

3. Discussion

TCM is generally classified by an acute and profound but reversible left ventricular dysfunction in the absence of significant coronary artery disease. The revised Mayo criteria are most commonly used currently to establish diagnosis of TCM which includes combination of clinical presentation, ECG, transthoracic echo, and angiographic finding [7]. It is often triggered by an acute emotional or physical stress [4]. TCM is associated with a catecholamine surge and adrenoceptor hyperactivity which can increase the cardiotoxicity leading to increased chances of complications. Increased levels of norepinephrine in the state of stress can cause localized ventricular wall motion abnormalities and ST segment changes [8]. In our case, we believe the rupture of the left ventricular wall was multifactorial and a consequence of increased afterload due to elevated blood pressure, probable increased catecholamine surge, and adrenoceptor hyperactivity in the setting of acute stress.

As per Kumar et al., the characteristics of patients with cardiac rupture in TCM when compared to patients with TCM who did not had cardiac rupture include the following: female gender, older age group, higher systolic and diastolic blood pressure, higher frequency of ST elevations in inferior lead, low ejection fraction (EF), and higher left ventricular peak systolic fraction [9]. Our patient portrayed a number of these characteristics including older age, female gender, higher systolic and diastolic pressures, and severely reduced EF.

As histopathological slides from our patient showed no thrombus and minimal atherosclerosis of coronary arteries, our case falls into the newly diagnosed category of MINOCA (myocardial infarction with nonobstructive coronary arteries). TCM is one of the categories of MINOCA; other categories include coronary spasm, coronary dissection, plaque disruption, spontaneous coronary emboli, myocarditis, and coronary microvasculature dysfunction [10]. Our pathological findings were classical for TCM, and apart from the area of rupture, no other area of infarction was seen. Although coronary spasm can also lead to infarction and subsequent death, hence we cannot exclude it definitively, but when our patient's histological slides are taken in consideration with clinical scenario, TCM is the more likely diagnosis.

A thorough literature review of 20 previous cases of TCM complicated with cardiac rupture is listed in Table 1. The characteristics of these patients include 95% females and mean age of 74.9 years. 16 patients presented with chest pain or discomfort (76%); 17 had ST segment elevations (81%); only 9 cases mentioned troponin levels and out of these, 8 showed increased troponin (89%). These findings further support that TCM mimics acute myocardial infarction. Including our case, a total of 17 patients died (81%). The location of rupture was reported in ten cases; six at the apex (60%), two involving the anterior wall (20%), and two involving the posterior wall (20%).

Table 1: Reported cases with cardiac rupture in takotsubo cardiomyopathy patients (Ovid MEDLINE, 2018).

Authors	Age (in years)	Gender	Clinical presentation	EKG finding	Troponin (ng/ml)	ECHO findings	Catheterization findings	Outcomes	Autopsy findings
Kumar et al. [9]	62	Female	Weakness and lightheadedness	ST elevation in I, II, and V5-V6	11.64	EF 30% and severely reduced LV systolic function in mid and distal segments and preserved at basal segments	Nonstentable 50-75% stenosis at mid LAD artery	Death	Slit-like rupture at the mid portion of the posterior ventricular wall
Zalewska-Adamiec et al. [11]	74	Female	Chest pain	Sinus rhythm with QS complex and ST segment elevation in V2-V6	2.041	Contractile disturbances in the apex and hyperkinesis of basal segments with EF 56% and cardiac tamponade	No significant stenosis	Surgical repair and good condition on discharge	Not applicable
Kudaiberdiev et al. [12]	63	Female	Chest pain, lightheadedness, dyspnea	Q waves in III and aVF, T wave inversions in lead II, III, and aVF, and ST-T abnormalities in V5-V6	0.0	LV dilatation EF (35%) moderate MR, hypoakinesia and thinning of LV inferolateral wall with rupture and cross-over blood shunt through two defects into the pericardium	Patent coronary arteries	Surgical repair and good condition on discharge	Not applicable
Sung et al. [13]	73	Female	Chest pain and dyspnea	ST elevation in V2-V5	1.3	Akinesis of mid to apical left ventricle with EF of 58%	Patent coronary arteries	Death	Not performed
Yoshida et al. [5]	78	Female	Chest pain and dyspnea	RBBB and ST elevation in V2-V6 with QS pattern	Not mentioned	Apical kinesis with wall thinning and massive pericardial effusion	Patent coronary arteries	In good condition after discharge	Not applicable
Indorato et al. [1]	70	Female	Chest pain and nausea	Not done	Not done	Not performed	Not performed	Death. Patient died en route to hospital	Hemorrhagic infarction of LV apex. 0.4 cm line of ruptured myocardium from anterior to posterior wall at the apex

Table 1: Continued.

Authors	Age (in years)	Gender	Clinical presentation	EKG finding	Troponin (ng/ml)	ECHO findings	Catheterization findings	Outcomes	Autopsy findings
Shams [14]	73	Male	Clinical features of pulmonary edema	Sinus tachycardia with Q waves and ST elevation in inferior leads and depression in anterolateral leads	2.840	Left ventriculography: akinesis in the middle and basal-inferior wall and in broad band of mid anterior, mid lateral, and mid septal parts of the left ventricle and hemopericardium. Bedside, limited echo shows cardiac tamponade	Stenosis of all three major arteries. No signs of coronary occlusion	Death	Hemopericardium, perforation of LV free wall at upper posterior part
Kurisu and Inoue [2]	81	Female	Unconsciousness	ST segment elevation in I, II, III, aVF, and V2-V6	Not mentioned	Apical akinesia and basal hyperkinesis	Patent coronary arteries	Death	Not performed
Sacha et al. [6]	81	Female	Chest pain	Diffuse ST elevation in the precordial and limb leads	1.55	Balloon-like LV motion abnormalities with akinesis from mid to apical portions and hyperkinesis of base	No coronary artery disease	Death	Hemopericardium with an LV free wall rupture measuring 10 mm in the apical region and no patent coronary arteries. Inside the heart, there was a mural thrombus in the apical area
Jaguszewski et al. [15]	82	Female	Chest pain	St segment elevation from V1 to V5	14.82	Abnormal LV contraction with apical ballooning pattern with EF of 55%	Patent coronary arteries	Death	Wide penetrating apical rupture as well as 1500 ml of thrombi and liquid blood in the pericardium
Shinozaki et al. [16]	90	Female	Chest pain	ST segment elevation in aVL and V1-V4	Not mentioned	LV apical akinesis and hyperkinesis of base	Intact coronary arteries	Death	Not mentioned
Akashi et al. [8]	70	Female	Chest discomfort	ST elevation in I, II, III, aVL, aVF, and V2-V6	Not mentioned	Apical akinesis and basal hyperkinesis with EF of 51%	Normal coronary arteries	Death	Not performed

Table 1: Continued.

Authors	Age (in years)	Gender	Clinical presentation	EKG finding	Troponin (ng/ml)	ECHO findings	Catheterization findings	Outcomes	Autopsy findings
Showkathali et al. [17]	86	Female	Chest pain	ST segment elevation in anterolateral and inferior leads	Not mentioned	Shows TCM and no intraventricular gradient	Normal RCA and mild atheromatous LAD artery	Death	Not mentioned
Yamada et al. [18]	71	Female	Shoulder and back pain	St segment elevation in leads V4-V6 and abnormal Q waves in leads V4-V5	Not mentioned	Left ventricular apical wall akinesis. Hyperkinesis in the basal wall with mitral valve systolic anterior wall motion	No coronary artery stenosis	Death	Not performed
Stöllberger et al. [19]	71	Female	Generalized tonic clonic seizure	ST segment elevation in II, II, avF, V5, and V6	Trop-T positive	Left ventricular apical wall, apical septum, and apical posterior wall akinesia and small pericardial effusion	Normal coronary arteries	Death	5 mm left ventricular rupture in the apicoposterior region
Ohara et al. [20]	79	Female	Chest pain	ST segment elevation in 1, aVL, and V1-V5; depression in leads III and avF; and abnormal Q wave in V1-V4	Not mentioned	Akinesis of the left ventricular apical wall	Patent coronary arteries	Death	Rupture in the anterior portion of the left ventricle, patent coronary arteries, and hemopericardium
Mafrici et al. [21]	87	Female	Chest pain and dyspnea	ST segment elevation in inferior leads and V2-V6	Trop-T: 20	Apical dyskinesis with hyperkinesis of left ventricular basal segment	Patent coronary arteries	Death	Not performed
Ishida et al. [22]	67	Female	Chest pain	ST segment elevation in I, avL, and V2-V5	Not mentioned	Apical ballooning, basal hyperkinesis, and left ventricular outflow pressure gradient of 110 mmHg associated with systolic anterior movement of anterior mitral leaflet	Extensive akinesis from the apex to mid portion	Surgical repair to correct the cardiac rupture slit	Not applicable

Table 1: Continued.

Authors	Age (in years)	Gender	Clinical presentation	EKG finding	Troponin (ng/ml)	ECHO findings	Catheterization findings	Outcomes	Autopsy findings
Leva et al. [23]	65	Female	Chest pain and dyspnea	ST segment elevation in anterior leads	Not mentioned	Akinesis from mid to apical LV and basal hyperkinesis, EF of 30%	No significant stenosis of epicardial coronary arteries	Death	Not mentioned
Iskander et al. [24]	77	Female	Unconsciousness, chest pain, and dyspnea	ST segment. Elevation in leads I, aVL, and V2-V6	Trop-T: 3.60	EF of 25%. Severe dyskinesis of anterolateral wall of LV, no LVOT obstruction	No coronary artery obstruction with slow flow down the LAD	Death	Fresh clot on epicardial surface, slit-like rupture on anteroapical surface of LV
Present case	75	Female	Chest pain and dyspnea	Sinus rhythm, no ST segment elevation, poor R wave progression	6.80	EF of 30-35%, severe hypokinesis of apical LV, and asymmetric hypertrophy of the basal septum	Not performed	Death	Hemopericardium, patent epicardial coronary arteries, slit-like 1 cm × 0.8 cm rupture of the anterior wall of LV

Abbreviations: LV: left ventricle; LAD: left anterior descending artery; RCA: right coronary artery; EF: ejection fraction; TCM, takotsubo cardiomyopathy; LVOT: left ventricular outflow tract obstruction; LAD: left anterior descending artery.

The prognosis of TCM is usually favourable, and left ventricular function improves in the majority of cases with conservative management. Currently, there is no standardised treatment protocol for the patients with TCM [24]. Although beta blockers have been suggested in studies to prevent the progression and recurrence of TCM [16], but recent TCM registry results show no survival benefit with beta blocker [4]. The same registry states that the use of angiotensin receptor blocker or angiotensin-converting enzyme was associated with improved survival [4]. Further studies are needed to delineate the role of beta blockers in TCM. The ST segment elevation in TCM is usually transient and recovers within few days; persistent ST elevation is a warning sign for continued myocardial injury and portend an impending ventricular free wall rupture [24]. The treatment of cardiac rupture in the setting of TCM is surgical repair [11]. It is unclear to date whether anticoagulation plays any role in TCM, but apical thrombus formation had been reported in patients with TCM [8].

4. Conclusion

Due to devastating complications of TCM, our case highlights the need for close monitoring of patients with TCM for the first few days. Special consideration should be paid to older female patients as they have higher rates of cardiac rupture.

Acknowledgments

We are really thankful to Dr. James L. Fishback (Chancellor's Club Distinguished Teaching Professor (Emeritus), Pathology and Lab Medicine) for his help in interpretation of the pathology slides.

References

[1] F. Indorato, Y. J. Akashi, C. Rossitto, C. Raffino, and G. Bartoloni, "Takotsubo cardiomyopathy associated with rupture of the left ventricular apex: assessment of histopathological features of a fatal case and literature review," *Forensic Science, Medicine, and Pathology*, vol. 11, no. 4, pp. 577–583, 2015.

[2] S. Kurisu and I. Inoue, "Cardiac rupture in tako-tsubo cardiomyopathy with persistent ST-segment elevation," *International Journal of Cardiology*, vol. 158, no. 1, pp. e5–e6, 2012.

[3] K. Singh, K. Carson, Z. Usmani, G. Sawhney, R. Shah, and J. Horowitz, "Systematic review and meta-analysis of incidence and correlates of recurrence of takotsubo cardiomyopathy, *International Journal of Cardiology*, vol. 174, no. 3, pp. 696–701, 2014.

[4] C. Templin, J. R. Ghadri, J. Diekmann et al., "Clinical features and outcomes of takotsubo (stress) cardiomyopathy," *The New England Journal of Medicine*, vol. 373, no. 10, pp. 929–938, 2015.

[5] S. Yoshida, K. Miwa, T. Matsubara et al., "Stress-induced takotsubo cardiomyopathy complicated with wall rupture and thrombus formation," *International Journal of Cardiology*, vol. 161, no. 1, pp. e18–e20, 2012.

[6] J. Sacha, J. Maselko, A. Wester, Z. Szudrowicz, and W. Pluta, "Left ventricular apical rupture caused by takotsubo cardiomyopathy-comprehensive pathological heart investigation," *Circulation Journal*, vol. 71, no. 6, pp. 982–985, 2007.

[7] D. C. Scantlebury and A. Prasad, "Diagnosis of takotsubo cardiomyopathy," *Circulation Journal*, vol. 78, no. 9, pp. 2129–2139, 2014.

[8] Y. J. Akashi, T. Tejima, H. Sakurada et al., "Left Ventricular Rupture Associated with Takotsubo Cardiomyopathy," *Mayo Clinic Proceedings*, vol. 79, no. 6, pp. 821–824, 2004.

[9] S. Kumar, S. Kaushik, A. Nautiyal et al., "Cardiac rupture in takotsubo cardiomyopathy: a systematic review," *Clinical cardiology*, vol. 34, no. 11, pp. 672–676, 2011.

[10] S. Pasupathy, R. Tavella, and J. F. Beltrame, "Myocardial infarction with nonobstructive coronary arteries (MINOCA): the past, present, and future management," *Circulation*, vol. 135, no. 16, pp. 1490–1493, 2017.

[11] M. Zalewska-Adamiec, H. Bachórzewska-Gajewska, M. Kozuch, F. Marek, T. Hirnle, and S. Dobrzycki, "Cardiac rupture in takotsubo cardiomyopathy treated surgically," *Advances in Interventional Cardiology*, vol. 3, pp. 278-279, 2016.

[12] T. Kudaiberdiev, I. Akhmedova, G. Imanalieva et al., "Surgical treatment of left ventricular wall rupture, regarded as a consequence of takotsubo cardiomyopathy," *SAGE Open Medical Case Reports*, vol. 5, 2017.

[13] J.-M. Sung, S.-J. Hong, I.-H. Chung et al., "Rupture of right ventricular free wall following ventricular septal rupture in takotsubo cardiomyopathy with right ventricular involvement," *Yonsei Medical Journal*, vol. 58, no. 1, pp. 248–251, 2017.

[14] S. Y-Hassan, "Cardiac rupture in a patient with takotsubo syndrome triggered by acute myocardial infarction: two messages," *International Journal of Cardiology*, vol. 177, no. 1, pp. 162–165, 2014.

[15] M. Jaguszewski, M. Fijalkowski, R. Nowak et al., "Ventricular rupture in takotsubo cardiomyopathy," *European Heart Journal*, vol. 33, no. 8, p. 1027, 2012.

[16] K. Shinozaki, A. Tamura, Y. Abe, S. Yano, and J. Kadota, "Left ventricular free wall rupture in takotsubo cardiomyopathy," *International Journal of Cardiology*, vol. 115, no. 1, pp. E3–E4, 2007.

[17] R. Showkathali, R. Dworakowski, and P. MacCarthy, "Catastrophic ruptured takotsubo cardiomyopathy," *Journal of Cardiovascular Medicine*, vol. 16, no. 9, pp. 644-645, 2015.

[18] R. Yamada, N. Watanabe, T. Kume et al., "Left ventricular rupture associated with takotsubo-like left ventricular dysfunction (apical ballooning)," *Journal of Echocardiography*, vol. 4, no. 2, pp. 59–62, 2006.

[19] C. Stöllberger, J. Huber, B. Enzelsberger, and J. Finsterer, "Fatal outcome of epileptic seizure-induced takotsubo syndrome with left ventricular rupture," *European Journal of Neurology*, vol. 16, no. 6, pp. e116–e117, 2009.

[20] Y. Ohara, Y. Hiasa, S. Hosokawa et al., "Left ventricular free wall rupture in transient left ventricular apical ballooning," *Circulation Journal*, vol. 69, no. 5, pp. 621–623, 2005.

[21] A. Mafrici, R. Proietti, R. Fusco, A. De Biase, and S. Klugmann, "Left ventricular free wall rupture in a Caucasian female with takotsubo syndrome: a case report and a brief literature review," *Journal of Cardiovascular Medicine*, vol. 7, no. 12, pp. 880–883, 2006.

[22] T. Ishida, T. Yasu, K. Arao, M. Kawakami, and M. Saito, "Bedside diagnosis of cardiac rupture by contrast echocardiography," *Circulation*, vol. 112, no. 24, pp. e354–e355, 2005.

[23] R. Ieva, M. Correale, N. D. Brunetti, and M. Di Biase, "A "bad" case of tako-tsubo syndrome," *Journal of Thrombosis and Thrombolysis*, vol. 28, no. 2, pp. 248–251, 2009.

[24] M. Iskander, A. Abugroun, K. Shehata, F. Iskander, and A. Iskander, "Takotsubo cardiomyopathy-induced cardiac free wall rupture: a case report and review of literature," *Cardiology Research*, vol. 9, no. 4, pp. 244–249, 2018.

4

Systemic Lupus Erythematosus Complicated with Hypertrophic Cardiomyopathy

Huihui Ma,[1,2] Xin Cao,[3] Jing Zhang,[1,2] Yongmei Zhou,[1,2] Rong Luo,[4] Tao He,[1,2] Jianhong Tao,[1,2] and Xiaoping Li[1,2]

[1]*Department of Cardiology, Sichuan Provincial People's Hospital, University of Electronic Science and Technology of China, Chengdu, Sichuan 610072, China*
[2]*Chinese Academy of Sciences Sichuan Translational Medicine Research Hospital, Chengdu 610072, China*
[3]*Chengdu University of Traditional Chinese Medicine, Chengdu, Sichuan 610075, China*
[4]*Institute of Geriatric Cardiovascular Disease, Chengdu Medical College, Chengdu, Sichuan 610500, China*

Correspondence should be addressed to Xiaoping Li; lixiaoping0119@163.com
Academic Editor: Ertugrul Ercan

A 32-year-old female with systemic lupus erythematosus (SLE) for more than 7 years, and long-term treatment with cyclophosphamide, cyclosporine, methotrexate, and tacrolimus, later found to be combined with hypertrophic cardiomyopathy (HCM) for one year. The patient denied a family history of cardiomyopathy and sudden cardiac death (SCD). Echocardiography suggested that uneven thickening of the left ventricle (LV), mainly in the lower middle segment. Cardiac magnetic resonance (CMR) showed that the walls of the left ventricular (LV) were significantly thickened, as about 21 mm, mainly in the middle and lower segments. Genetic tests showed no known or suspected pathogenic variations were found and no significant enhancement in CMR, so secondary HCM was diagnosed clinically. After symptomatic treatment, the patient was discharged, and long-term follow-up was conducted. The diagnosis of HCM, which combined with SLE or second to usage of tacrolimus, was based on symptoms, echocardiography, and CMR; no endomyocardial biopsies were performed.

1. Introduction

Hypertrophic cardiomyopathy (HCM) is a disease characterized by cardiac hypertrophy, which is usually manifested as left ventricular hypertrophy [1, 2]. HCM can be diagnosed by left ventricular wall or septal thickness ≥ 15 mm measured by two-dimensional echocardiography or ≥13 mm in patients with a definite family history [1–4]. Systemic lupus erythematosus (SLE) is an autoimmune disease, and the etiology is not completely clear. It is characterized by autoantibodies and immune complexes, which can cause multiple system damage [5]. Cardiovascular system is one of the most frequently involved systems, and cardiovascular events are also an important cause of death in lupus patients [6–12]. Up to 9% of patients with SLE are reported to have cardiac manifestations, including myocarditis, cardiomyopathy (CM), and/or heart failure (HF) [13]. Whether there is cardiomyopathy directly caused by lupus is not clear [13]. We present the 10th case of HCM associated with SLE and discuss the possible causes of cardiac hypertrophy in this patient.

2. Clinical Data

2.1. Case Report. A 32-year-old female was admitted to the emergency department for 6-day history of fever accompanied by abdominal pain and diarrhea. The highest body temperature was about 39.4°C, with obvious chill and Raynaud's phenomenon. The local clinic provided anti-inflammatory, antiviral, and antipyretic treatments such as "Cephalosporins, Ribavirin and Lysine Acetylsalicylate", but the body temperature was not significantly decreased. After that, the patient continued to have fever; the body temperature was monitored at 37.8-38.5°C, so she was admitted to our emergency department.

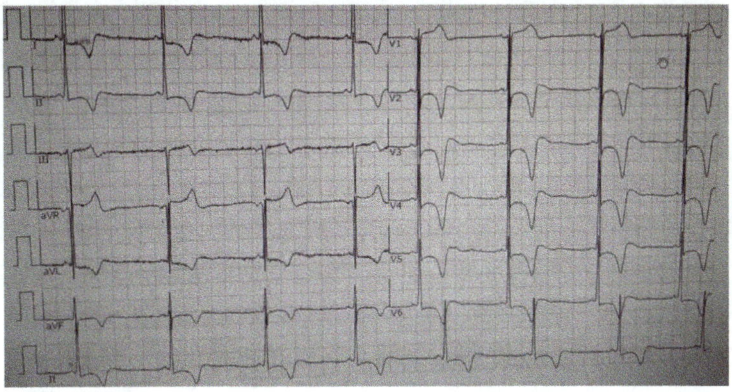

FIGURE 1: Electrocardiogram showing significant sinus bradycardia, with normal electric axis, short PR interval, high left ventricular voltage, and ST-T change; V2-V6 leads T-wave inversion.

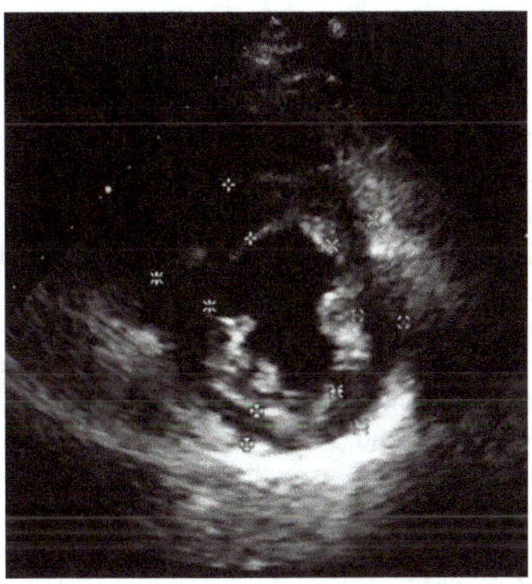

FIGURE 2: Echocardiography showing the thickened walls in the middle and lower segments.

The patient was diagnosed with SLE for more than 7 years. After that, she was hospitalized in our hospital for several times due to recurrent fever accompanied by abdominal pain, diarrhea, nausea, vomiting, etc., and received anti-infection and immune regulation treatment (long-term use of cyclophosphamide, cyclosporine, methotrexate, and tacrolimus).

2.2. Physical and Laboratory Examination. After admission, the patient presented with Cushing's syndrome. Bone friction was positive, and there was no cardiac murmur.

Laboratory evaluations revealed the following: leukocyte count was 7.160×10^9/L, neutrophil count was 6.480×10^9 /L, platelet count was 188×10^9/L, and hemoglobin level was 131 g/L. Brain natriuretic peptide (BNP) was 752 pg/mL. Procalcitonin was 0.08 ng/mL. Erythrocyte sedimentation rate was 27 mm/h. Carbohydrate antigen 19-9 (CA19-9) was 63.86 U/nL. Complement C3 was 0.313 g/L; complement C4 was 0.078 g/L. The results of anti-Nrnp/Sm antibody, anti-dsDNA antibody, and anti-nucleosome antibody (ANUA) were all positive (+++). Anti-histone antibody (AHA) was also postive (++), and meanwhile, anti-ribosome P-protein antibody (ARPA) and anti-nuclear anti-

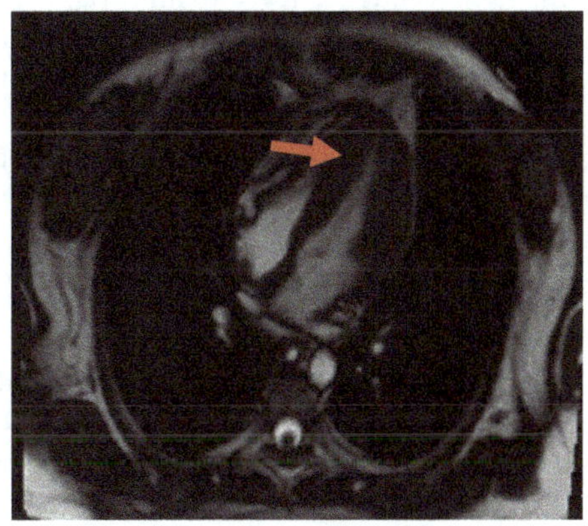

FIGURE 3: Cardiac magnetic resonance showing the walls of the left ventricle were significantly thickened, mainly in the middle and lower segments (T2-weighted image).

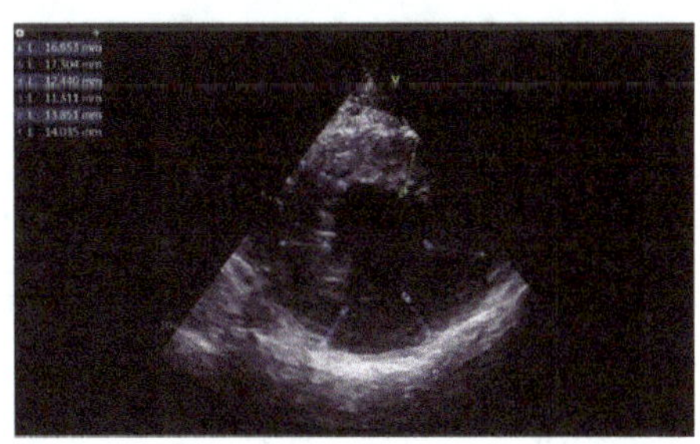

FIGURE 4: Echocardiography on reexamination showing little thickening of the left ventricular wall.

body (ANA) were postive (+), too. Nuclear homogeneous type was 1 : 3200, and nuclear particle type was 1 : 1000.

2.3. Electrocardiogram. The electrocardiogram of the patient showed significant sinus bradycardia, with normal electrical axis, short PR interval, high left ventricular voltage, and ST-T change. V2-V6 leads T-wave inversion (Figure 1).

2.4. Echocardiography. The echocardiography showed left ventricular diastolic dysfunction, and the left ventricular ejection fraction (LVEF) of the heart was 67%. The cardiac

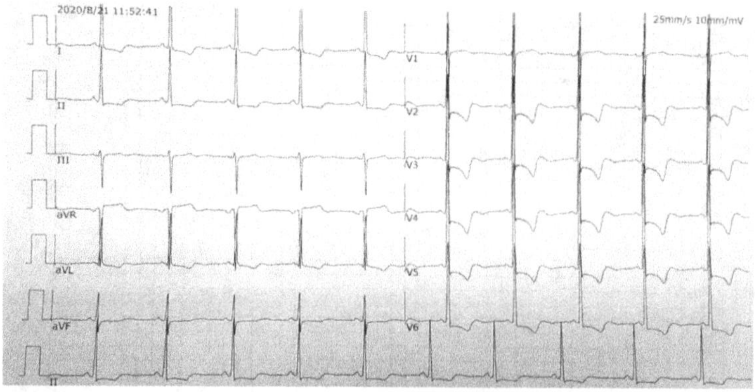

FIGURE 5: Electrocardiogram on reexamination showing sinus rhythm; T-wave inversion was significantly improved than before.

diameter was normal (left atrial, LA = 25 mm; left ventricle, LV = 45 mm; right ventricle, RV = 18 mm; right atrial, RA = 34 × 27 mm). The left ventricular myocardium was unevenly thickened, especially in the middle and lower segments up to 15 mm. Left ventricular diastolic function decreased, E/A = 0.9. Systolic anterior motion (SAM) syndrome was slightly positive. The systolic and diastolic pulmonary blood pressures were about 24 mmHg and 11 mmHg, respectively, with an average of about 16 mmHg (Figure 2).

2.5. CMR. CMR confirmed left ventricular diastolic dysfunction. The walls of the left ventricle were significantly thickened, mainly in the middle and lower segments. The diastolic period thickness was about 21 mm. There was no obstruction in the LVOT and late gadolinium enhancement (LGE) of the myocardial wall. No obvious thickening of the pericardium and effusion was found. On the basis of these data, HCM was diagnosed (Figure 3).

3. Genetic Testing

To exclude primary HCM, we used a blood DNA extraction kit to extract genomic DNA from peripheral blood samples. We targeted and enriched for the exons and neighboring introns (within 50 bp) of the 130 genes associated with cardiomyopathy. Based on the guideline for the interpretation of sequence variants: a joint consensus recommendation of the American College of Medical Genetics and Genomics and the Association for Molecular Pathology [14], no known or suspected pathogenic variants consistent with the phenotype were found.

4. Outcome and Follow-Up

At a follow-up visit in August 2020, the patient described occasional chest tightness, but the symptoms were not apparent, and the drug was not taken. Echocardiography showed no significant change in ventricular wall thickness from that recorded 1 year earlier (Figure 4), but ECG showed that the T-wave inversion of the V2-V6 leads improved (Figure 5).

5. Discussion

We have described a patient with SLE in combination with HCM. The patient had a 7-year history of SLE but no history of myocardial hypertrophy in the previous 6 years. Only nine cases of SLE with HCM have been described, and the underlying mechanisms linking them, if present, are unknown. Therefore, we investigated whether our patient had SLE coincident with primary HCM or HCM secondary to SLE, drug treatment, or unknown cause.

The majority of HCM cases are caused by gene mutations, but it can also occur secondary to other diseases or to long-term use of certain drugs, such as anabolic steroids, tacrolimus, and hydroxychloroquine [15–17]. SLE is a multisystem connective tissue disease that can affect all organs of the body. More than 50% of SLE patients have cardiac involvement, and lesions can involve the pericardium, myocardium, endocardium, valve, conduction system, and coronary arteries [8]. The pericardium is commonly the first site to be involved and occurs in 11%–54% of cases according to electrocardiographic studies [9]. Autopsy findings suggest that about 62% of SLE patients have pericardium involvement [10]. Myocarditis is the most typical feature of myocardial involvement in SLE, and it can progress to ventricular dysfunction, dilated cardiomyopathy (DCM), and HF [11, 12]. Coronary heart disease (CAD) is the most common cause of death in patients with late-onset or long-term SLE [11–13].

The patient described here had received a diagnosis of SLE 7 years before presentation, but she had no family history of HCM or SCD and denied a history of hypertension. Echocardiography and CMR imaging supported a diagnosis of nonobstructive HCM. To exclude idiopathic HCM, we performed next-generation sequencing and analysis with a focus on 130 genes known to be associated with cardiomyopathy. The patient had no known or suspected pathogenic variants consistent with the phenotype, which exclude mostly idiopathic cardiomyopathy and instead suggested HCM secondary to another cause(s).

As noted, the cardiovascular system is commonly involved in SLE [9–12], which initially suggested that SLE may have been the direct cause of HCM. However, HCM has not been clearly linked to SLE to date, and cases of SLE

TABLE 1: Case report about patients with SLE and HCM.

Cases	Age (years)	Gender	Symptom	Drugs	Diagnostic methods (HCM)	References
Asherson et al., 1992	51	Female	Palpitations, chest pain	Steroids, immunosuppressant, warfarin, antidepressant	Echocardiography	[18]
Asherson et al., 1992	45	Female	Palpitations, dyspnea	Propranolol, mexiletine, digoxin, amiodarone	Echocardiography	[18]
Ara et al., 1998	45	Female	Intermittent palpitations, grade II dyspnea, orthopnoea	Hydroxychloroquine	Echocardiography	[19]
Dongji and Yuan, 1998	35	Female	Chest distress, syncope	Hormone, β-blocker, calcium antagonist	Echocardiography	[20]
Anastasiadis et al., 2001	32	Female	Arthralgias, malar rush, intermittent palpitations membranoproliferative nephritis	N	Echocardiography	[21]
Anastasiadis et al., 2001	37	Female	Physical and laboratory findings similar to those found in case 1	N	Echocardiography	[21]
Anastasiadis et al., 2001	19	Male	Liver failure due to Budd-Chiari syndrome antiphospholipid syndrome	N	Echocardiography	[21]
Maezawa Linghua, 2002	23	Female	Palpitations	Steroid		[22]
Kotani et al., 2005	37	Female	Exertional chest pain nephrotic syndrome	Prednisolone, cyclophosphamide, mizoribine, β-blocker	Echocardiography, pathological biopsy	[23]
The present study	32	Female	Fever accompanied by abdominal pain and diarrhea	Cyclophosphamide, cyclosporin, methotrexate tacrolimus	Echocardiography, CMR	

N: not mentioned in the article; CMR: cardiac magnetic resonance.

complicated with HCM are rare (Table 1) [18–23]. Among the nine reported cases, eight (89%) were female, and two reported a family history of SCD ($n = 1$) and HCM ($n = 1$) [18, 20]. As shown in Table 1, the patients were relatively young (mean age 36.0 ± 10.4 years) and had a history of systemic disease for many years. HCM was mainly diagnosed by echocardiography, with only one patient undergoing echocardiography and pathological biopsy [23]. The findings of the present study are similar to the previously reported cases. Of note, both SLE and SLE with HCM predominantly affect women.

We considered whether our patient's long-term use of medications such as tacrolimus might be the cause of HCM, especially because her echocardiography and ECG were normal prior to 2019. Diffuse thickening is a key characteristic of drug-induced cardiomyopathy, but it can also manifest as heterogeneous thickening [17, 24], as may have been the case with our patient. Tacrolimus is an effective immunosuppressant most commonly used in patients with kidney, liver, or heart transplants [25]. However, tacrolimus has been reported to have toxic side effects, including cardiotoxicity [17, 26]. Tacrolimus-induced HCM has been described mainly, but not exclusively, in children [11, 27, 28]. And the change is reversible [17]. During follow-up, the patient studied here ceased to take tacrolimus, and although echocardiography showed no significant change in wall thickness, the T-wave inversion of the ECG leads was improved. The patient had no family history of hypertension, HCM, or other cardiovascular disease. Taking these observations into account, we suspected that HCM in our patient was most likely caused by tacrolimus. However, longer follow-up may be needed to prove it.

The goal of this report is to provide further information about the clinical presentation of SLE with HCM and to provide some clues for the study of the relationship between them. Although the concomitant occurrence of the two pathologies may be purely coincidental, advances in molecular biology techniques may shed light on the direct underlying mechanisms linking SLE and HCM.

6. Conclusion

To the best of our knowledge, our patient is the 10th reported case of SLE combined with HCM. The specific mechanism linking SLE and HCM is not yet clear, but a significant gender bias is present, with 89% of the reported cases being female. Patients with SLE should be cautioned about the potential for cardiovascular complications.

Authors' Contributions

Huihui Ma, Jing Zhang, Yongmei Zhou, and Rong Luo collected previous study of systemic lupus erythematosus (SLE) and hypertrophic cardiomyopathy (HCM). Xiaoping Li, Xin Cao, Tao He, and Jianhong Tao conceived and designed the study. Huihui Ma wrote the paper. All authors read and approved the manuscript.

Acknowledgments

This work was supported by the National Natural Science Foundation of China (No. 81770379, No. 81500297, and No. 81470521).

References

[1] Chinese Society of Cardiology, Chinese adult hypertrophic cardiomyopathy diagnosis and treatment guidelines preparation group, Editorial Board of Chinese Journal of Cardiology, "Guidelines for the diagnosis and treatment for Chinese adult patients with hypertrophic cardiomyopathy," *Chinese Journal of Cardiology*, vol. 45, no. 12, pp. 1015–1032, 2017.

[2] C. M. Wolf, "Hypertrophic cardiomyopathy: genetics and clinical perspectives," *Cardiovascular diagnosis and therapy*, vol. 9, no. S2, pp. S388–S415, 2019.

[3] B. J. Maron, "Clinical course and management of hypertrophic cardiomyopathy," *The New England Journal of Medicine*, vol. 379, no. 7, pp. 655–668, 2018.

[4] M. Shah, "Hypertrophic cardiomyopathy," *Cardiology in the Young*, vol. 27, no. S1, pp. S25–S30, 2017.

[5] K. Oku and T. Atsumi, "Systemic lupus erythematosus: nothing stale her infinite variety," *Modern Rheumatology*, vol. 28, no. 5, pp. 758–765, 2018.

[6] A. I. Diadyk, G. G. Taradin, A. E. Bagriĭ, N. F. Iarovaia, and T. V. Taradina, "Cardiac involvement in systemic lupus erythematosus [J]," *Mayo Clinic Proceedings*, vol. 74, no. 3, pp. 275–284, 1999.

[7] J. Chen, Y. Tang, M. Zhu, and A. Xu, "Heart involvement in systemic lupus erythematosus: a systemic review and meta-analysis," *Clinical Rheumatology*, vol. 35, no. 10, pp. 2437–2448, 2016.

[8] K. Tselios and M. B. Urowitz, "Cardiovascular and pulmonary manifestations of systemic lupus erythematosus," *Current Rheumatology Reviews*, vol. 13, no. 3, pp. 206–218, 2017.

[9] N. E. Doherty and R. J. Siegel, "Cardiovascular manifestations of systemic lupus erythematosus," *American Heart Journal*, vol. 110, no. 6, pp. 1257–1265, 1985.

[10] A. Doria, L. Iaccarino, P. Sarzi-Puttini, F. Atzeni, M. Turriel, and M. Petri, "Cardiac involvement in systemic lupus erythematosus," *Lupus*, vol. 14, no. 9, pp. 683–686, 2005.

[11] C. Usalan, H. Buyukhatipoglu, and O. Tiryaki, "Systemic lupus erythematosus complicated by dilated cardiomyopathy and severe heart failure," *Clinical Rheumatology*, vol. 26, no. 1, pp. 125–127, 2007.

[12] J. J. Miner and A. H. Kim, "Cardiac manifestations of systemic lupus erythematosus," *Rheumatic Diseases Clinics of North America*, vol. 40, no. 1, pp. 51–60, 2014.

[13] M. L. Ishimori, M. Agarwal, R. Beigel et al., "Systemic lupus erythematosus cardiomyopathy—a case series demonstrating a reversible form of left ventricular dysfunction," *Echocardiography*, vol. 31, no. 5, pp. 563–568, 2014.

[14] on behalf of the ACMG Laboratory Quality Assurance Committee, S. Richards, N. Aziz et al., "Standards and guidelines for the interpretation of sequence variants: a joint consensus recommendation of the American College of Medical Genetics and Genomics and the Association for Molecular Pathology," *Genetics in Medicine*, vol. 17, no. 5, pp. 405–423, 2015.

[15] E. Joyce, A. Fabre, and N. Mahon, "Hydroxychloroquine cardiotoxicity presenting as a rapidly evolving biventricular cardiomyopathy: key diagnostic features and literature review," *European Heart Journal Acute Cardiovascular Care*, vol. 2, no. 1, pp. 77–83, 2013.

[16] A. Frustaci, E. Morgante, D. Antuzzi, M. A. Russo, and C. Chimenti, "Inhibition of cardiomyocyte lysosomal activity in hydroxychloroquine cardiomyopathy," *International Journal of Cardiology*, vol. 157, no. 1, pp. 117–119, 2012.

[17] K. Noda, T. Ukichi, K. Furuya et al., "Tacrolimus-induced hypertrophic cardiomyopathy in a patient with dermatomyositis," *Rheumatology (Oxford, England)*, vol. 56, no. 11, pp. 2037-2038, 2017.

[18] R. A. Asherson, D. Ames, J. Coltart, C. Byrne, and G. R. Hughes, "Hypertrophic cardiomyopathy in systemic lupus erythematosus and "lupus-like" disease. Chance association? A report of 2 cases," *The Journal of Rheumatology*, vol. 19, no. 12, pp. 1973–1977, 1992.

[19] J. Ara, J. Vivancos, J. Soler-Carrillo, J. C. Paré, R. Cervera, and J. Font, "Hypertrophic cardiomyopathy and systemic lupus erythematosus," *Clinical Rheumatology*, vol. 17, no. 6, pp. 531–533, 1998.

[20] D. An and F. Yuan, "A case of systemic lupus erythematosus with hypertrophic obstructive cardiomyopathy [J]," *Journal of Clinical Internal Medicine*, vol. 3, p. 144, 1998.

[21] G. P. Anastasiadis, I. Moyssakis, K. Boki, and M. Kyriakidis, "Hypertrophic cardiomyopathy in systemic lupus erythematosus," *Mayo Clinic Proceedings*, vol. 76, no. 1, p. 111, 2001.

[22] M. Linghua, "Systemic lupus erythematosus with hypertrophic cardiomyopathy improved by steroid therapy: a case report [J]," *Kanto rheumatism*, vol. 36, pp. 77–86, 2002.

[23] T. KOTANI, T. TAKEUCHI, M. SAKAMOTO et al., "A case of systemic lupus erythematosus associated with hypertrophic cardiomyopathy," *Nihon Rinshō Men'eki Gakkai Kaishi*, vol. 28, no. 6, pp. 413–417, 2005.

[24] M. U. Dogar, N. N. Shah, S. Ishtiaq et al., "Hydroxychloroquine-induced restrictive cardiomyopathy: a case report," *Postgraduate Medical Journal*, vol. 94, no. 1109, pp. 185-186, 2018.

[25] L. Szabó, N. Szentandrássy, K. Kistamás et al., "Effects of tacrolimus on action potential configuration and transmembrane ion currents in canine ventricular cells," *Naunyn-Schmiedeberg's Archives of Pharmacology*, vol. 386, no. 3, pp. 239–246, 2013.

[26] S. M. Dehghani, M. Haghighat, M. H. Imanieh et al., "Tacrolimus related hypertrophic cardiomyopathy in liver transplant recipients," *Archives of Iranian Medicine*, vol. 13, no. 2, pp. 116–119, 2010.

[27] T. M. Jarzembowski, E. John, F. Panaro et al., "Reversal of tacrolimus-related hypertrophic obstructive cardiomyopathy 5 years after kidney transplant in a 6-year-old recipient," *Pediatric Transplantation*, vol. 9, no. 1, pp. 117–121, 2005.

[28] R. K. Chang, S. V. McDiarmid, J. C. Alejos, S. E. Drant, and T. S. Klitzner, "Echocardiographic findings of hypertrophic cardiomyopathy in children after orthotopic liver transplantation," *Pediatric Transplantation*, vol. 5, no. 3, pp. 187–191, 2001.

5

Takotsubo Cardiomyopathy Secondary to Adrenal Insufficiency

Ian Garrahy,[1] Peter Nicholas III,[1] Oreoluwa Oladiran,[1] and Salik Nazir[2]

[1]*Department of Internal Medicine, Reading Hospital and Medical Center, Tower Health, West Reading, PA, USA*
[2]*Department of Cardiology, University of Toledo Medical Center, Toledo, Ohio, USA*

Correspondence should be addressed to Ian Garrahy; ian.garrahy@gmail.com
Academic Editor: Takatoshi Kasai

We report a case of a middle-aged female who presented with altered mental status, hypotension, and hypoglycemia and was diagnosed with secondary adrenal insufficiency. She was also found to have elevated troponin I on initial evaluation with diffuse T wave inversions on electrocardiogram. Transthoracic echocardiogram revealed ejection fraction of 38% with apical akinesia. Subsequent left heart catheterization revealed clean coronary arteries. She was diagnosed with typical Takotsubo cardiomyopathy secondary to adrenal insufficiency. She was managed with IV hydrocortisone with resolution of symptoms. This article adds to the select few cases in the literature of the association of Takotsubo cardiomyopathy resulting from secondary adrenal insufficiency.

1. Introduction

Stress-induced cardiomyopathy, also known as Takotsubo cardiomyopathy (TCM), apical ballooning syndrome, and broken heart syndrome, is an increasingly reported form of nonischemic cardiomyopathy characterized by reversible left ventricular dysfunction in the absence of anatomically corresponding angiographically significant coronary artery lesion [1], dyskinesia with hyperkinesia of the midventricular and/or apical segments of the left ventricle (termed "basal ballooning variant" or "reverse TC"), and a focal dyskinesia of any segment of the left ventricle ("focal variant") [2]. The disorder is a commoner in postmenopausal women and usually precipitated by intense physical and emotional stress [2]. In rare cases, it is reported to be associated with adrenal insufficiency. We aim to report a similar case of TCM associated with adrenal insufficiency and review the existing literature on this association.

2. Case Description

A 55-year-old female with a history of eczema on topical steroids was admitted with altered mental status, hypotension, and hypoglycemia. She presented with a blood glucose of 29 mg/dL which was corrected with IV dextrose. She was started on norepinephrine for her hypotension that was unresponsive with crystalloids. On physical exam, blood pressure was 100/67 (78) on norepinephrine and she was lethargic but arousable to sternal rub. The patient reported that she applied desoximetasone 0.25% cream 2 times daily over her whole body for eczema over the past decade.

Labs were remarkable for morning cortisol of 2.8 mcg/dL, ACTH < 5 pg/mL, and sodium 132 mEq/L. The ACTH stimulation test yielded inadequate cortisol responses of 8.1 and 12.0 mcg/dL, before and 90 minutes after the ACTH, respectively. Given these laboratory findings, it was concluded that she had secondary adrenal insufficiency due to her chronic topical steroid use. She was treated with IV hydrocortisone 100 mg every 8 hours which quickly resolved all her electrolyte derangements (including hypoglycemia) and hypotension and improved her encephalopathy.

Concurrently, the patient was noted to have an elevated troponin, which peaked at 0.37 ng/mL. The patient denied chest pain, dyspnea, lightheadedness, or palpitations. Her EKG exhibited diffuse T wave inversions (Figure 1). Transthoracic echocardiogram revealed an ejection fraction of

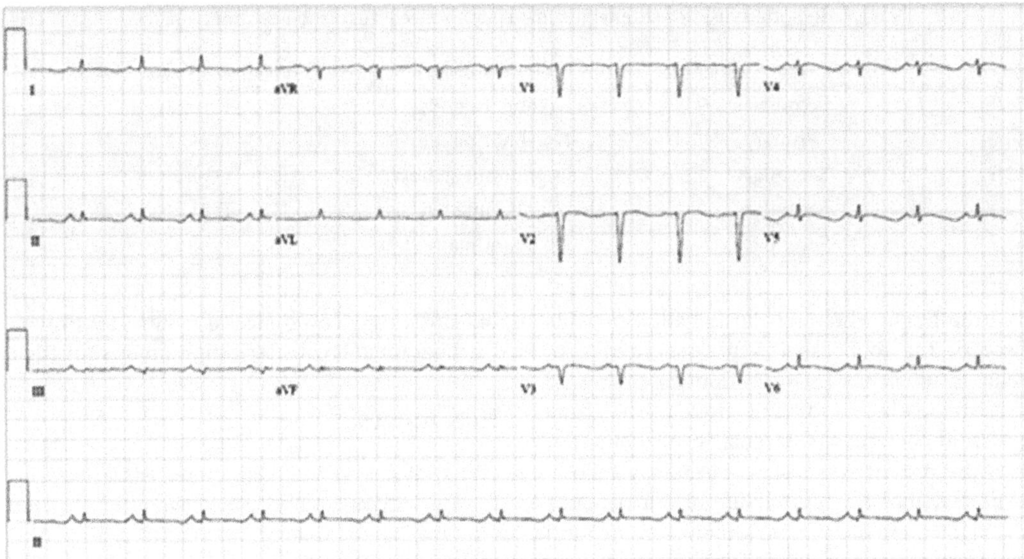

FIGURE 1: EKG.

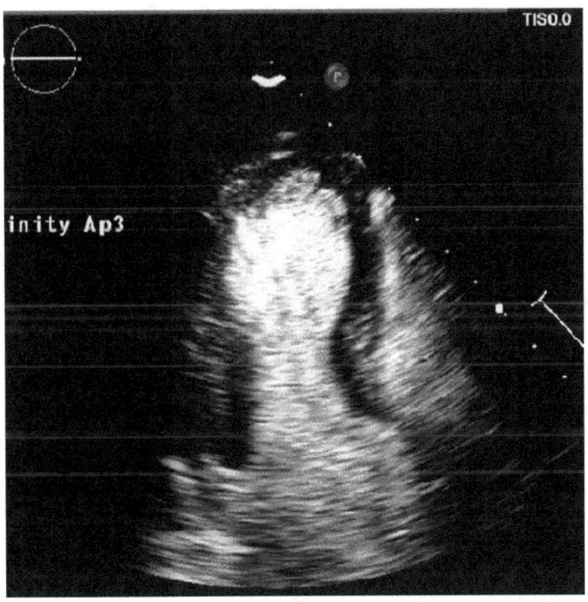

FIGURE 2: Apical 2 chamber echocardiogram with definity contrast.

38% with apical akinesis (Figure 2) concerning for typical TCM. Given that the patient was asymptomatic, we discussed a nuclear stress test versus left heart catheterization with the patient, and it was mutually decided to proceed with a nuclear stress test which demonstrated reversible apical inferior perfusion defect and apical inferior wall motion abnormality. Eventually, the patient underwent a left heart catheterization which showed clean coronaries (Figure 3). Based on these findings, she was diagnosed with typical TCM secondary to adrenal insufficiency due to exogenous steroid use. Her troponin subsequently trended down, her IV hydrocortisone was tapered to oral hydrocortisone, and she was discharged in stable condition with endocrine and cardiology outpatient follow-up.

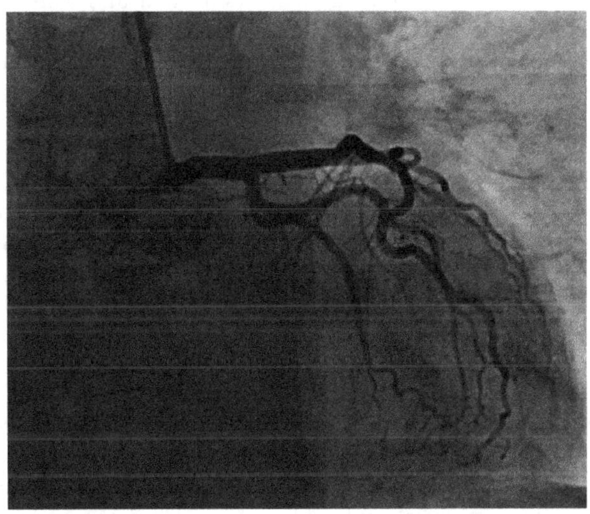

FIGURE 3: Cardiac catheterization of the left coronary artery.

3. Discussion

Patients with Takotsubo cardiomyopathy typically suffer from an acute stressor. In the present case, we attribute the Takotsubo cardiomyopathy to secondary adrenal insufficiency as evidenced by the decreased ACTH, cortisol, and the lack of adequate response of cortisol levels to ACTH administration. Although Takotsubo cardiomyopathy may have been caused by other causes such as the hyponatremia and hypoglycemia, it is more likely that adrenal insufficiency was the cause as it is a unifying diagnosis for hyponatremia, hypotension, and hypoglycemia. We therefore made a diagnosis of Takotsubo cardiomyopathy due to secondary adrenal insufficiency.

Most cases of Takotsubo cardiomyopathy associated with adrenal insufficiency are documented in the pediatric age group [3–5]. To our knowledge, only four cases of Takotsubo cardiomyopathy associated with adrenal insufficiency have

Table 1: Reported cases of adrenal insufficiency-induced Takotsubo cardiomyopathy.

Case	Age/sex	Primary vs. secondary AI	Coronary angiogram	Typical vs. atypical TCM	Author
1	74/F	Secondary	No abnormalities	Typical	Iga et al.
2	64/F	Primary	No abnormalities	Typical	Iga et al.
3	62/F	Secondary	No significant stenosis	Typical	Eto et al.
4	53/F	Secondary	No significant stenosis	Typical	Sakihara et al.
5	55/F	Secondary	No abnormalities	Typical	Garrahy et al.

been reported in the English literature in the adult patients (Table 1). Three of the four cases were associated with secondary adrenal insufficiency [6–8]. All four cases showed reversible cardiomyopathy and improved myocardial function with steroid therapy for adrenal insufficiency. In the present case, the patient was lost to cardiology follow-up, so there is no evidence for reversibility of our patient's cardiomyopathy. However, the patient's hypoglycemia and hypotension improved quickly with IV hydrocortisone, highlighting the importance of early supplemental hydrocortisone in these patients.

The cause of left ventricular dysfunction in Takotsubo cardiomyopathy is still unknown. It may represent catecholamine-induced myocardial stunning that results from a combination of myocardial ischemia related to diffuse microvascular dysfunction and multivessel epicardial spasm [9]. Although the evidence is strong that catecholamines play a large role in the acute reversible myocardial injury, it is still unclear why the apical segment is more affected than the basal segment [10]. The most plausible explanation is the increased volume of adrenergic receptors in the apex of the heart [11].

While it is known that treatment of the underlying condition/removal of the stressor is the cornerstone for management of TCM which in this case was glucocorticoid therapy, studies have also shown that glucocorticoids are important for the maintenance of membrane calcium transport function in the cardiac sarcoplasmic reticulum and, thus, for myocardial contractility [12]. Glucocorticoids also reduce ischemia-reperfusion-induced myocardial apoptosis [13]. Furthermore, intracellular calcium concentration is affected by glucocorticoids. The authors also showed that microsomal phosphorylase activity in the myocardium was depleted by adrenalectomy [14]. The decreased phosphorylase activity may impair glycogenolysis and the excitation-contraction coupling of the heart [15–17]. Considering all these effects, it can be concluded that glucocorticoids can rescue myocyte apoptosis and improve cardiac function.

This present case reports the rare finding of Takotsubo cardiomyopathy caused by secondary adrenal insufficiency. Treatment of the inciting etiology along with careful monitoring of cardiac function coupled with appropriate guideline-directed treatment of cardiomyopathy can reverse the left ventricular dysfunction.

Acknowledgments

The authors would like to thank Dr. Peter Will, Department of Cardiology, Tower Health System, for providing the echocardiogram and catheterization images for the manuscript.

References

[1] C. Walker and W. Butt, "A case of cardiovascular collapse due to adrenal insufficiency," *Journal of Paediatrics and Child Health*, vol. 24, no. 3, pp. 197-198, 1988.

[2] C. Templin, J. R. Ghadri, J. Diekmann et al., "Clinical features and outcomes of Takotsubo (stress) cardiomyopathy," *New England Journal of Medicine*, vol. 373, no. 10, pp. 929–938, 2015.

[3] B. A. Boston, C. DeGroff, C. E. Hanna, and M. Reller, "Reversible cardiomyopathy in an infant with unrecognized congenital adrenal hyperplasia," *The Journal of Pediatrics*, vol. 124, no. 6, pp. 936–938, 1994.

[4] M. Derish, K. Eckert, and C. Chin, "Reversible cardiomyopathy in a child with Addison's disease," *Intensive Care Medicine*, vol. 22, no. 5, pp. 460–463, 1996.

[5] A. Afzal and F. Khaja, "Reversible cardiomyopathy associated with Addison's disease," *The Canadian Journal of Cardiology*, vol. 16, no. 3, pp. 377–379, 2000.

[6] K. Iga, K. Hori, and H. Gen, "Deep negative T waves associated with reversible left ventricular dysfunction in acute adrenal crisis," *Heart and Vessels*, vol. 7, no. 2, pp. 107–111, 1992.

[7] K. Eto, T. Koga, A. Sakamoto, N. Kawazoe, S. Sadoshima, and K. Onoyama, "Adult reversible cardiomyopathy with pituitary adrenal insufficiency caused by empty sella – a case report," *Angiology*, vol. 51, no. 4, pp. 319–323, 2000.

[8] S. Sakihara, K. Kageyama, T. Nigawara, Y. Kidani, and T. Suda, "Ampulla (Takotsubo) cardiomyopathy caused by secondary adrenal insufficiency in ACTH isolated deficiency," *Endocrine Journal*, vol. 54, no. 4, pp. 631–636, 2007.

[9] K. Oki, W. Matsuura, J. Koide et al., "Ampulla cardiomyopathy associated with adrenal insufficiency and hypothyroidism," *International Journal of Cardiology*, vol. 108, no. 3, pp. 391-392, 2006.

[10] S. Nazir, S. Lohani, N. Tachamo, S. Ghimire, D. R. Poudel, and A. Donato, "Takotsubo cardiomyopathy associated with epinephrine use: a systematic review and meta-analysis," *International Journal of Cardiology*, vol. 229, pp. 67–70, 2017.

[11] K. A. Bybee, T. Kara, A. Prasad et al., "Systematic review: transient left ventricular apical ballooning: a syndrome that mimics ST-segment elevation myocardial infarction," *Annals of Internal Medicine*, vol. 141, no. 11, pp. 858–865, 2004.

[12] H. Mori, S. Ishikawa, S. Kojima et al., "Increased responsiveness of left ventricular apical myocardium to adrenergic stimuli," *Cardiovascular Research*, vol. 27, no. 2, pp. 192–198, 1993.

[13] N. Narayan, "Effects of adrenalectomy and in vivo administration of dexamethasone on ATP- dependent calcium accumulation by sarcoplasmic reticulum from rat heart," *Journal of*

Molecular and Cellular Cardiology, vol. 15, no. 1, pp. 7–15, 1983.

[14] J. M. Pearl, D. P. Nelson, S. M. Schwartz et al., "Glucocorticoids reduce ischemia-reperfusion-induced myocardial apoptosis in immature hearts," *The Annals of Thoracic Surgery*, vol. 74, no. 3, pp. 830–837, 2002.

[15] N. Narayanan and R. L. Khandelwal, "Microsomal phosphorylase in rat heart: depletion following adrenalectomy and restoration byin vivoadministration of dexamethasone*," *Endocrinology*, vol. 117, no. 4, pp. 1544–1549, 1985.

[16] Z. J. Penefsky and F. V. McCann, "Electrical properties of developing rat heart. Effects of dexamethasone," *Journal of Developmental Physiology*, vol. 12, no. 1, pp. 27–33, 1989.

[17] K. Machida, R. Ishibashi, T. Hara, A. Ohtsuka, and K. Hayashi, "Effects of corticosterone on Ca2+ uptake and myofibrillar disassembly in primary muscle cell culture," *Bioscience, Biotechnology, and Biochemistry*, vol. 67, pp. 244–249, 2003.

6

Complete Heart Block Complicating Takotsubo Syndrome

Michael J. McGee, [1,2,3] William Yu, [2] Joshua McCarthy, [2] Malcolm Barlow, [2] and Rosemary Hackworthy [2]

[1] *School of Medicine and Public Health, University of Newcastle, Newcastle, NSW, Australia*
[2] *Cardiovascular Department, John Hunter Hospital, Newcastle, NSW, Australia*
[3] *Hunter Medical Research Institute, Newcastle, NSW, Australia*

Correspondence should be addressed to Michael J. McGee; michael.mcgee@health.nsw.gov.au

Academic Editor: Manabu Shirotani

An 81-year-old woman presents with shortness of breath resulting in a diagnosis of picornavirus and complete heart block. Troponin was elevated and there was concern about acute coronary syndrome. The final diagnosis after echocardiogram and coronary angiogram was Takotsubo syndrome in addition to the heart block which required pacemaker insertion.

1. History of Presentation

An 81-year-old woman presented to a peripheral emergency department with a two-week history of shortness of breath. She had been commenced on oral antibiotics for a lower respiratory tract infection in the community.

1.1. Past Medical History. The patient has a history of hypertension, dyslipidaemia, osteoporosis, anxiety, and gastrooesophageal reflux disease.

1.2. Medications at Admission. Irbesartan 300 mg daily, hydrochlorothiazide 12.5 mg daily, thyroxine 50 mcg daily, rosuvastatin 10 mg daily, sertraline 25 mg daily, aspirin 100 mg daily, metoprolol 12.5 mg twice daily were the medications for the patients.

1.3. Clinical Course. On assessment in the emergency department, the patient was found to be in complete heart block (CHB) with a ventricular escape of 48 bpm (Figure 1). She denied chest pain on presentation or recently. High sensitivity troponin was found to be elevated at 525 ng/L (<16). The patient was transported to the local tertiary hospital for the management of acute coronary syndrome and complete heart block. A respiratory viral PCR swab was sent prior to transport. The swab later returned positive for picornavirus. B-type natriuretic peptide (BNP) was elevated at 1174 ng/L (<266) and subsequent troponins fell.

Echocardiogram after transfer revealed a large area of left ventricular apical hypokinesis, moderate atrial dilatation, and tricuspid regurgitation in the context of the known complete heart block (Figure 2 and supplementary figure 1).

Cardiac catheterisation was delayed secondary to inability to lie flat as a result of the respiratory infection, with cough fits and agitation without desaturation. This was performed on day 9 postpresentation. The coronary angiogram revealed nonobstructive coronary artery disease, with a focal 50% stenosis in the midleft circumflex coronary artery (supplemental figure 2). The left ventriculogram performed revealed near normalisation of the apical hypokinesis and an elevated end diastolic pressure of 20 mmHg (Figure 3). Laboratory findings are listed in Table 1.

1.4. Management. The complete heart block continued after cessation of the metoprolol. The patient was initially managed conservatively as the ventricular escape was greater than 40 bpm without hypotension. The patient did have

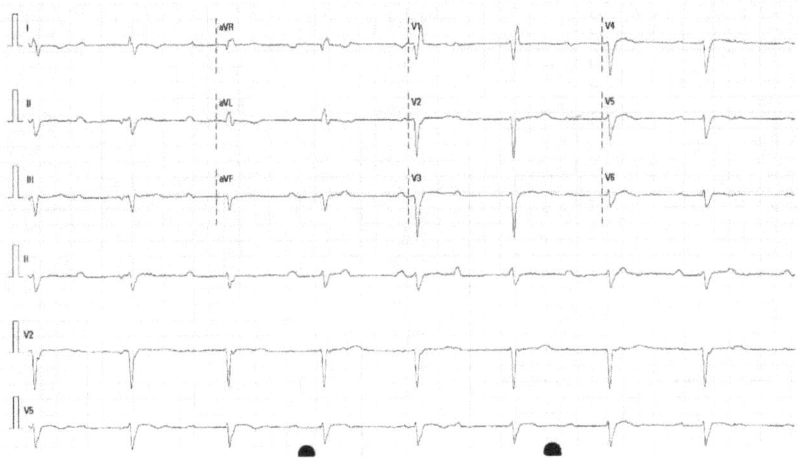

Figure 1: Electrocardiogram revealing complete heart block with a ventricular escape at approximately 48 beats per minute.

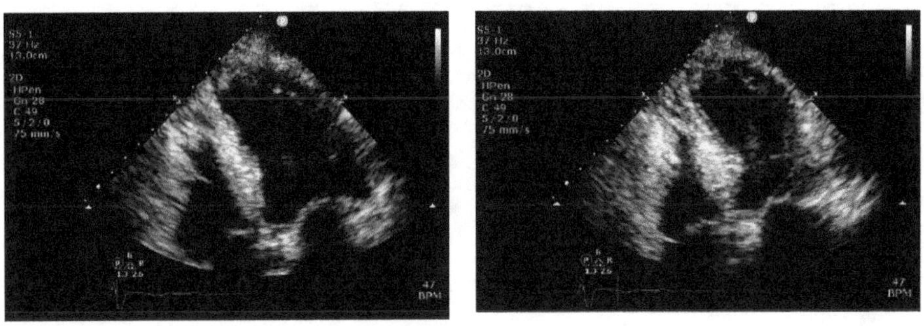

(a) (b)

Figure 2: Transthoracic echocardiogram performed on presentation. Apical 4 chamber view, at end diastole (a) and end systolic (b) demonstrating left ventricular apical hypokinesis.

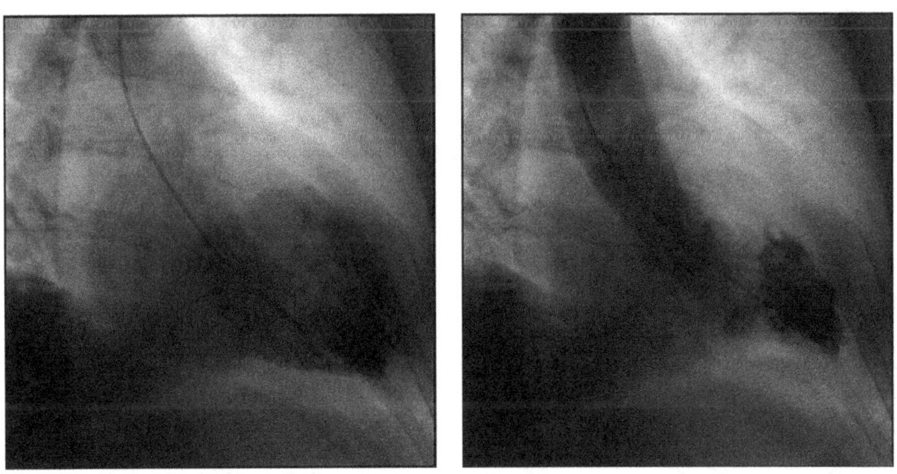

(a) (b)

Figure 3: Cardiac catheterisation performed on day 9, left ventriculogram at end diastole (a) and end systole (b) demonstrating resolution of the apical hypokinesis.

exacerbations of coughing and agitation when lying flat, which could be attributed to either heart failure or respiratory tract infection. Chest X-ray on presentation was not consistent with heart failure despite the raised BNP. The picornavirus infection was managed conservatively. Nine days after presentation, once the patient was able to lie flat without incident, a dual chamber Biotronik pacemaker was implanted, DDD 60–130 (Figure 4). The patient was discharged on aspirin, irbesartan, rosuvastatin, and sertraline.

1.5. Follow-Up. Interrogation of the pacemaker 6 weeks post-implantation revealed underlying complete heart block with

Table 1

Value	Initial	Peak	Reference range
Troponin I	525	525	<16 ng/L
TSH	2.84		0.40-5.00 mIU/L
Sodium	131	139	135–145 mmol/L
Potassium	4.4	5.5	3.5–5.2 mmol/L
Creatinine	82	121	45-90μmol/L
Calcium (corrected)	2.56	2.71	2.10-2.60 mmol/L
BNP	1174		<266 ng/L
CRP	38	49	<5 mg/L
WCC	11.5	14.1	4.0-11.0 × 10^9/L
Haemoglobin	123	131	115-165 g/L

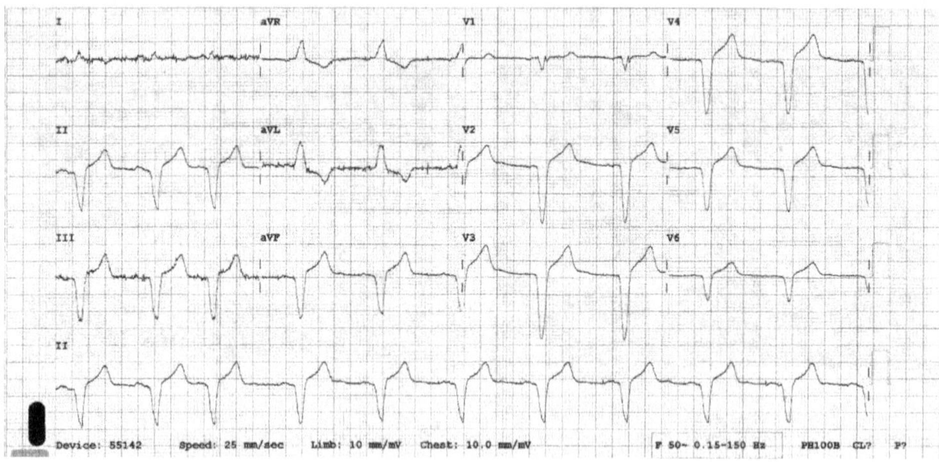

Figure 4: Electrocardiogram following implantation of a dual chamber pacemaker with atrial sensed, ventricular paced complexes.

100% ventricular pacing, no tachyarrhythmias, and satisfactory device parameters. The patient remains independent in the community 6 months following discharge.

2. Discussion

The patient had previously been referred to a cardiologist as an outpatient due to concerns regarding cardiomegaly on chest X-ray and resistant hypertension. Investigations completed 6 months prior to the patient's hospitalisation revealed normal left ventricular size and systolic function on an echocardiogram and right bundle branch block on an electrocardiogram.

It appears that the Takotsubo syndrome (TTS) in our patient's case was precipitated by the lower respiratory tract infection with picornavirus. This phenomenon of an emotional or physiological insult as a trigger for TTS has been well described. This case is unusual given the presence of complete heart block in association with TTS at time of presentation. It is unclear when the patient developed complete heart block as the ventricular escape was robust and was well tolerated hemodynamically. There was preexisting right bundle branch block, and the possibility of progressive conduction disease is high.

The alternative diagnoses for this case include acute coronary syndrome and viral-induced myocarditis. Picornavirus family has been associated with viral myocarditis in other cases and series [1]. Cardiac magnetic resonance imaging could help distinguish in cases were the diagnosis is unclear. We felt the characteristics of the echocardiogram and angiogram were consistent with TTS, and subsequently, cardiac magnetic resonance imaging and cardiac biopsy were not pursued.

Acute coronary syndrome was another possible diagnosis, with spontaneous recanalization. We felt this was unlikely given that the extensive wall motion abnormality was beyond a single coronary artery territory (the patient did not have a left anterior descending that wrapped around the apex) and was disproportionate to the peak troponin.

Several case reports of TTS and CHB exist [2–4]. The clinical challenges are twofold: firstly, determining which precipitates the other, and secondly, determining the need for a cardiac implantable electronic device (CIED). If the TTS is secondary to CHB, then pacing will be required; however, if the CHB is secondary to TTS, then there is the possibility of recovery and a CIED can be avoided. Cases of both scenarios have been reported in the literature [5, 6].

CIED implantation is not a benign procedure with recent research documenting a high complication rate of

Table 2

Case	Year	Author	Age	Sex	TTS and CHB	CIED	F/U period (months)	Resolved
1	2004	Saito et al. [12]	86	F	1	Yes	NR	Unknown
2	2006	Nef et al. [13]	58	M	1	Yes	3	Yes
3	2006	Lee et al. [14]	72	F	1	No	<1	Yes
4	2007	Nault et al. [2]	62	F	1	Yes	24	Yes
5	2008	Kurisu et al. [9]	78	M	1	Yes	<1	Unknown
6			87	F	1	Yes	NR	Unknown
7	2009	Inoue et al. [3]	82	F	1	Yes	3	Unknown
8	2009	Kodama et al. [15]	57	F	1	Yes	NR	Unknown
9			39	F	1	Yes	NR	Unknown
10	2011	Siry et al. [16]	70	F	1	Yes	NR	Unknown
11	2012	Benouda et al. [17]	81	F	1	Yes	NR	Unknown
12	2012	Shanmugasundar et al. [4]	72	F	1	Yes	NR	Unknown
13	2013	Chadha et al. [18]	61	F	1	No	12	Yes
14	2013	Wakiya et al. [19]	86	F	1	Yes	12	No
15	2013	Sugiura et al. [5]	63	F	1	No	NR	Unknown
16	2015	Stiermaier et al. [6]	NR	NR	1	Yes	NR	Unknown
17			NR	NR	1	Yes	NR	Unknown
18			NR	NR	1	Yes	NR	Unknown
19			NR	NR	1	No	NR	Unknown
20	2015	Korantzopoulos et al. [20]	71	F	1	Yes	6	No
21	2017	Inayat et al. [11]	59	F	1	Yes	6	No
22	2018	Afzal et al. [21]	62	F	1	Yes	6	No
23	2019	Sakul et al. [10]	73	F	1	Yes	20	No
24	2020	McGee	81	F	1	Yes	3	No

NR: not reported.

approximately 10% [7]. There are case reports of TTS occurring post CIED implantation [8]. Case reports of TTS and CHB have described implantation of dual chamber pacemakers, biventricular pacemakers, and defibrillator for the treatment of CHB [9–11]. One of the largest consecutive series of TTS reported a CHB prevalence of 2.2% [6]. Including our case, we were able to identify 24 reported cases of CHB complicating TTS. In four of the cases, a CIED was not implanted due to the resolution of the heart block. In further two cases, the AV block resolved postimplantation of the CIED (Table 2).

3. Conclusion

TTS is not a benign condition and presents a number of clinical challenges. An association with complete heart block is not uncommon and often requires CIED implantation.

Take-home messages and learning objectives are as follows:

(i) Takotsubo syndrome can result in a wide range of dangerous arrhythmias, both brady and tachycardic

(ii) Takotsubo syndrome can complicate other cardiovascular disease entities

(iii) Most, but not all patients who have complete heart block and Takotsubo syndrome require a pacemaker

Abbreviations

CIED: Cardiac implantable electronic device
CHB: Complete heart block (third-degree atrioventricular block)
TTS: Takotsubo syndrome.

Disclosure

During the time of drafting, all authors were employed by Hunter New England Health. The employer had no role in drafting or reviewing the manuscript.

Supplementary Materials

Supplementary 1. Supplemental Figure 1: Transthoracic echocardiogram performed on presentation. Apical 2 chamber view, at end diastole (left) and end systolic (right) demonstrating left ventricular apical hypokinesis. Supplemental figure 2: Coronary angiography, with the left coronary artery (left) and the right coronary artery (right) demonstrating non-obstructive coronary artery disease.

Supplementary 2. Supplemental Videos: Video 1: Transthoracic echocardiogram performed on presentation. Apical 2 chamber view demonstrating apical hypokinesis with preserved basal function consistent with takotsubo syndrome. Video 2: Transthoracic echocardiogram performed on presentation. Apical 3 chamber view demonstrating apical hypokinesis with preserved basal function consistent with takotsubo syndrome. Video 3: Transthoracic echocardiogram performed on presentation. Apical 4 chamber view demonstrating apical hypokinesis with preserved basal function consistent with takotsubo syndrome. Video 4: Cardiac catheterisation performed on day 9, left ventriculogram demonstrating resolution of the apical hypokinesis.

References

[1] E. Arbustini, E. Porcu, O. Bellini et al., "Enteroviral infection causing fatal myocarditis and subclinical myopathy," *Heart*, vol. 83, no. 1, pp. 86–90, 2000.

[2] M. A. Nault, A. Baranchuk, C. S. Simpson, and D. P. Redfearn, "Takotsubo cardiomyopathy: a novel "proarrhythmic" disease," *Anadolu Kardiyoloji Dergisi*, vol. 7, pp. 101–103, 2007.

[3] M. Inoue, H. Kanaya, T. Matsubara, Y. Uno, T. Yasuda, and K. Miwa, "Complete atrioventricular block associated with Takotsubo cardiomyopathy," *Circulation Journal*, vol. 73, no. 3, pp. 589–592, 2009.

[4] R. Shanmugasundaram, K. Tamilarasu, G. Rajendiran, and A. Murali, "An uncommon presentation of a rare disease - high-degree AV block with Takotsubo cardiomyopathy," *Indian Heart Journal*, vol. 64, no. 5, pp. 511–514, 2012.

[5] T. Sugiura, Y. Dohi, S. Yamashita et al., "Midventricular ballooning Takotsubo cardiomyopathy complicated by transient complete atrioventricular block," *Internal Medicine*, vol. 52, no. 17, pp. 1919–1921, 2013.

[6] T. Stiermaier, C. Eitel, S. Denef et al., "Prevalence and clinical significance of life-threatening arrhythmias in Takotsubo cardiomyopathy," *Journal of the American College of Cardiology*, vol. 65, no. 19, pp. 2148–2150, 2015.

[7] I. Ranasinghe, C. Labrosciano, D. Horton et al., "Institutional variation in quality of cardiovascular implantable electronic device implantation: a cohort study," *Annals of Internal Medicine*, vol. 171, no. 5, pp. 309–317, 2019.

[8] S. G. Chun, V. Kwok, D. K. Pang, and T. K. Lau, "Transient left ventricular apical ballooning syndrome (Takotsubo cardiomyopathy) as a complication of permanent pacemaker implantation," *International Journal of Cardiology*, vol. 117, no. 1, pp. e27–e30, 2007.

[9] S. Kurisu, I. Inoue, T. Kawagoe et al., "Torsade de pointes associated with bradycardia and Takotsubo cardiomyopathy," *The Canadian Journal of Cardiology*, vol. 24, no. 8, pp. 640–642, 2008.

[10] N. F. N. Sakul, S. Shrestha, N. Balabbigari, and S. Talati, "Complete heart block: a rare complication of Takotsubo syndrome," *Case Reports in Cardiology*, vol. 2019, Article ID 2576373, 5 pages, 2019.

[11] F. Inayat, H. U. H. Virk, W. Ullah, and I. Riaz, "Takotsubo cardiomyopathy-related complete heart block and torsades de pointes," *BML Case Reports*, vol. 2017, 2017.

[12] M. Saito, Y. Hayashi, O. Sasaki, M. Inoue, S. Fujioka, and M. Kouno, "A case of foxhole-shaped left ventricular abnormality induced by complete atrioventricular block with delayed recovery of wall motion," *Nihon Ronen Igakkai Zasshi.*, vol. 41, no. 5, pp. 546–551, 2004.

[13] H. M. Nef, H. Möllmann, J. Sperzel et al., "Temporary third-degree atrioventricular block in a case of apical ballooning syndrome," *International Journal of Cardiology*, vol. 113, no. 2, pp. e33–e35, 2006.

[14] W. L. Lee, L. F. Miao, H. W. Chan, and M. Z. Chen, "Takotsubo syndrome with transient complete atrioventricular block," *Chinese Medical Journal*, vol. 119, no. 1, pp. 73–76, 2006.

[15] S. Kodama, K. Miyoshi, Y. Shiga et al., "Takotsubo cardiomyopathy complicated by high-grade atrioventricular block: a report of two cases," *Experimental and Clinical Cardiology*, vol. 14, no. 2, pp. e35–e38, 2009.

[16] M. Siry, N. Scheffold, D. Wimmert-Roidl, and G. Konig, "A rare complication of Takotsubo cardiomyopathy," *DMW - Deutsche Medizinische Wochenschrift*, vol. 136, no. 4, pp. 129–132, 2011.

[17] L. Benouda, V. Roule, A. Foucault, Z. Dahdouh, A. Lebon, and P. Milliez, "Conduction disturbances in Takotsubo cardiomyopathy: a cause or a consequence?," *International Journal of Cardiology*, vol. 159, no. 1, pp. 61-62, 2012.

[18] S. Chadha, A. Lodha, V. Shetty, A. Sadiq, G. Hollander, and J. Shani, "Complete heart block in Takotsubo cardiomyopathy," *Heart & Lung*, vol. 42, no. 1, pp. 48–50, 2013.

[19] M. Wakiya, H. Hara, M. Iwano et al., "Complete atrioventricular block associated with not apical but midventricular ballooning," *Journal of Cardiology Cases*, vol. 7, no. 4, pp. e109–e113, 2013.

[20] K. Panagiotis, N. Nikas Dimitrios, L. Konstantinos et al., "High-grade atrioventricular block and Takotsubo cardiomyopathy: case report and review of the literature," *International Cardiovascular Research Journal*, vol. 9, no. 2, article e11407, 2017.

[21] A. Afzal, J. Watson, J. W. Choi, J. M. Schussler, and M. D. Assar, "Takotsubo cardiomyopathy in the setting of complete heart block," *Baylor University Medical Center Proceedings*, vol. 31, no. 4, pp. 502–505, 2018.

7

A Rare Case of Takotsubo Syndrome and Acute Coronary Syndrome of the Right Coronary Artery

Nicholas Mencer,[1] **Larry Todd Justice**,[1] **William Black**,[2] **and Kayleigh Litton**[2]

[1]*Department of Interventional Cardiology Methodist Medical Center, Oak Ridge, Tennessee 37748, USA*
[2]*Department of Interventional Cardiology, The University of Tennessee Knoxville, Knoxville, Tennessee 37996, USA*

Correspondence should be addressed to Nicholas Mencer; nicholas.mencer@lmunet.edu
Academic Editor: Assad Movahed

Takotsubo syndrome (TTS) is an increasingly recognized heart disease that was initially regarded as a benign condition, but since has proven to cause irreversible myocardial damage, resembling that of acute coronary syndrome (ACS). The etiology of TTS is still uncertain but may be associated with catecholamine elevations during times of emotional or physical stress. Catecholamines are also understood to have prothrombotic properties, which could lead to ACS. With these similarities, differentiating these two pathologies can be difficult, especially when TTS and ACS occur simultaneously.

1. Introduction

The pathogenesis of takotsubo syndrome (TTS) is not completely understood. Proposed mechanisms involve catecholamine excess during times of physical or emotional stress that lead to left ventricular myocardial dysfunction by direct catecholamine-associated toxicity and microvascular spasm [1, 2]. Although TTS may sometimes present as an ST elevation myocardial infarction (STEMI), angiography typically reveals no occlusive lesion within the coronary arteries. We present a case of a postmenopausal Caucasian female with TTS and coexisting critical stenosis of the right coronary artery (RCA).

2. Case Report

A previously healthy 89-year-old female presented to the emergency department complaining of midsternal chest discomfort that radiated to her back. Her chest discomfort began the day prior to presentation, but she initially attributed it to indigestion and thus waited to seek medical attention. Her chest pain persisted however, which prompted her to seek evaluation in the emergency department. Upon arrival, she was given aspirin with resolution of her symptoms. Laboratory analysis revealed an elevated troponin I level of 0.319 and initial creatine kinase (CK) of 12.7. Brain natriuretic peptide level on presentation was not checked. Electrocardiogram (ECG) was notable for diffuse T-wave inversions demonstrating inferior, as well as anterolateral ischemia, and a prolonged QTc of 503 ms (Figure 1). Echocardiogram demonstrated moderate left ventricular dysfunction (ejection fraction of 35%-40%) with mid to distal anteroseptal, anterolateral, and apical akinesis (Figure 2). The patient was taken to the catheterization suite and underwent emergent left heart catheterization. Angiography revealed 90% stenosis in the mid right coronary artery (RCA) which was believed to be the culprit lesion. There were no significant obstructive lesions noted in the left anterior descending or left circumflex arteries. She underwent percutaneous coronary intervention (PCI) with successful stent placement to the RCA (Figure 3). She was then started on appropriate guideline-directed medical therapy and observed in the intensive care unit where her chest pain resolved. Repeat laboratory analysis revealed that CK had decreased to 6.4. ECG obtained following PCI revealed interval improvement of the inferior T-wave inversions, with sustained T-wave abnormalities in the anterolateral leads (Figure 4). Cardiac magnetic resonance imaging is

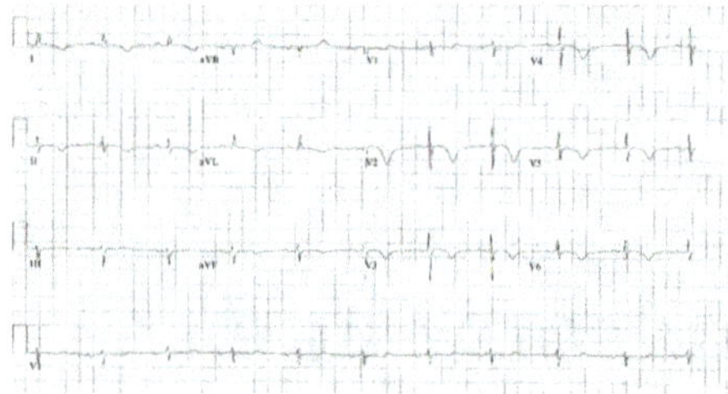

Figure 1: ECG on admission demonstrating diffuse T-wave inversions.

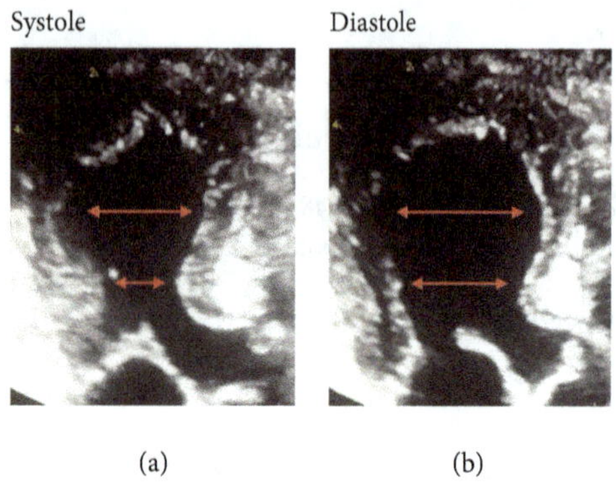

Figure 2: Apical three chamber echocardiogram demonstrating left ventricular apical ballooning and basal hyperkinesis consistent with takotsubo syndrome.

not available at our facility and was not performed. The remainder of her hospitalization proceeded without incident, and she was discharged home in stable condition three days later.

The patient was evaluated two weeks after discharge in an outpatient clinic and was feeling well. She again denied any stressors prior to the onset of pain but reported that the development of chest pain caused her a great deal of emotional distress. Repeat echocardiogram was obtained which revealed normal left ventricular systolic function (Figure 5).

3. Discussion

There have been numerous case reports of patients presenting with profound left ventricular dysfunction after suffering severe emotional or physical stress. This syndrome was first described in Japan in 1990 and is commonly referred to as transient apical ballooning syndrome or takotsubo syndrome [3–8]. Takotsubo syndrome is often associated with emotional triggers but has frequently been described in association with physical triggers. A large registry of patients with TTS found that physical triggers were more common than emotional triggers—women were more likely to have emotional triggers whereas men were more likely to have a physical trigger [9]. Although the diagnosis of TTS has historically been based on the presence of angiographically normal coronary arteries, there have been multiple reports of TTS occurring in the setting of physiological stress from acute coronary syndrome (ACS) [10]. The prevalence of TTS is estimated to be 2%-3% in patients who present with ACS and may be

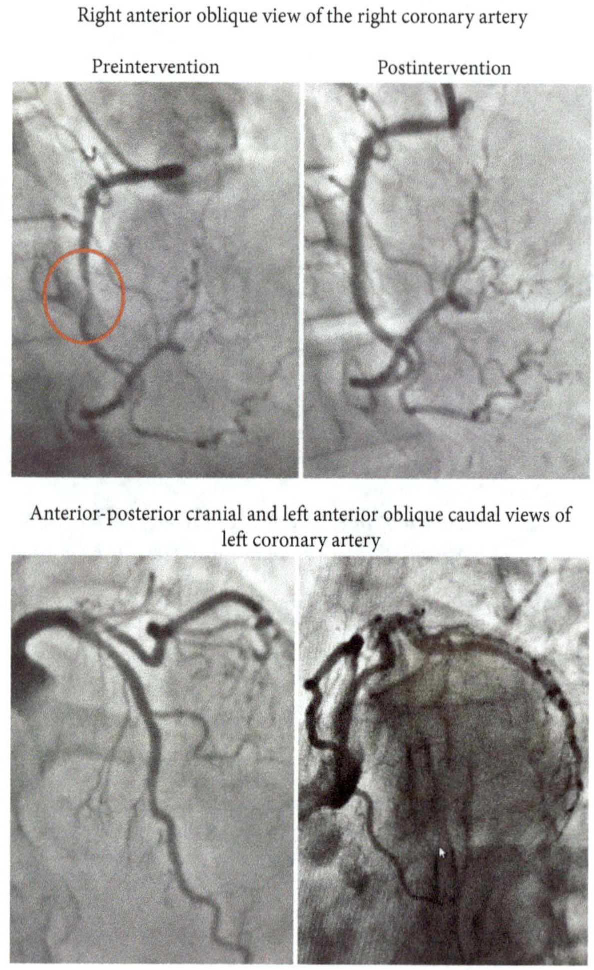

Figure 3: Angiographical images obtained during cardiac catheterization.

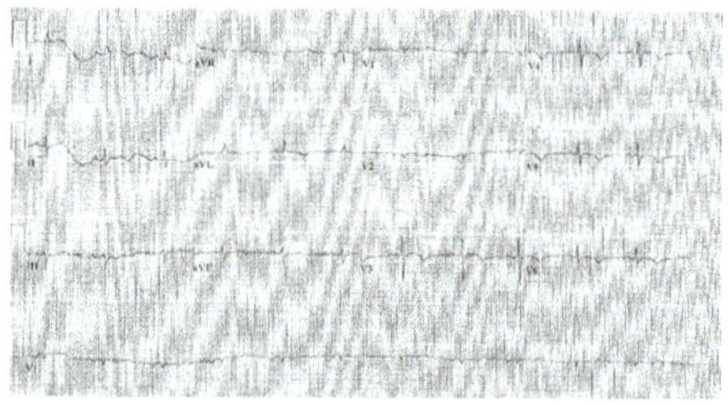

Figure 4: ECG post-PCI demonstrating interval improvement of inferior T-wave inversions and sustained T-wave abnormalities in the anterolateral leads.

underestimated in individuals with coexisting coronary artery disease [11]. The recently updated International Takotsubo Diagnostic Criteria (InterTAK Diagnostic Criteria) specifically states that "significant coronary artery disease is not a contraindication in takotsubo syndrome" [1]. The exact pathophysiology of myocardial dysfunction due to sympathetic stimulation is unknown, but numerous mechanisms have been proposed. One potential mechanism is direct myocardial ischemia due to coronary arterial spasm—it has been shown that increased mental stress can cause vasoconstriction in patients without coronary artery disease

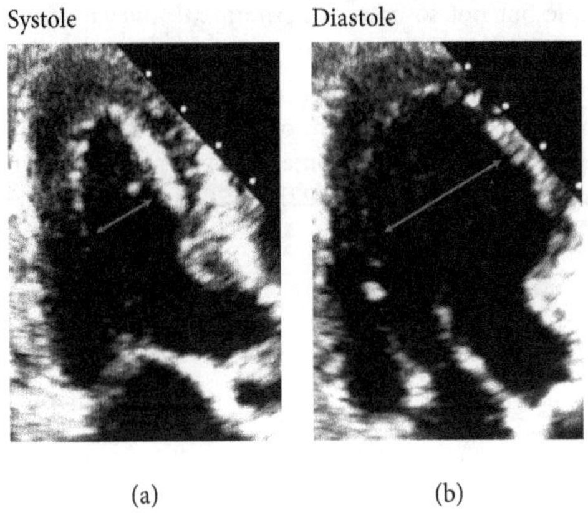

FIGURE 5: Apical three chamber echocardiogram obtained two weeks following revascularization of the RCA demonstrating no residual left ventricular dysfunction.

[12]. Another potential mechanism is sympathetically mediated microvascular dysfunction resulting in abnormal coronary blood flow in the absence of obstructive disease [13]. A third potential mechanism is direct myocyte injury due to increased levels of circulating catecholamines which have been shown to cause contraction band necrosis. Similar injury patterns have been reported with catecholamine excess due to pheochromocytoma and subarachnoid hemorrhage [14, 15].

However, recent review suggests that although catecholamine excess may be linked to TTS, there is no direct causality [16].

This case poses two interesting questions: is the physiologic and emotional stress of chest pain enough to cause TTS? Can the catecholamine excess from TTS cause ACS? Catecholamines have been demonstrated to have prothrombotic properties in coronary arteries. Lin and Young demonstrated that by raising the plasma epinephrine concentration to approximately 27 nmol/L, the incidence of cyclic blood flow reductions in the coronary arteries of canines increased by 60% [17]. Catecholamine levels in takotsubo patients are 2-3 times higher than myocardial infarction patients 1-2 days after the onset of symptoms and 20 times higher than normal adults [18]. Additionally, the catecholamine levels in takotsubo patients remain elevated over myocardial infarction levels for 7-9 days [19]. With the known prothrombotic properties of catecholamines and the suspected rise in catecholamines associated with TTS, it is possible that TTS could have occurred first in our patient, leading to ACS of the RCA. This could have occurred either by thrombosis in our patient's native coronary artery or with the acute left ventricular (LV) systolic dysfunction associated TTS, an embolic event from a LV thrombus. However, extensive review of our patient's history, cardiac imaging, laboratory findings, and medical record failed to elucidate a possible cause for TTS other than her ACS.

Based on her description of symptoms and failure to identify another cause, we hypothesize that she initially developed ACS of the RCA, and the emotional distress from this event is likely the etiology of her TTS. Previous case series have reported that postischemic myocardial stunning has features typical of TTS and suggested that ACS may trigger TTS [20]. It can be difficult to distinguish between TTS and ACS as they have similar clinical presentations, and both can cause transient wall motion abnormalities [21]. Cardiac magnetic resonance imaging (CMR) can help distinguish TTS from myocardial infarction when there is diagnostic uncertainty, but unfortunately, we were unable to perform this in our patient [22].

4. Conclusion

The diagnosis of TTS has historically been a diagnosis of exclusion that required the presence of normal coronary arteries, but recent expert consensus has been updated to remove CAD as an exclusion criterion. Previous case reports have described cases of TTS coexisting with ACS as well as cases of ACS triggering TTS. This case contributes to the growing body of case reports that suggest that TTS and ACS can occur concomitantly.

Disclosure

Nicholas Mencer, DO, Larry Todd Justice, MD, William Black, MD, and Kayleigh Litton, DO certify that they have no affiliations with or involvement in any organization or entity with any financial interest (such as honoraria; educational grants; participation in speakers' bureaus; membership, employment, consultancies, stock ownership, or other equity interest; and expert testimony or patent-licensing arrangements) or nonfinancial interest (such as personal or professional relationships, affiliations, knowledge, or beliefs) in the subject matter or materials discussed in this manuscript.

Authors' Contributions

All authors had access to all data and a role in writing this manuscript.

References

[1] J.-R. Ghadri, I. S. Wittstein, A. Prasad et al., "International expert consensus document on takotsubo syndrome (part I): clinical characteristics, diagnostic criteria, and pathophysiology," *European Heart Journal*, vol. 39, no. 22, pp. 2032–2046, 2018.

[2] H. M. Nef, H. Mollmann, S. Kostin et al., "Tako-Tsubo cardiomyopathy: intraindividual structural analysis in the acute phase and after functional recovery," *European Heart Journal*, vol. 28, no. 20, pp. 2456–2464, 2007.

[3] D. Pavin, H. Le Breton, and C. Daubert, "Human stress cardiomyopathy mimicking acute myocardial syndrome," *Heart*, vol. 78, no. 5, pp. 509–511, 1997.

[4] S. Kawai, H. Suzuki, H. Yamaguchi et al., "Ampulla cardiomyopathy ('takotsubo' cardiomyopathy) – reversible left ventricular dysfunction: with ST segment elevation," *Japanese Circulation Journal*, vol. 64, 2000.

[5] R. P. Villareal, A. Achari, S. Wilansky, and J. M. Wilson, "Anteroapical stunning and left ventricular outflow tract obstruction," *Mayo Clinic Proceedings*, vol. 76, no. 1, pp. 79–83, 2001.

[6] H. Z. Brandspiegel, R. A. Marinchak, S. J. Rials, and P. R. Kowey, "A broken heart," *Circulation*, vol. 98, no. 13, pp. 1349–1349, 1998.

[7] K. Tsuchihashi, K. Ueshima, T. Uchida et al., "Transient left ventricular apical ballooning without coronary artery stenosis: a novel heart syndrome mimicking acute myocardial infarction," *Journal of the American College of Cardiology*, vol. 38, no. 1, pp. 11–18, 2001.

[8] S. Kurisu, H. Sato, T. Kawagoe et al., "Tako-tsubo-like left ventricular dysfunction with ST-segment elevation: a novel cardiac syndrome mimicking acute myocardial infarction," *American Heart Journal*, vol. 143, no. 3, pp. 448–455, 2002.

[9] C. Templin, J. R. Ghadri, J. Diekmann et al., "Clinical features and outcomes of takotsubo (stress) cardiomyopathy," *The New England Journal of Medicine*, vol. 373, no. 10, pp. 929–938, 2015.

[10] S. Y-Hassan, "Acute coronary syndrome or takotsubo syndrome: most probably both of them, the first has triggered the second," *International Journal of Cardiology*, vol. 190, pp. 367-368, 2015.

[11] K. Kato, A. R. Lyon, J. R. Ghadri, and C. Templin, "Takotsubo syndrome: aetiology, presentation and treatment," *Heart*, vol. 103, no. 18, pp. 1461–1469, 2017.

[12] C. R. Lacy, R. J. Contrada, M. L. Robbins et al., "Coronary vasoconstriction induced by mental stress (simulated public speaking)," *The American Journal of Cardiology*, vol. 75, no. 7, pp. 503–505, 1995.

[13] K. A. Bybee, A. Prasad, G. W. Barsness et al., "Clinical characteristics and thrombolysis in myocardial infarction frame counts in women with transient left ventricular apical ballooning syndrome," *The American Journal of Cardiology*, vol. 94, no. 3, pp. 343–346, 2004.

[14] C. Wilkenfeld, M. Cohen, S. L. Lansman et al., "Heart transplantation for end-stage cardiomyopathy caused by an occult pheochromocytoma," *The Journal of Heart and Lung Transplantation*, vol. 11, pp. 363–366, 1992.

[15] G. Neil-Dwyer, P. Walter, J. M. Cruickshank, B. Doshi, and P. O'Gorman, "Effect of propranolol and phentolamine on myocardial necrosis after subarachnoid haemorrhage," *BMJ*, vol. 2, no. 6143, pp. 990–992, 1978.

[16] S. Y-Hassan, "Plasma epinephrine levels and its causal link to takotsubo syndrome revisited: critical review with a diverse conclusion," *Cardiovascular Revascularization Medicine*, 2018.

[17] H. Lin and D. B. Young, "Opposing effects of plasma epinephrine and norepinephrine on coronary thrombosis in vivo," *Circulation*, vol. 91, no. 4, pp. 1135–1142, 1995.

[18] I. S. Wittstein, D. R. Thiemann, J. A. C. Lima et al., "Neurohumoral features of myocardial stunning due to sudden emotional stress," *The New England Journal of Medicine*, vol. 352, no. 6, pp. 539–548, 2005.

[19] E. Kazakauskaitė, A. Jankauskas, T. Lapinskas, R. Ordienė, and E. Ereminienė, "Takotsubo cardiomyopathy: the challenging diagnosis in clinical routine," *Medicina*, vol. 50, no. 1, pp. 1–7, 2014.

[20] S. Y-Hassan, "Takotsubo syndrome triggered by acute coronary syndrome in a cohort of 20 patients: an often missed diagnosis," *International Journal of Cardiology and Research*, vol. 2, pp. 28–33, 2015.

[21] L. C. Napp, J. R. Ghadri, V. L. Cammann, J. Bauersachs, and C. Templin, "Takotsubo cardiomyopathy: completely simple but not so easy," *International Journal of Cardiology*, vol. 197, pp. 257–259, 2015.

[22] J. R. Ghadri, I. S. Wittstein, A. Prasad et al., "International expert consensus document on takotsubo syndrome (Part II): diagnostic workup, outcome, and management," *European Heart Journal*, vol. 39, no. 22, pp. 2047–2062, 2018.

8

A Case of Lymphocytic Myocarditis with Eosinophilic Degranulation Successfully Treated with Steroid Therapy

Tomoko Inoue,[1,2] Fusako Sera,[1] Shunsuke Nishimura,[1] Kei Nakamoto,[1] Yasumasa Tsukamoto,[1] Isamu Mizote,[1] Tomohito Ohtani,[1] Shungo Hikoso,[1] Yoshihiko Ikeda,[3] Yumiko Hori,[4] Hatsue Ishibashi-Ueda,[3] Eiichi Morii,[4] Tetsuo Minamino,[2] and Yasushi Sakata[1]

[1]*Department of Cardiovascular Medicine, Osaka University Graduate School of Medicine, Osaka, Japan*
[2]*Department of Cardiorenal and Cerebrovascular Medicine, Faculty of Medicine, Kagawa University, Kagawa, Japan*
[3]*Department of Pathology, National Cardiovascular Center, Osaka, Japan*
[4]*Department of Pathology, Osaka University Graduate School of Medicine, Osaka, Japan*

Correspondence should be addressed to Fusako Sera; sera@cardiology.med.osaka-u.ac.jp
Academic Editor: Assad Movahed

A 49-year-old woman was admitted with suspicion of acute myocarditis. On the next day after admission, her serum troponin I level continued to rise, indicating progression of myocardial damage. Moreover, her symptoms persisted, and left ventricular ejection fraction did not improve. Because of a predominant infiltration of lymphocytes in the myocardial specimens, lymphocytic myocarditis was diagnosed. However, a close observation of the specimens revealed eosinophil degranulation. Based on this finding, intravenous steroid therapy was initiated. High-dose methylprednisolone led to rapid and appreciable improvements in symptoms and left ventricular function within 12 hours after the first administration, which was followed by normalization of serum troponin I level. Steroid therapy was switched to oral administration and tapered carefully. There was no recurrence of left ventricular dysfunction or elevation of serum troponin I level. In eosinophilic myocarditis, eosinophil degranulation has been recognized as an important finding associated with progression of inflammation and myocardial damage. However, no attention has been paid to the presence and clinical implications of eosinophil degranulation in lymphocytic myocarditis. This case indicates that eosinophil degranulation in lymphocytic myocarditis may be an important finding associated with a high therapeutic response to steroid therapy.

1. Introduction

Acute myocarditis has a broad spectrum of clinical presentations, ranging from mild symptoms to severe heart failure and lethal arrhythmia requiring mechanical circulatory support [1]. In some cases, delayed diagnosis and intervention may result in fatal hemodynamic deterioration. The therapeutic strategy for acute myocarditis varies according to histological changes; therefore, early endomyocardial biopsy should be considered to guide cause-specific treatment [2]. Immunosuppressive therapy such as steroids plays an important role in eosinophilic and giant cell myocarditis; however, its efficacy remains controversial in lymphocytic myocarditis [3].

We herein report a case of acute lymphocytic myocarditis successfully treated with steroid therapy, in which a predominantly lymphocytic infiltration of the myocardium was accompanied by eosinophil degranulation.

2. Case Presentation

A 49-year-old woman presented to our hospital with arthralgia, nausea, and fever lasting for seven days and chest pain over a

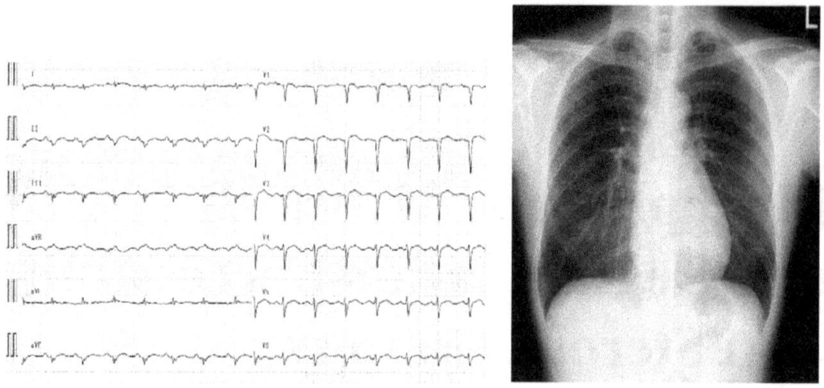

(a) (b)

FIGURE 1: Electrocardiography and thoracic radiography findings on admission. (a) Electrocardiogram shows a sinus rhythm with poor R progression in precordial leads; (b) postero-anterior thoracic radiogram shows no features of heart failure.

few days. Laboratory data showed elevated serum troponin I level. Echocardiography showed reduced left ventricular (LV) ejection fraction (LVEF) with anterior wall motion abnormalities. The patient was admitted to our hospital because myocardial infarction or myocarditis was suspected.

She had no significant medical history or known drug allergies. On admission, chest pain, nausea, and inappetence persisted. Although blood pressure values were normal, she had physical fatigue and sinus tachycardia with minimal exertion. Laboratory data on admission showed a white blood cell count of 4460/μL, including 7.2% eosinophils (eosinophil count: 321/μL), serum creatine kinase (CK) level of 147 U/L (CK-MB: 3.7 ng/mL), troponin I level of 0.47 ng/mL, and B-type natriuretic peptide (BNP) level of 109 pg/mL. The levels of immunoglobulin and autoantibody were within normal limits.

The electrocardiogram showed sinus rhythm with low voltage in limb leads and poor R progression in precordial leads (Figure 1(a)). Thoracic radiography excluded cardiomegaly, pleural effusion, or pulmonary congestion (Figure 1(b)). Echocardiography revealed a LV end-diastolic diameter of 50 mm and LVEF of 42% with hypokinesis in the LV anterior region.

Coronary angiography showed no significant stenosis. Three endomyocardial biopsy specimens were obtained from the right interventricular septum. Myocardial specimens showed abundant lymphocytic infiltration with interstitial edema and slight perivascular fibrosis (Figure 2(a)). Very few eosinophils and no giant cells were found in the specimens. Based on these findings, she was pathologically diagnosed with acute lymphocytic myocarditis. However, a close observation of the specimens revealed eosinophils with degranulation (Figure 2(b)). Eosinophil degranulation was also confirmed by direct fast scarlet stain (DFS) and immunostaining for major basic protein (MBP) (Figures 2(c) and 2(d)).

On the next day after admission, peripheral blood eosinophil count decreased from 321/μL to 162/μL, whereas serum troponin I level continued to rise from 0.47 ng/μL to 1.007 ng/μL. Her symptoms (chest pain, nausea, and inappetence) persisted, and LVEF remained 45%. Although she was diagnosed with lymphocytic myocarditis, we decided to initiate steroid therapy because of the presence of eosinophil degranulation in the biopsy specimens. Methylprednisolone was administered at a dose of 1,000 mg/day for 3 days. Echocardiography performed 12 hours after the first administration of methylprednisolone showed marked improvement of LVEF from 45% to 65% (Figure 3) and normalization of regional wall motion. The pulse rate decreased and symptoms improved. On the following day, serum troponin I level decreased from 1.007 ng/μL to 0.152 ng/μL (Figure 3). Because of a dramatic response to high-dose steroid therapy, methylprednisolone was changed to oral prednisolone at a dose of 30 mg/day and tapered carefully. The troponin I level normalized by the eighth day after the first administration. The patient was discharged 20 days after admission with a normal LVEF and BNP level of 6.4 pg/mL. Paired serum viral antibodies for adenovirus, influenza virus, coxsackievirus, and enterovirus were all negative. The dose of oral prednisolone was tapered over 6 months to 2.5 mg/day and finally discontinued. There was no further recurrence of LV dysfunction or elevation of serum troponin I level.

3. Discussion

This report presents a case of acute lymphocytic myocarditis successfully treated with steroid therapy, in which eosinophil degranulation was observed in the abundant infiltration of lymphocytes into the myocardium. This case indicates that eosinophil degranulation in lymphocytic myocarditis may be an important finding associated with a high therapeutic response to steroid administration. Treatment strategy for acute myocarditis mainly focuses on supportive care to prevent heart failure or other fatal complications using inotropic agents or mechanical circulatory support [2, 4]. As for other pharmacological therapies, immunosuppressive therapy is thought to be effective for eosinophilic and giant cell myocarditis, which often has a fulminant presentation with abrupt impairment of LV function and lethal arrhythmia [1]. On the other hand, the benefits of immunosuppressive therapy in lymphocytic myocarditis still remain controversial [3]. In previous randomized controlled studies [5], immunosuppressive therapy did not

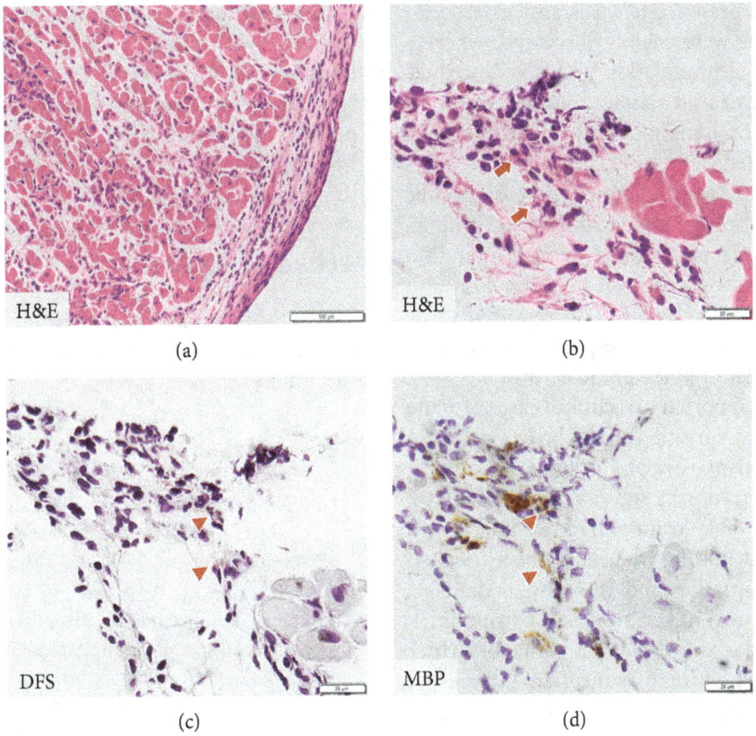

FIGURE 2: Right ventricular myocardial biopsy specimen. (a) Extensive inflammatory cell infiltration (consisting of lymphocytes and no giant cells) with little necrosis (hematoxylin-eosin (H&E) staining); (b) a few eosinophils (red arrow) with degranulation can be observed (H&E staining); (c, d) eosinophil degranulation (red arrowhead) confirmed by direct fast scarlet (DFS) staining and immunostaining for major basic protein (MBP).

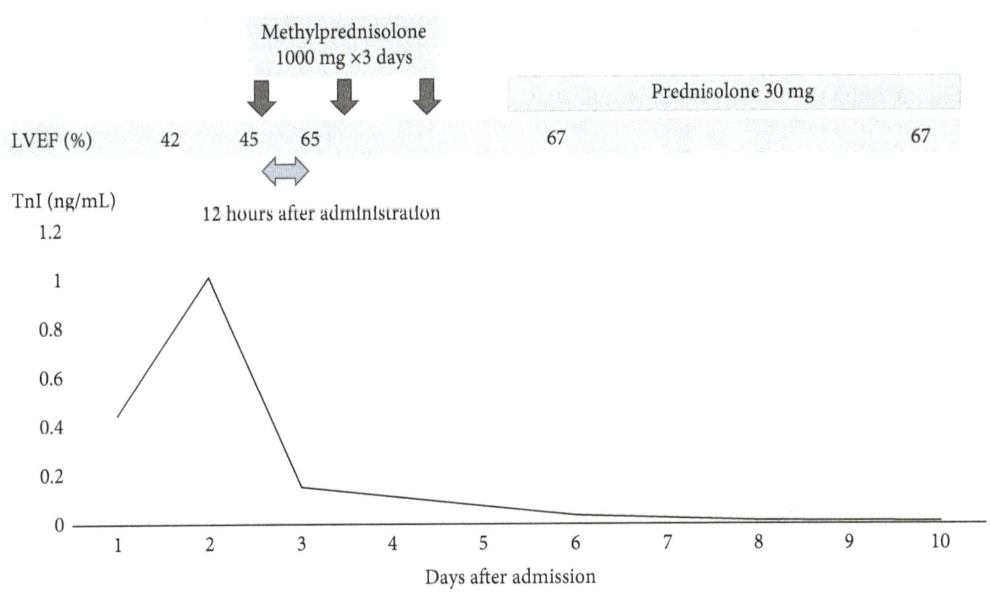

FIGURE 3: Changes in troponin I (TnI) level and left ventricular ejection fraction (LVEF) before and after steroid therapy. Rapid improvements in TnI and LVEF were found after the steroid administration.

improve the prognosis of acute lymphocytic myocarditis; therefore, routine steroid therapy is not recommended for lymphocytic myocarditis by the European Society of Cardiology guideline [2]. In contrast, several reports showed the effectiveness of steroid therapy in lymphocytic myocarditis. Reiff and Missov recently reported a case of fulminant lymphocytic myocarditis successfully treated with immunosuppressive therapy [6]. Weitsman et al. also reported on the effectiveness of early immunosuppressive therapy in acute lymphocytic myocarditis with persistent heart failure [7]. In these previous reports, the presence of virus and its association with clinical outcomes were mainly discussed, whereas the presence of eosinophil degranulation was not described. Furthermore, the presence and clinical implications of eosinophil degranulation in lymphocytic myocarditis have not been previously reported.

Previous in vitro studies have indicated that eosinophilic granule proteins, such as collagenase, major basic protein, and eosinophilic cationic protein, induce further migration of eosinophils and lead to progression of inflammation and myocardial damage [8]. Mast cells were also reported to be involved in inflammatory and fibrous response in the heart and be activated by eosinophilic granule proteins [9]. Furthermore, deMello et al. reported two clinical cases of acute necrotizing eosinophilic myocarditis in which deposition of the major basic protein of the eosinophil granule was identified within necrotic myocardium in autopsy specimens [10]. Therefore, we considered that eosinophil degranulation in myocarditis is an important finding which may be associated with progression of inflammation and myocardial damage. Because of the continuous rise in serum level of troponin I, which is an important marker of myocardial damage, further deterioration of cardiac function was of concern in the present case. Steroid therapy resulted in rapid and appreciable improvements not only in symptoms and vital signs, but also in cardiac function. Therefore, this can be considered a case of acute lymphocytic myocarditis with a high therapeutic response to steroid therapy. There may be several possible explanations for our findings. Combined lymphocytic and eosinophilic immune-mediated process may have been associated with progression of myocardial injury, in which early steroid administration may have regulated the eosinophilic immune-mediated process. Although viral infections have been considered the most important triggers of lymphocytic myocarditis, they may also cause eosinophilic myocarditis. In fact, Murphy et al. reported a case of eosinophilic-lymphocytic myocarditis after smallpox vaccination [11]. Another possibility is that eosinophil degranulation in the present case was an early sign of eosinophilic myocarditis and that early steroid therapy may have prevented progression of inflammation and myocyte necrosis due to further migration and degranulation of eosinophils. Eosinophilic myocarditis generally progresses from acute necrotic stage, marked by infiltration and extracellular deposition of eosinophils, to the fibrotic stage [12]. Myocyte necrosis has been known to be associated with eosinophil degranulation [8]. Myocardial specimens of our patient showed eosinophil degranulation with very little myocyte necrosis, which may have indicated that she was in a very early stage of eosinophilic myocarditis before myocardial necrosis developed.

Early diagnosis of eosinophilic myocarditis is sometimes difficult when endomyocardial biopsy specimens show no appreciable eosinophil infiltration. The presence of degranulation may be an initial important finding associated with the eosinophilic inflammatory process. It is noteworthy that a case of eosinophilia complicated by eosinophilic endomyocardial disease with deposition of eosinophil granule proteins in cardiac tissues in the virtual absence of eosinophil infiltration was previously reported [13].

In conclusion, early endomyocardial biopsy provides clinicians with valuable information about treatment strategy in patients with myocarditis. A close observation of biopsy specimens for eosinophil degranulation may help identify patients with lymphocytic myocarditis who may benefit from immunosuppressive therapy. Further investigation is required to pursue this possibility.

Acknowledgments

The authors thank Masami Koutaka and Takako Sawamura for technical assistance in histological staining of myocardial specimens.

References

[1] I. Kindermann, C. Barth, F. Mahfoud et al., "Update on myocarditis," *Journal of the American College of Cardiology*, vol. 59, no. 9, pp. 779–792, 2012.

[2] A. L. Caforio, S. Pankuweit, E. Arbustini et al., "Current state of knowledge on aetiology, diagnosis, management, and therapy of myocarditis: a position statement of the European Society of Cardiology Working Group on Myocardial and Pericardial Diseases," *European Heart Journal*, vol. 34, no. 33, pp. 2636–2648, 2013.

[3] M. P. Winter, P. Sulzgruber, L. Koller, P. Bartko, G. Goliasch, and A. Niessner, "Immunomodulatory treatment for lymphocytic myocarditis-a systematic review and meta-analysis," *Heart Failure Reviews*, vol. 23, no. 4, pp. 573–581, 2018.

[4] P. Atluri, B. W. Ullery, J. W. MacArthur et al., "Rapid onset of fulminant myocarditis portends a favourable prognosis and the ability to bridge mechanical circulatory support to recovery," *European Journal of Cardio-Thoracic Surgery*, vol. 43, no. 2, pp. 379–382, 2013.

[5] B. Maisch and P. Alter, "Treatment options in myocarditis and inflammatory cardiomyopathy," *Herz*, vol. 43, no. 5, pp. 423–430, 2018.

[6] C. Reiff and E. Missov, "A case of fulminant lymphocytic myocarditis responsive to immunosuppression," *The American Journal of Medicine*, vol. 131, no. 11, pp. e465–e466, 2018.

[7] T. Weitsman, G. Weisz, A. Keren, and T. Hasin, "Prompt benefit of early immunosuppressive therapy in acute lymphocytic myocarditis with persistent heart failure," *Clinical Research in Cardiology*, vol. 105, no. 9, pp. 794–796, 2016.

[8] P. C. Tai, D. J. Hayes, J. B. Clark, and C. J. F. Spry, "Toxic effects of human eosinophil products on isolated rat heart cells in vitro," *The Biochemical Journal*, vol. 204, no. 1, pp. 75–80, 1982.

[9] V. Patella, G. de Crescenzo, I. Marinò et al., "Eosinophil granule proteins activate human heart mast cells," *Journal of Immunology*, vol. 157, no. 3, pp. 1219–1225, 1996.

[10] D. E. deMello, H. Liapis, S. Jureidini, S. Nouri, G. M. Kephart, and G. J. Gleich, "Cardiac localization of eosinophil-granule major basic protein in acute necrotizing myocarditis," *The New England Journal of Medicine*, vol. 323, no. 22, pp. 1542–1545, 1990.

[11] J. G. Murphy, R. S. Wright, G. K. Bruce et al., "Eosinophilic-lymphocytic myocarditis after smallpox vaccination," *The Lancet*, vol. 362, no. 9393, pp. 1378–1380, 2003.

[12] A. M. Al Ali, L. P. Straatman, M. F. Allard, and A. P. Ignaszewski, "La myocardite a eosinophiles : Serie de cas et

analyse bibliographique," *The Canadian Journal of Cardiology*, vol. 22, no. 14, pp. 1233–1237, 2006.

[13] B. L. Wright, K. M. Leiferman, and G. J. Gleich, "Eosinophil granule protein localization in eosinophilic endomyocardial disease," *The New England Journal of Medicine*, vol. 365, no. 2, pp. 187-188, 2011.

9

Reverse Takutsubo Cardiomyopathy in a Patient with Phlegmasia Cerulea Dolens

Gift Echefu[1], **Daniel Hammett**[1], **Amir Ausef**[2] and **Lance LaMotte**[3]

[1]*Baton Rouge General Medical Center Internal Medicine Residency Program, Baton Rouge, LA, USA*
[2]*Hospital Medicine Group, Baton Rouge General Medical Center, Baton Rouge, LA, USA*
[3]*Baton Rouge Cardiology Center, Baton Rouge, LA, USA*

Correspondence should be addressed to Gift Echefu; gift.echefu@brgeneral.org

Academic Editor: Yigit Canga

Reverse takotsubo cardiomyopathy (rTTC) is a rare variant of takotsubo cardiomyopathy (TTC) which is characterized by reversible left ventricular (LV) dysfunction. Emotional and physical stress have been implicated in triggering TTC especially in postmenopausal women. TTC and its variants are becoming more recognized due to the widespread adoption of early coronary angiography in the setting of acute coronary syndromes. A man in his late 50s presented to the emergency department with left lower extremity pain, swelling, and cyanosis. Clinical assessment was consistent with phlegmasia cerulea dolens, with deep venous thrombosis detected by venous duplex ultrasound. During his admission, he developed clinical and EKG findings suggestive of acute coronary syndrome. Emergent coronary angiography and ventriculography revealed basal and midventricular hypokinesis with hyperdynamic left ventricular apex, depressed LV dysfunction without coronary artery obstruction diagnostic of reverse takotsubo cardiomyopathy. Venous thromboembolism is a rare finding but has been associated with takotsubo cardiomyopathy and should be considered in the appropriate setting.

1. Background

Takotsubo cardiomyopathy (TTC) is a type of stress-induced cardiomyopathy characterized by reversible left ventricular dysfunction and ballooning in the apical and/or midventricular areas in the absence of actual stenosis detected by coronary angiography [1]. Takotsubo cardiomyopathy is usually associated with intense emotional or physical stress with higher incidence in postmenopausal women [2]. It is estimated to affect 1-2% of all patients who present with an acute myocardial infarction [3]. The presentation can mimic acute coronary syndrome with chest pain, dyspnea, and even cardiogenic shock, but is often associated with recovery to normal cardiac systolic function [3]. TTC can be classified based on the region of the left ventricle involved, into the classic apical ballooning variant, accounting for nearly 80% of cases, and the less occurring atypical variants [4]. The atypical variants include the basal or reverse (rTTC), midventricular (mTTC), and localized. Reverse and midventricular takotsubo cardiomyopathies are variants of takotsubo cardiomyopathy that, respectively, involve the basal or the midventricular walls while retaining the contractility of the apical segments.

The exact pathogenesis of reverse takotsubo cardiomyopathy is not completely understood; however, etiologies such as catecholamine excess, coronary artery spasm and microvascular dysfunction have been described [5]. Venous thromboembolism, specifically pulmonary embolism, has been reported in association with stress-induced cardiomyopathy [6]. Phlegmasia cerulea dolens (PCD) is a rare but potentially fatal complication of acute massive deep venous thromboembolism characterized by severe pain, swelling, and cyanosis in affected extremities. We present a case of a middle-aged male admitted for thrombolytic management of PCD who ultimately developed cardiogenic shock from rTTC.

2. Case Presentation

A 55-year-old man with history of fifty pack-year tobacco use and severe malnutrition presented to our hospital with left lower extremity pain, associated with swelling and purplish-blue discoloration that began a day prior to admission. He reported cough productive of yellowish-brown sputum, progressive shortness of breath at rest, as well as orthopnea that began 2 weeks prior to presentation. In the months prior to presentation, he had anorexia, poor oral intake, 22 lbs. weight loss, and generalized weakness. He had no chest pain, palpitations, fever, night sweats, joint pain, or skin rash. He did not seek medical care for these symptoms in the months preceding presentation. He had no significant past medical history and was not on routine home medications including supplements or hormonal therapy.

Physical exam revealed hypotension (92/60 mmHg), tachycardic (106 beat per minute), afebrile, respiratory rate was 16 cycles per minute, and oxygen saturated on room air was 97%. He appeared cachectic and older than stated age. Lung auscultation revealed decreased breath sounds on the right posterior lung fields, without wheezing or crackles. Heart rate and rhythm were fast and regular; he had no jugular venous distension or abnormal heart sounds. Extremity exam revealed an erythematous, tender, left lower extremity cool to touch and cyanotic to the midthigh without palpable distal pulses. Other physical exam findings were normal.

Initial workup revealed normocytic anemia, leukocytosis, and multiple electrolyte derangements: hypokalemia, hyponatremia, hypomagnesemia, anion gap metabolic acidosis, and severe protein caloric malnutrition (Table 1). Lower extremity venous duplex ultrasound revealed completely occluded left-sided superficial and deep vein thrombosis involving the external iliac vein, common femoral vein, and all its tributaries, popliteal to midposterior tibial veins. CT angiography of the chest ruled out pulmonary embolism but revealed multiple cavitary masses in the right lower and upper lobes with the largest measuring 9.7 × 9.1 × 11.8 cm. Differentials for the incidental pulmonary lesions included mycobacterial or fungal infections and malignancy. Initial troponin was normal 0.002 ng/mL (<0.045), and electrocardiogram revealed sinus tachycardia and ventricular rate of 121 with no repolarization abnormalities (Figure 1).

Vital signs improved with initial aggressive IV fluid hydration. Heparin drip was initiated, and vascular surgery team was consulted for possible thrombectomy. Due to initial investigations suggesting an infectious process and/or malnutrition, blood and urine cultures were obtained, and cefepime and azithromycin were initiated for pneumonia. Blood and urine cultures yielded no growth at five days. Viral respiratory panel was negative for respiratory viruses; sputum culture yielded light growth of pan-sensitive *Pseudomonas fluorescens/putida.* Repeat sputum culture on admission day two yielded no growth. He underwent catheter directed thrombolysis for phlegmasia cerulea dolens. He was improving clinically, with stable hemodynamics not previously requiring pressor support. However, on admission day three, he developed new onset atrial fibrillation with rapid ventricular response, chest pain, refractory hypotension, and EKG indicating anterior ST-elevation myocardial infarction (Figure 2). Troponin was elevated at 16 ng/mL (reference < 0.015 ng/mL) and BNP 370 pg/mL (reference < 99 pg/mL). Bedside transthoracic echocardiogram revealed severely depressed left ventricular systolic function (ejection fraction-20%) with basal hypokinesis. Due to hemodynamic compromise and atrial fibrillation, norepinephrine and amiodarone infusion was initiated. He underwent emergent cardiac catheterization. Coronary angiography with ventriculography revealed normal coronaries, basal and midventricular hypokinesis with hyperdynamic left ventricular apex, and ejection fraction of 35%, indicating reverse and midventricular takotsubo cardiomyopathy (Figures 3(a)–3(c)).

TABLE 1: Initial laboratory findings.

Laboratory findings		Reference range
Hemoglobin	9.5	13.7-17.0 g/dL
White blood count	23.25	4.0-11.0 K/μL
Platelet count	272	150-400 K/μL
Sodium	123	136-145 mmol/L
Potassium	2.4	3.5-5.1 mmol/L
Bicarbonate (serum)	14	21-32 mmol/L
Creatinine	1.20	0.70-1.30 mg/dL
Albumin	1.2	3.4-5.0 g/dL
Magnesium	1.5	1.8-2.4 mg/dL
International normalized ratio	1.4	0.8-1.2 IU
Prothrombin time	17.3	12.3-14.6 sec
Partial thromboplastin time	29	23-36 sec
Fibrinogen activity	304	225-450 mg/dL
Troponin	<0.015	<0.015 ng/mL
BNP	36.4	<99 pg/mL

He continued to clinically decline despite supportive measures with worsening hypoxemic respiratory failure requiring oxygen supplementation and cardiogenic shock. CT angiography of the chest did not reveal acute pulmonary embolism or aortic syndromes. On admission day 4, patient and family decided to pursue comfort care declining further life prolonging measures. He declined mechanical ventilation, pressor support was withdrawn, and he transitioned to palliative care, expiring on admission day 5.

3. Discussion

Takotsubo cardiomyopathy (TTC) is a sudden onset but often reversible heart failure syndrome that was initially described in Japanese postmenopausal women by Sato and Uchida [7]. TTC is distinguished by the characteristic of transient left ventricular apical hypokinesis and basal hyperkinesis, which often resolves spontaneously after a few days or weeks. Presentation can mimic acute coronary syndrome with chest pain, elevated troponin, localized T wave, and ST segment changes on electrocardiogram but with absence of obstructive coronary disease on angiography [3, 8, 9].

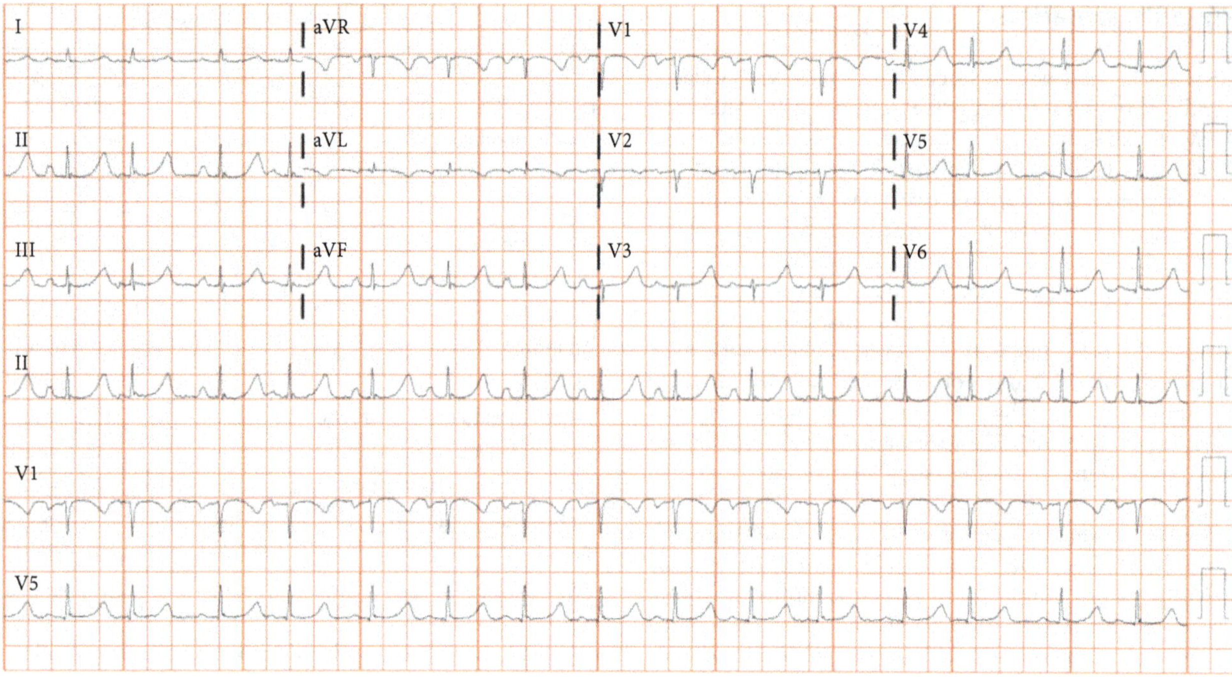

FIGURE 1: Electrocardiogram at presentation.

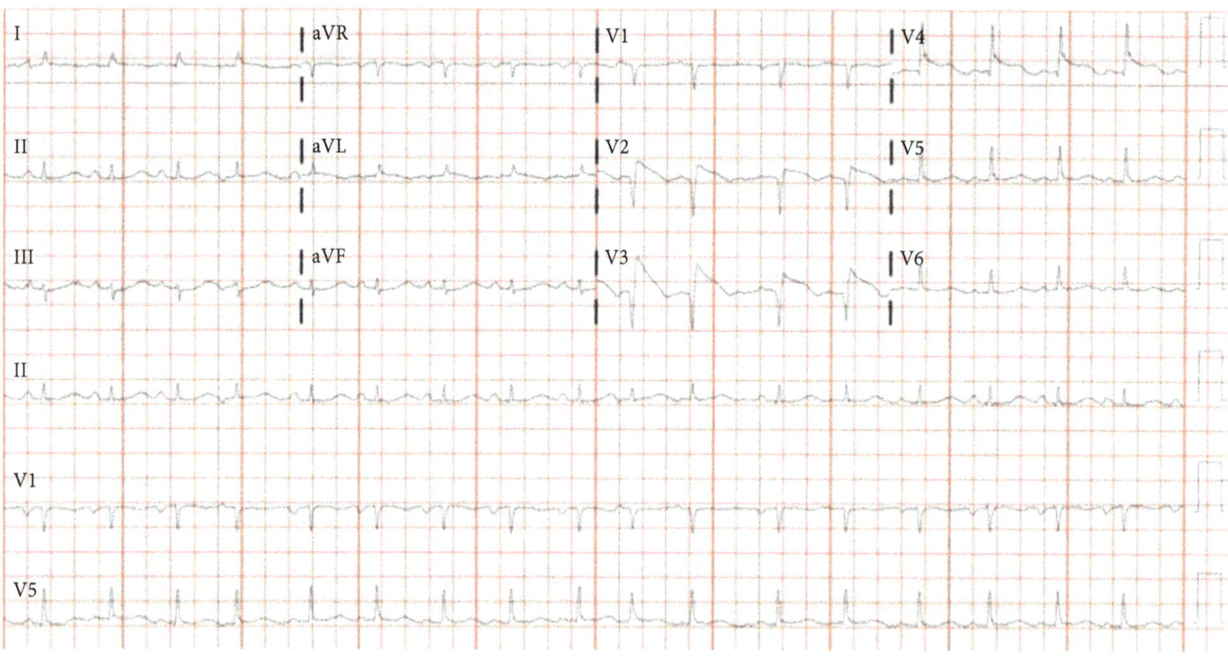

FIGURE 2: Electrocardiogram on admission day 3.

Several variants have been described on the basis of location of ventricular wall motion abnormality. These include the midventricular, reverse, and localized variants [10].

Reverse or inverted takotsubo cardiomyopathy (rTTC) is characterized by circumferential basal hypokinesia and apical hypercontractility. The precise pathophysiology of reverse takotsubo remains unclear [11, 12]. Existing theory is that catecholamine surge due to intense physiological or mental stress results in myocardial stunning, as well as multivessel coronary artery spasm and indirect myocardial damage [5]. It has been linked to excessive catecholamine release associated with catecholamine-secreting tumors such as pheochromocytoma and paraganglioma [13]. There are reports of rTTC in patients with head injury and intracranial bleed, elucidating a neurologic stress-related LV dysfunction syndrome [14, 15]. Cerebrocortical damage is believed to induce immense sympathetic excitation of the myocardium and coronary vasoconstriction [16]. Cases of intravenous administration of catecholamines and other receptor agonists have also been linked to rTTC [17–21].

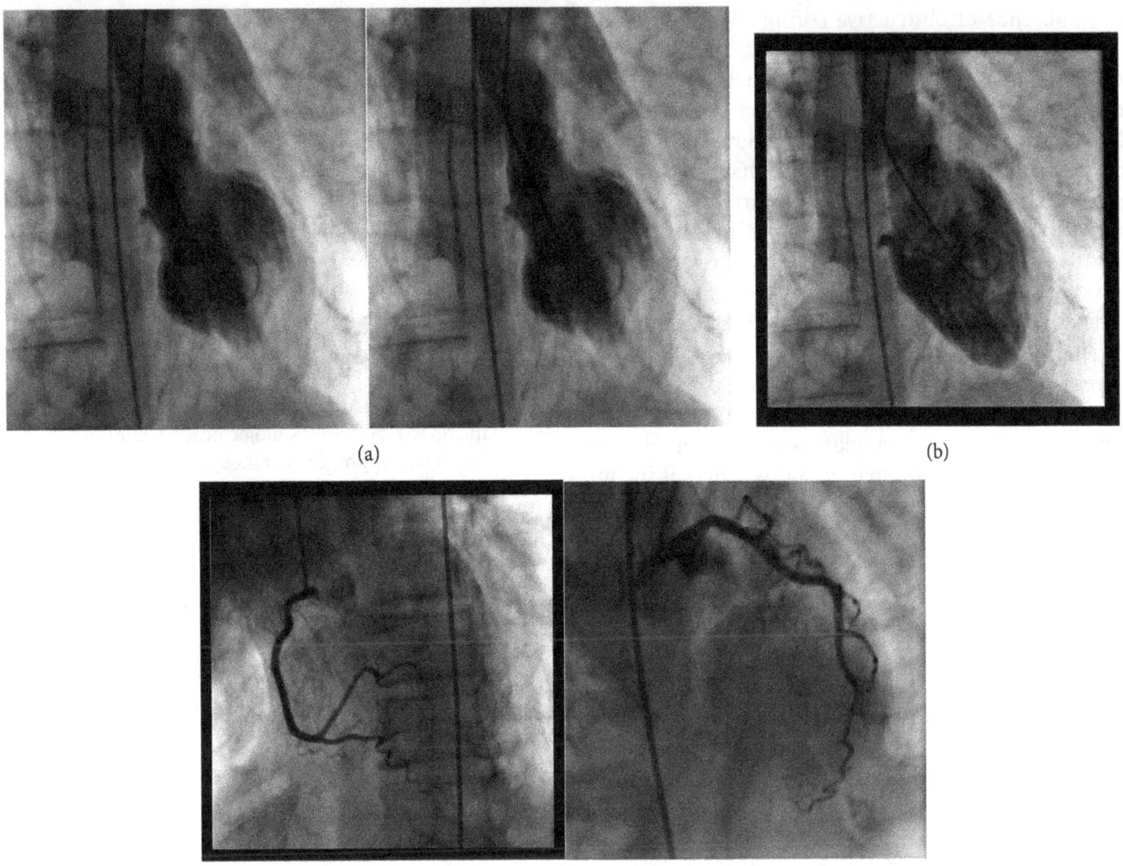

(c)

FIGURE 3: (a) Ventriculography of the left ventricle in systole showing basal and midventricular hypokinesis. (b) Ventriculography of the left ventricle in diastole. (c) Coronary angiography showing normal coronaries.

TTC has been reported in association with venous thromboembolism (VTE) such as pulmonary embolism [6], but the precise mechanism underlying this link remains unclear. Pulmonary embolism is a possible complication in about 12-40% of cases; this was not detected in our patient [22]. Our patient presented with malnutrition, hemodynamic circulatory compromise from phlegmasia cerulea dolens, incidental lung masses on imaging, and subsequently developed rTTC culminating in cardiogenic shock. Phlegmasia cerulea dolens is a life-threatening complication of acute deep venous thrombosis with risk of vascular ischemia, circulatory collapse, and shock [23]. Acute venous outflow obstruction associated with PCD results in disequilibrium of the Starling forces favoring development of massive interstitial edema with potential to progress to circulatory shock. In our patient, the trigger for rTCC was likely due to intense catecholamine surge from physical stress due to severe pain, vascular dysfunction, and hemodynamic compromise associated with PCD. Notably, severe pain has been reported as a potential trigger in VTE-associated TTC [24]. The mechanism may be related to intense sympathetic response inducing coronary vasospasm in the setting of increased myocardial work and oxygen demand, depressing myocardial function. PCD portends poor prognosis with potential to be fatal in a more critical setting such as present case. A systematic review by Chinsakchai et al. [25] reported that malignancy conferred the highest risk of PCD, as well as higher mortality risk of 55% in this subset of patients. Further research is needed to elucidate the pathophysiological mechanisms for various ventricular morphologies of stress-induced cardiomyopathies.

In addition to the characteristic pattern of left ventricular dysfunction on echocardiography, clinicopathologic features of reverse takotsubo cardiomyopathy differ significantly from those of other variants. The density of cardiac adrenoreceptors is the highest at the base in younger patients and with advancing age shifts from base to apex, explaining why majority of rTTC cases are relatively young [26]. rTTC is linked to higher mental and physical stress than emotional stress seen in the classic variant [26]. Troponin level is reportedly higher in rTTC than in other TTC variants [27]. This is attributed to the larger muscle mass in the base of the heart, typically involved in rTTC. Conversely, brain natriuretic peptide (BNP) is higher in apical and midventricular variants, which could explain the relatively severe heart failure symptoms seen in other variants at presentation [10, 27, 28]. This pattern was particularly consistent in this case, with comparatively higher troponin than BNP (Table 1). However, our patient had more florid heart failure symptoms than previously reported in literature for rTTC variant.

Diagnosis of TTC is based on the revised Mayo criteria which includes transient LV dyskinesis, regional wall motion abnormalities involving more than an epicardial vascular distribution, absence of obstructive coronary artery disease on coronary angiography, new electrocardiographic findings, troponin elevation, absence of pheochromocytoma, and myocarditis. Coronary angiography with ventriculography is considered gold standard [29, 30]. Several inpatient studies on hospitalized patients with rTTC have shown that men appear to be younger with a higher mortality rate. This has been attributed to a higher prevalence of cardiogenic shock, cardiac arrest, and respiratory failure requiring mechanical ventilation in this population [8, 31]. In our case, the patient was male, critically ill, in respiratory failure, and in cardiogenic shock.

Management of TTC is individualized and centers on supportive therapy with beta blocker and angiotensin converting enzyme inhibitors or angiotensin receptor blocker depending on patient's hemodynamic status. There is inconclusive evidence in the prophylactic cardioprotective benefit in the use of these medicines on the risk of developing TTC [32, 33]. Symptomatic hypotension can be safely managed with vasopressors in the absence of left ventricular outflow obstruction. Anticoagulant is indicated in patients with left ventricular thrombi or those with large areas of cardiac hypokinesis [30].

Prognostic indicators for poor outcomes and mortality in TTC in hospitalized patients include low ejection fraction, hemodynamic instability, atrial fibrillation, acute neurological and psychiatric manifestation, significantly increased troponin, and physical trigger [30, 34–36].

Increasing investigations have shown that short- and long-term mortalities are actually higher than initially believed for this condition with presumed good prognosis [33]. The in-hospital mortality in the acute stage is reported to be between 4 and 6%, comparable to the mortality from ST-segment-elevation myocardial infarction even with increasing access to primary percutaneous coronary interventions [31, 32, 34, 37]. Mortality in men is significantly higher, even after adjusting for differences in baseline characteristics [8, 31, 34]. Sharkey et al. in their cohort of 136 patients reported high mortality among TTC patients was highest within the first year of diagnosis with malignancy conferring the highest risk [33]. This is comparable to the report by Song et al., reporting greater than 50% mortality in the first year among patients with malignancy [37].

4. Conclusion

This is the first case of phlegmasia cerulean dolens reported in a patient with reverse takotsubo cardiomyopathy. Adrenergic storm and circulatory compromise associated with venous thromboembolism such as PCD increases the risk of stress induced cardiomyopathy. Physical stressors have been reported to cause rTTC rather than emotional stress seen with the classic variant. Critically ill males admitted to the intensive care unit with respiratory failure and cardiogenic shock are at highest risk of mortality from ensuing cardiogenic failure. Stress-induced cardiomyopathy should be suspected in patients with PCD who develop cardiogenic shock.

References

[1] T. M. Pilgrim and T. R. Wyss, "Takotsubo cardiomyopathy or transient left ventricular apical ballooning syndrome: a systematic review," *International journal of cardiology*, vol. 124, no. 3, pp. 283–292, 2008.

[2] A. S. Dande, L. I. Fisher, and M. K. Warshofsky, "Inverted takotsubo cardiomyopathy," *The Journal of Invasive Cardiology*, vol. 23, no. 4, pp. E76–E78, 2011.

[3] A. Prasad, A. Lerman, and C. S. Rihal, "Apical ballooning syndrome (Tako-Tsubo or stress cardiomyopathy): a mimic of acute myocardial infarction," *American Heart Journal*, vol. 155, no. 3, pp. 408–417, 2008.

[4] R. Ono and L. M. Falcão, "Takotsubo cardiomyopathy systematic review: pathophysiologic process, clinical presentation and diagnostic approach to takotsubo cardiomyopathy," *International Journal of Cardiology*, vol. 209, pp. 196–205, 2016.

[5] F. Pelliccia, J. C. Kaski, F. Crea, and P. G. Camici, "Pathophysiology of takotsubo syndrome," *Circulation*, vol. 135, no. 24, pp. 2426–2441, 2017.

[6] Q. Jin, Q. Luo, Z. Zhao et al., "Takotsubo syndrome with pulmonary embolism: a case report and literature review," *BMC Cardiovascular Disorders*, vol. 18, no. 1, p. 229, 2018.

[7] H. T. H. Sato and T. Uchida, *Stunned Myocardium with Specific Left Ventricular Configuration Due to Multivessel Spasm*, 1990.

[8] R. Khera, K. Light-McGroary, F. Zahr, P. A. Horwitz, and S. Girotra, "Trends in hospitalization for takotsubo cardiomyopathy in the United States," *American Heart Journal*, vol. 172, pp. 53–63, 2016.

[9] M. Gianni, F. Dentali, A. M. Grandi, G. Sumner, R. Hiralal, and E. Lonn, "Apical ballooning syndrome or takotsubo cardiomyopathy: a systematic review," *European Heart Journal*, vol. 27, no. 13, pp. 1523–1529, 2006.

[10] S. Piérard, M. Vinetti, and P. Hantson, "Inverted (reverse) takotsubo cardiomyopathy following cerebellar hemorrhage," *Case Reports in Cardiology*, vol. 2014, Article ID 781926, 2014.

[11] K. Tsuchihashi, K. Ueshima, T. Uchida et al., "Transient left ventricular apical ballooning without coronary artery stenosis: a novel heart syndrome mimicking acute myocardial infarction," *Journal of the American College of Cardiology*, vol. 38, no. 1, pp. 11–18, 2001.

[12] H. H. Awad, A. R. McNeal, and H. Goyal, "Reverse takotsubo cardiomyopathy: a comprehensive review," *Annals of translational medicine*, vol. 6, no. 23, p. 460, 2018.

[13] Y. L. Chiang, P. C. Chen, C. C. Lee, and S. K. Chua, "Adrenal pheochromocytoma presenting with Takotsubo-pattern cardiomyopathy and acute heart failure: a case report and literature review," *Medicine*, vol. 95, no. 36, article e4846, 2016.

[14] S. Maréchaux, P. Fornes, S. Petit et al., "Pathology of inverted takotsubo cardiomyopathy," *Cardiovascular Pathology*, vol. 17, no. 4, pp. 241–243, 2008.

[15] A. Manzanal, L. Ruiz, J. Madrazo, M. Makan, and J. Perez, "Inverted takotsubo cardiomyopathy and the fundamental diagnostic role of echocardiography," *Texas Heart Institute Journal*, vol. 40, no. 1, pp. 56–59, 2013.

[16] P. V. Ennezat, D. Pesenti-Rossi, J. M. Aubert et al., "Transient left ventricular basal dysfunction without coronary stenosis in acute cerebral disorders: a novel heart syndrome (inverted takotsubo)," *Echocardiography*, vol. 22, no. 7, pp. 599–602, 2005.

[17] A. Kaoukis, V. Panagopoulou, H. R. Mojibian, and D. Jacoby, "Reverse takotsubo cardiomyopathy associated with the consumption of an energy drink," *Circulation*, vol. 125, no. 12, pp. 1584-1585, 2012.

[18] T. Härle, K. Kronberg, H. Nef, H. Möllmann, and A. Elsässer, "Inverted takotsubo cardiomyopathy following accidental intravenous administration of epinephrine in a young woman," *Clinical Research in Cardiology*, vol. 100, no. 5, pp. 471–473, 2011.

[19] P. Esnault, L. Née, T. Signouret, N. Jaussaud, and F. Kerbaul, "Reverse takotsubo cardiomyopathy after iatrogenic epinephrine injection requiring percutaneous extracorporeal membrane oxygenation," *Canadian Journal of Anaesthesia*, vol. 61, no. 12, pp. 1093–1097, 2014.

[20] D. Belliveau and S. De, "Reverse takotsubo cardiomyopathy following exogenous epinephrine administration in the early postpartum period," *Echocardiography*, vol. 33, no. 7, pp. 1089–1091, 2016.

[21] G. Khoueiry, N. Abi Rafeh, B. Azab et al., "Reverse takotsubo cardiomyopathy in the setting of anaphylaxis treated with high-dose intravenous epinephrine," *The Journal of Emergency Medicine*, vol. 44, no. 1, pp. 96–99, 2013.

[22] J. M. Perkins, T. R. Magee, and R. B. Galland, "Phlegmasia caerulea dolens and venous gangrene," *The British Journal of Surgery*, vol. 83, no. 1, pp. 19–23, 2005.

[23] C. B. Lewis, M. K. Hensley, J. E. Barrett, S. B. Van Norman, A. S. Taylor, and J. C. Horowitz, "Phlegmasia cerulea dolens: a rare cause of shock," *Respirology Case Reports*, vol. 7, no. 5, article e00424, 2019.

[24] S. Challa, J. L. Ganji, A. Raizada, M. Q. Najib, P. M. Panse, and H. P. Chaliki, "Takotsubo cardiomyopathy in a patient with pulmonary embolism," *European Journal of Echocardiography*, vol. 12, no. 10, p. E39, 2011.

[25] K. Chinsakchai, K. Ten Duis, F. L. Moll, and G. J. de Borst, "Trends in management of phlegmasia cerulea dolens," *Vascular and Endovascular Surgery*, vol. 45, no. 1, pp. 5–14, 2011.

[26] R. Ramaraj and M. R. Movahed, "Reverse or inverted takotsubo cardiomyopathy (reverse left ventricular apical ballooning syndrome) presents at a younger age compared with the mid or apical variant and is always associated with triggering stress," *Congestive Heart Failure*, vol. 16, no. 6, pp. 284–286, 2010.

[27] B. G. Song, W. J. Chun, Y. H. Park et al., "The clinical characteristics, laboratory parameters, electrocardiographic, and echocardiographic findings of reverse or inverted takotsubo cardiomyopathy: comparison with mid or apical variant," *Clinical Cardiology*, vol. 34, no. 11, pp. 693–699, 2011.

[28] M. R. Movahed and K. Mostafizi, "Reverse or inverted left ventricular apical ballooning syndrome (reverse takotsubo cardiomyopathy) in a young woman in the setting of amphetamine use," *Echocardiography*, vol. 25, no. 4, pp. 429–432, 2008.

[29] S. Kawai, A. Kitabatake, H. Tomoike, and Group TC, "Guidelines for diagnosis of takotsubo (ampulla) cardiomyopathy," *Circulation Journal*, vol. 71, no. 6, pp. 990–992, 2007.

[30] H. Medina de Chazal, M. G. Del Buono, L. Keyser-Marcus et al., "Stress cardiomyopathy diagnosis and treatment: JACC state-of-the-art review," *Journal of the American College of Cardiology*, vol. 72, no. 16, pp. 1955–1971, 2018.

[31] K. Singh, K. Carson, R. Shah et al., "Meta-analysis of clinical correlates of acute mortality in takotsubo cardiomyopathy," *The American journal of cardiology*, vol. 113, no. 8, pp. 1420–1428, 2014.

[32] P. Tornvall, O. Collste, E. Ehrenborg, and H. Järnbert-Petterson, "A case-control study of risk markers and mortality in takotsubo stress cardiomyopathy," *Journal of the American College of Cardiology*, vol. 67, no. 16, pp. 1931–1936, 2016.

[33] S. W. Sharkey, D. C. Windenburg, J. R. Lesser et al., "Natural history and expansive clinical profile of stress (tako-tsubo) cardiomyopathy," *Journal of the American College of Cardiology*, vol. 55, no. 4, pp. 333–341, 2010.

[34] C. Templin, J. R. Ghadri, J. Diekmann et al., "Clinical features and outcomes of takotsubo (stress) cardiomyopathy," *New England Journal of Medicine*, vol. 373, no. 10, pp. 929–938, 2015.

[35] T. Stiermaier, F. Santoro, C. Eitel et al., "Prevalence and prognostic relevance of atrial fibrillation in patients with takotsubo syndrome," *International Journal of Cardiology*, vol. 245, pp. 156–161, 2017.

[36] I. El-Battrawy, S. Lang, U. Ansari et al., "Impact of concomitant atrial fibrillation on the prognosis of takotsubo cardiomyopathy," *Ep Europace*, vol. 19, no. 8, pp. 1288–1292, 2017.

[37] B. G. Song, H. S. Yang, H. K. Hwang et al., "The impact of stressor patterns on clinical features in patients with takotsubo cardiomyopathy: experiences of two tertiary cardiovascular centers," *Clinical Cardiology*, vol. 35, no. 11, pp. E6–13, 2012.

10

Acute Coronary Syndrome Mimicking Takotsubo Cardiomyopathy or Takotsubo Cardiomyopathy Mimicking Acute Coronary Syndrome?

Martin Chaumont[1] **Marc Blaimont,**[2] **Rachid Briki,**[1] **Philippe Unger,**[1] **and Nadia Debbas**[1]

[1]*Cardiology Department, CHU Saint-Pierre, 322 rue Haute, B-1000 Brussels, Belgium*
[2]*Cardiology Department, Hôpital de Jolimont, 7100 La Louvière, Belgium*

Correspondence should be addressed to Martin Chaumont; martin.chaumont2012@gmail.com

Academic Editor: Filippo M. Sarullo

A healthy 66-year-old female presented to the emergency department with acute chest pain, T-wave inversion in the anterior leads, and elevated troponin-I. Coronary angiography showed a stenosis in the midportion of the left anterior descending coronary artery (LAD), which did not wrap the left ventricle (LV) apex. LV angiography demonstrated a large LV apical akinetic systolic ballooning with a 45% ejection fraction. Fractional flow reserve (FFR) of LAD lesion was 0.71. Percutaneous intervention was performed. At six months, transthoracic echocardiography was normal. Fifteen months later, the patient presented with chest pain and a small rise in troponin-I. Coronary angiogram was unchanged. Repeat FFR in distal LAD was 0.86 and left ventriculography was normal. Diagnostic criteria for Takotsubo cardiomyopathy (TTC) require the absence of obstructive coronary artery disease. In the present case, TTC was highly suspected on the basis of typical LV apex ballooning. However, significant ischemia in the same territory was demonstrated by positive FFR, which could not be falsely positive in this context. Current TTC diagnostic criteria increase specificity for diagnosing TTC. This case reminds us that it is at the price of reduced sensitivity, since there is no reason to believe that coronary lesions may protect from TTC.

1. Introduction

We herein present a typical case of Takotsubo cardiomyopathy (TTC) with an atypical feature: a positive fractional flow reserve in the hypokinetic territory.

2. Presentation of the Case

In March 2014, a 66-year-old exsmoker female presented to the emergency department with acute chest pain, shortness of breath for three hours and anterior non-ST-segment elevation myocardial infarction (NSTEMI), T-wave inversion > 3 mm in the anterior leads without significant ST shifts, and a major increase of troponin-I (150 ng/ml; normal < 14 ng/ml). She reported a medical history of hypertension and hypercholesterolemia treated with angiotensin-converting-enzyme-inhibitor and statin, respectively. Physical examination on admission was unremarkable. Loading doses of clopidogrel (600 mg), acetylsalicylic acid (300 mg), and enoxaparin (60 mg) were given; then, she immediately underwent a coronary angiography via a right radial artery approach.

Coronary angiography showed a diffusely diseased and calcified left anterior descending artery (LAD) with a single intermediate lesion in its midportion as assessed by quantitative coronary angiography (Figure 1, Moving image 1). The left circumflex artery (LCx) and the dominant right coronary arteries were also calcified but without significant lesion (<20% at angiography). Left ventriculography demonstrated a large akinesia of apical and midportions of the left ventricle (LV) inducing apex ballooning in the systole (Figure 2, Moving image 2) with an ejection fraction of 45%.

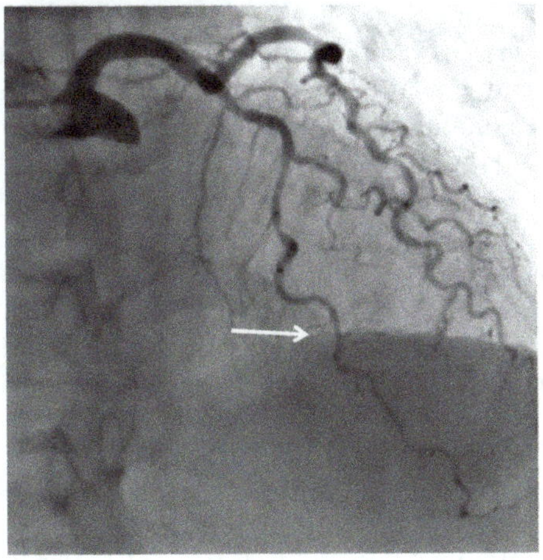

FIGURE 1: Diagnostic coronary angiogram. Intermediate lesion in the midportion of the left anterior descending artery (arrow) (right anterior oblique cranial).

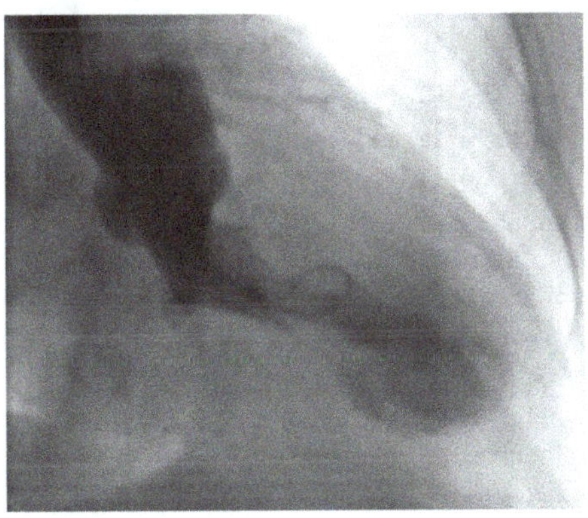

FIGURE 2: Left ventricle (right anterior oblique cranial). Large apical dyskinesia.

In order to differentiate between a TTC and a NSTEMI resulting from the culprit mid-LAD lesion, the ischemic significance of the latter was tested with fractional flow reserve (FFR) assessment. A 6Fr FL4 guiding catheter (Boston Scientific, USA) was positioned in the left main ostium, intracoronary nitroglycerine (200 μg) was injected, and PressureWire™ Certus (St. Jude Medical, USA) was advanced distally to the LAD lesion. At rest, Pd (mean blood pressure distal to the stenosis) over Pa (mean aortic pressure) was 0.83. Steady state hyperaemia was induced by continuous intravenous administration of adenosine through a 4Fr sheath placed in the humeral vein. The infusion was kept at 140 μg/kg/min for 180 seconds. The patient complained of "typical" adenosine-induced symptoms, and the Pd curve displayed the U shape. FFR proved to be positive for ischemia at 0.71 in the distal LAD, and pull back revealed a pressure jump proximal to the mid-LAD lesion (Figure 3).

Should we consider this presentation to be an acute coronary syndrome (ACS) related to the mid-LAD unstable plaque being the culprit lesion and implement percutaneous

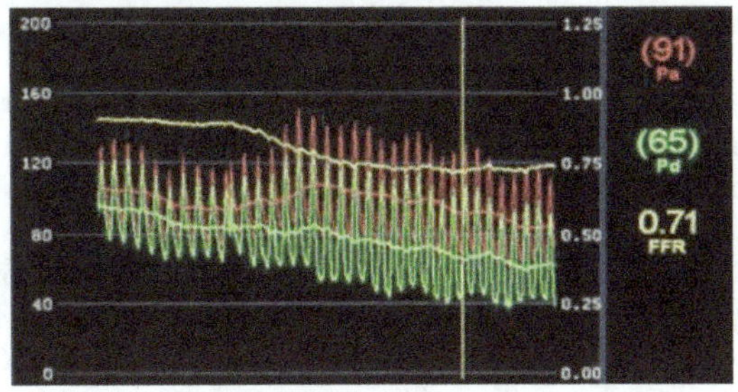

FIGURE 3: Fractional flow reserve in the midleft anterior descending artery.

intervention (PCI), which in turn carries some risk, particularly in complex cases [1, 2]? Or a TTC with a typical apical ballooning [3, 4]—which pathogenic mechanism is believed to be linked to microvascular dysfunction [5] and catecholamine cardiotoxicity [6]—with a significant but innocent concomitant mid-LAD coronary artery disease and therefore treat medically?

3. Actual Treatment and Management of the Case

PCI was elected; a Maverick® balloon catheter (2.0 × 15 mm, Boston Scientific, USA) was advanced to the mid-LAD lesion over the FFR wire. This proved difficult, warranting deep throat catheter engagement in the left main and proximal LAD. Several long balloon inflations achieved a very good "stent-like" result at the PCI site (Moving image 3). However, a retrograde dissection of the proximal LAD occurred into the left main trunk, the aortic cusp, and the proximal LCx (Moving image 4).

At this time, the patient reported chest pain and ST elevation in the anterior leads but was haemodynamically and rhythmically stable. The LCx was immediately wired with a Luge™ (Boston Scientific, USA). We proceeded to direct stenting of the proximal LAD, covering the retrograde dissection entry, into the left main to its ostium with a 3.5 × 28 mm drug-eluting stent (Synergy™, Boston Scientific, USA). After a proximal optimisation technique (4.5 × 8 mm Maverick® balloon catheter, Boston Scientific, USA) in the left main trunk and a final kissing into LAD and LCx arteries, complete disappearance of all contrast extravasation was obtained. Decision was made to leave LCx unstented as it had a good TIMI3 flow (Moving image 5). The patient recovered rapidly and was discharged three days later on full medical therapy.

Fifteen months later, the patient presented in the setting of a hypertensive crisis with chest pain, a small rise in troponin-I, and no ECG changes. Coronary angiogram was unchanged, with diffusely diseased coronary arteries, complete healing of the left main, proximal LAD, and LCx arteries, without in-stent restenosis (Moving image 6). There was no mid-LAD focal lesion, and the FFR in distal LAD was negative for ischemia (0.86). Left ventriculography was normal (Moving image 7).

4. Discussion

TTC and ACS involving the LAD can both induce reversible LV apical akinesia/dyskinesia [3, 4] reflecting myocardial stunning [7] and affect patients in the same age group and with similar risk factors [6].

Unlike in ACS, there is usually no significant coronary artery obstruction or acute plaque rupture [6] in TTC. However, true TTC may occur in the presence of significant CAD or even ACS, but this combination, when affecting LV apex, is particularly tricky [6, 8]. The current NSTEMI presentation supported by the positive FFR at the level of the mid-LAD partial occlusion can induce transient apical LV stunning and ballooning through several mechanisms, including coronary microvascular dysfunction which is encountered similarly in TTC and in ACS [5].

The age and gender, the postmenopausal context, and the transient large apical and midventricular segments wall motion dysfunctions, thus extending beyond a single epicardial coronary distribution may favor the diagnosis of TTC [6]. However, the lack of history of stressful event, the normal corrected QT interval, the high troponin-I level [6], and the long LAD anatomy encompassing anterior-apical and inferior-apical territories support the NSTEMI diagnosis. Moreover, according to the current cardiology society criteria, the positive FFR value in the mid-LAD allows to rule out the latter diagnosis [6]. Blunted coronary vasodilation in ACS and in TTC may decrease the sensitivity but certainly not the specificity of the FFR [2]. Moreover, the excellent angiographic result of sole balloon angioplasty of the culprit lesion supports the ACS diagnosis [1]. Of note, FFR measurement is safe in patients following NSTEMI [9].

When complications occurred, haemodynamic stability as well as proximal location of the dissection in a large vessel prompted us to proceed with interventional treatment rather than surgery despite the involvement of left main and aortic cusp. The mid-LAD culprit lesion was left unstented—with an angiographic "stent-like" result and complete revascularisation—because of the potential difficulty foreseen in advancing a stent to cover it. Complete healing 15 months later further confirms the treatment adequacy.

5. Conclusion

This case emphasizes an uncommon diagnostic challenge the clinician may be facing. In this setting, FFR was crucial to assess the functional significance and the aetiological role of the focal mid-LAD lesion, although a combined aetiology (ACS followed by TTC or the reverse) cannot be ruled out.

Supplementary Materials

Moving Image 1: diagnostic coronary angiogram (right anterior oblique cranial). Moving Image 2: diagnostic left ventriculography (right anterior oblique). Moving Image 3: percutaneous intervention (right anterior oblique cranial). Moving Image 4: left anterior descending artery dissection (right anterior oblique cranial). Moving Image 5: (A) percutaneous treatment of the left anterior descending artery, left main, and aortic cusp dissection; (B) final result (right anterior oblique cranial (A) and caudal (B)). Moving Image 6: fifteen months later (right anterior oblique cranial (A) and caudal (B)). Moving Image 7: ventriculography fifteen months later (right anterior oblique cranial). *(Supplementary Materials)*

References

[1] M. Roffi, C. Patrono, J.-P. Collet et al., "2015 ESC Guidelines for the management of acute coronary syndromes in patients presenting without persistent ST-segment Elevation," *European Heart Journal*, vol. 37, no. 3, pp. 267–315, 2016.

[2] C. Berry, D. Corcoran, B. Hennigan, S. Watkins, J. Layland, and K. G. Oldroyd, "Fractional flow reserve-guided management in stable coronary disease and acute myocardial infarction: recent developments," *European heart journal*, vol. 36, no. 45, pp. 3155–3164, 2015.

[3] W. Desmet, J. Bennett, B. Ferdinande et al., "The apical nipple sign: a useful tool for discriminating between anterior infarction and transient left ventricular ballooning syndrome," *European Heart Journal Acute Cardiovascular Care*, vol. 3, no. 3, pp. 264–267, 2014.

[4] S. Cisneros, R. Duarte, G. C. Fernandez-Perez et al., "Left ventricular apical diseases," *Insights into Imaging*, vol. 2, no. 4, pp. 471–482, 2011.

[5] H. S. Kim, J. A. Tremmel, C. W. Nam et al., "Quantitative comparison of microcirculatory dysfunction in patients with stress cardiomyopathy and ST-segment elevation myocardial infarction," *Journal of the American College of Cardiology*, vol. 58, no. 23, pp. 2430-2431, 2011.

[6] C. Templin, J. R. Ghadri, J. Diekmann et al., "Clinical features and outcomes of takotsubo (stress) cardiomyopathy," *New England Journal of Medicine*, vol. 373, no. 10, pp. 929–938, 2015.

[7] B. Shivalkar, W. Flameng, M. Szilard, S. Pislaru, M. Borgers, and J. Vanhaecke, "Repeated stunning precedes myocardial hibernation in progressive multiple coronary artery obstruction," *Journal of the American College of Cardiology*, vol. 34, no. 7, pp. 2126–2136, 1999.

[8] A. Prasad, G. Dangas, M. Srinivasan et al., "Incidence and angiographic characteristics of patients with apical ballooning syndrome (takotsubo/stress cardiomyopathy) in the HORIZONS-AMI trial: an analysis from a multicenter, international study of ST-elevation myocardial infarction," *Catheterization and Cardiovascular Interventions*, vol. 83, no. 3, pp. 343–348, 2014.

[9] J. Layland, K. G. Oldroyd, N. Curzen et al., "Fractional flow reserve vs. angiography in guiding management to optimize outcomes in non-ST-segment elevation myocardial infarction: the British Heart Foundation FAMOUS-NSTEMI randomized trial," *European Heart Journal*, vol. 36, no. 2, pp. 100–111, 2015.

11

Myocarditis in the Setting of Recent COVID-19 Vaccination

Laura Onderko, Benjamin Starobin, Amy E. Riviere, Patrick K. Hohl, Colin T. Phillips, Roisin B. Morgan, Aimee Welsh, Sanjeev A. Francis, and Maxwell Eyram Afari

Cardiovascular Disease Service Line, Maine Medical Center, Portland, Maine, USA

Correspondence should be addressed to Maxwell Eyram Afari; maxieafari@yahoo.co.uk
Academic Editor: Luigi Sciarra

We report three patients who presented with chest pain after receiving either the BNT162b2 Pfizer/BioNTech or mRNA-1273 Moderna/NIH vaccine. Clinical presentation, biomarker, and cardiac MRI supported myocarditis. It is imperative that potential side effects of COVID-19 vaccine are reported to improve our knowledge about COVID-19 and mRNA vaccines.

1. Introduction

The severe acute respiratory syndrome coronavirus 2 (SARS-CoV-2) is the causative agent of the Coronavirus Disease-2019 (COVID-19) pandemic. The global impact of the COVID-19 pandemic continues since initial descriptions of the COVID-19 syndrome in December 2019. Rapid development and administration of COVID-19 vaccines promise to mitigate COVID-19 fatalities. Early studies show that vaccination against COVID-19 is highly effective and safe [1]. We present three cases of myocarditis that occurred with close temporal relationship to recent COVID-19 vaccine administration with three cases of male patients aged 25-36 years diagnosed with myocarditis several days after receiving the second mRNA vaccine.

2. Case Reports

2.1. Case 1. A 25-year-old male with well-controlled Crohn's disease (not prescribed any medications) presented to the emergency department with chest pain. The chest pain began the day prior to presentation, worse with inspiration and with associated jaw pain. He reported that he received his second dose of the COVID-19 vaccine (BNT162b2 Pfizer/BioNTech) four days prior to presentation. He experienced malaise and myalgias that resolved within twenty-four hours after receiving the vaccine. Labs were significant for a Troponin T that peaked at 0.74 ng/ml (reference < 0.2 ng/ml). Tick panel (for Lyme, anaplasmosis, babesiosis, and ehrlichiosis) was negative since these are part of the differential work-up of myocarditis in the New England region of the United States. His electrocardiogram did not show any ischemic changes, and echocardiogram was significant for low normal left ventricular ejection fraction (LVEF) of 50%. He was admitted for further work-up and started on colchicine and ibuprofen for presumed myopericarditis. He underwent cardiac MRI which showed a left ventricular fraction of 56% and findings consistent with myocarditis with myocardial edema seen by T2 mapping and myocardial injury with focal late gadolinium enhancement (LGE) with multiple foci in the midwall. He did not have evidence of pericardial inflammation. He did not undergo endomyocardial biopsy. COVID-19 polymerase chain reaction (PCR) was negative. During his hospital stay, he was monitored on telemetry without any arrhythmias observed. He was discharged on low-dose beta-blocker with plans for repeat outpatient echocardiogram and cardiac monitor to screen for any arrhythmias as well as activity restriction.

2.2. Case 2. A 28-year-old male with a medical history significant for obesity presented with chest pain and lateral ST elevation myocardial infarction by electrocardiogram. He was taken to the catheterization laboratory, and coronary angiogram showed no luminal irregularities. On interview, he reported receiving his second dose of COVID-19 vaccine (NT162b2 Pfizer/BioNTech) three days prior to presentation.

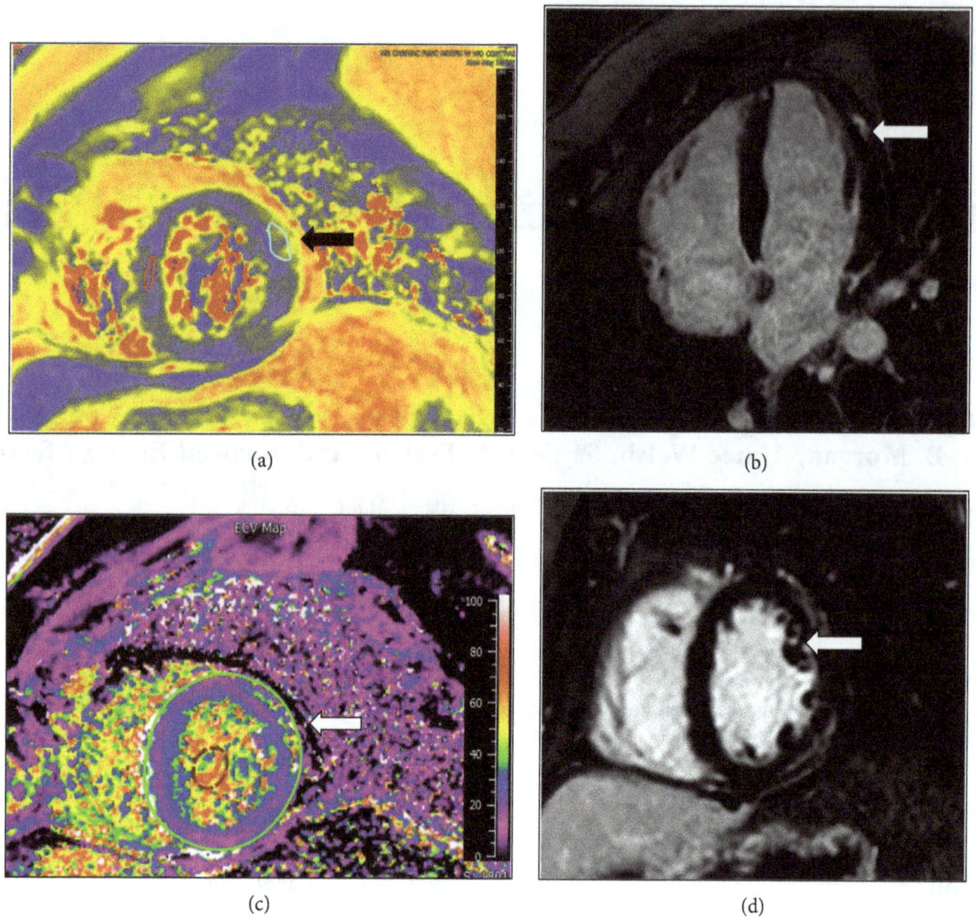

Figure 1: Cardiac MRI of patient C: (a) T2 map demonstrating increased T2 signal consistent with edema in epicardium of the apical lateral wall; (b) four-chamber view showing late gadolinium enhancement in the apical lateral wall; (c) ECV map showing increased signal consistent with edema in the midanterolateral segments; (d) short axis with late gadolinium enhancements in the midanterolateral segments.

After receiving the vaccine, he experienced fatigue, chills, and myalgias that resolved the day before presentation. Labs were significant for Troponin T peak of 1.42 ng/ml, C-reactive protein (CRP) peak of 68.6 mg/l (reference < 8.0 mg/l), and Erythrocyte Sedimentation Rate (ESR) of 19 mm/h (reference < 15 mm/h). He underwent cardiac MRI which showed a left ventricular ejection fraction of 56% and evidence of myocarditis with myocardial edema demonstrated on T2 mapping and myocardial injury with focal LGE in the basal inferior, mid- to distal lateral/inferolateral walls (Figure 1). He also did not undergo endomyocardial biopsy, and COVID-19 PCR was negative. During his hospital stay, he was monitored on telemetry without any arrhythmias observed. He was discharged on low-dose beta blocker and activity restriction with plan for continued outpatient follow-up.

2.3. *Case 3.* A 36-year-old male with a past medical history significant for gastroesophageal reflux disease (not prescribed any medications) who presented with chest pain and lateral ST elevations consistent with ST elevation myocardial infarction. He was taken to the cardiac catheterization laboratory, and coronary angiogram showed no luminal irregularities. On interview, he reported receiving the second dose of the mRNA-1273 Moderna/NIH vaccine two days prior to presentation. His Troponin T peaked at 0.35 ng/ml, CRP 49.7 mg/l, and ESR of 24 mm/h. Echocardiogram showed a left ventricular ejection fraction of 55-60%. Cardiac MRI was again consistent with myocarditis with LVEF of 56% and myocardial edema by T2 mapping and myocardial injury with focal LGE in the mid- to distal inferolateral and lateral walls (Figure 2). Again, no endomyocardial biopsy was obtained, and COVID-19 PCR was negative. During his hospital stay, he was monitored on telemetry without any arrhythmias observed. He was also discharged with low-dose beta-blocker, advice on activity restrictions, and outpatient follow-up.

3. Discussion

We describe three cases of myocarditis in young, healthy patients following COVID-19 vaccine administration (Table 1). The temporal timing of our cases correlates with similar reports in literature of myocarditis occurring 12-96 hours following immunization with an mRNA COVID-19 vaccine [2, 3]. These cases demonstrate a similar temporal relationship, increasing the likelihood of causality. This safety signal was not clinically apparent in the early vaccine experience, raising the possibility that the association is

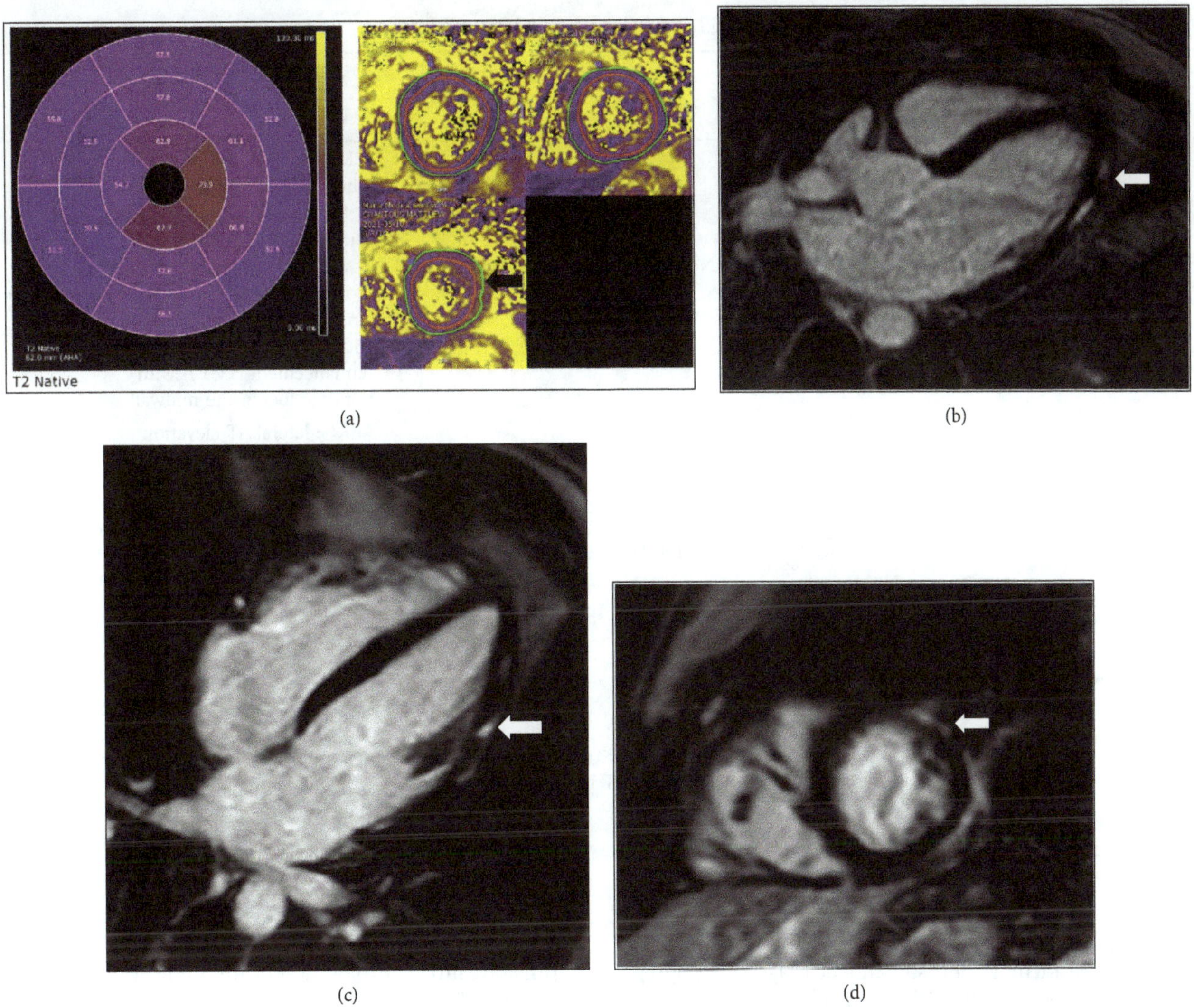

Figure 2: Patient D cardiac MRI: (a) T2 map demonstrating increased T2 signal consistent with edema in the epicardium of the apical lateral wall; (b–d) 3-chamber, 4-chamber, and apical short axis delayed images, respectively, demonstrating epicardial late gadolinium enhancement (LGE) corresponding to area of edema on T2 map.

purely coincidental as viruses responsible for myocarditis follow a seasonal distribution [4].

All three patients were ruled out for COVID-19 infection using the Centers for Disease Control and Prevention-(CDC-) approved gold standard test: polymerase chain reaction (PCR). Previous reports had demonstrated an association between COVID-19 infection and myocarditis [5]. Routine antigen or antibody testing is not part of our clinical work flow, and some have questioned the utility of antibody testing in the postvaccination cohort [6].

In case 1, we considered the possibility of Crohn's disease being a confounding factor for myocardial injury. On review of available case reports in the literature, episodes of myocarditis associated to Crohn's disease occur most often in the context of a disease flare or secondary to disease-modifying medication and remain an extremely rare extraintestinal manifestation of Crohn's disease [7].

Importantly, none of these patients developed malignant manifestations of myocarditis. They maintained normal systolic function and did not have any symptoms of clinical heart failure, arrhythmias, or conduction abnormalities. In addition, for the number of vaccinations that have been administered in our hospital catchment area, these cases would be exceedingly rare. At the time these patients presented to our institution, the Maine CDC reported vaccine administration of 661,051 initial doses and 612,781 second doses. Taking both these factors into consideration and knowing the morbidity and mortality of COVID-19 infection, the overall benefit of the COVID-19 vaccine outweighs this potential risk.

Proposed mechanisms of a COVID-19 vaccine-associated myocarditis are speculative. Both the BNT162b2 Pfizer/BioNTech and mRNA-1273 Moderna/NIH vaccines produced high-affinity neutralizing antibody in the early phases [8]. This raises the possibility of an inappropriate adaptive immune response causing clinical myocarditis. Serologic testing of the early phase I subjects demonstrated a robust T cell response, and specific cytokines were tracked [8]. It is plausible that the T cell immunity in these cases became dysregulated resulting in abnormal cytokine release.

Table 1: Patient characteristics and results.

Patient	Age	Sex	Medical history	Symptom onset	Vaccine	Troponin T reference < 0.02 ng/ml	Imaging	Ischemic work-up
A	25	Male	Crohn's disease (no medications)	Chest pain 4-day post-2nd vaccine	BNT162b2 Pfizer/ BioNTech	Troponin T = 0.74 ng/ml	EKG: no ischemic changes Echo: left ventricular ejection fraction (LVEF) = 50% Cardiac MRI (cMRI): LVEF = 56%, consistent with myocardial edema (T2 mapping) and myocardial injury (focal late gadolinium enhancement (LGE)) with multiple foci in the midwall	Not applicable
B	28	Male	Obesity	Chest pain 3-day post-2nd vaccine	BNT162b2 Pfizer/ BioNTech	Troponin T = 1.42 ng/ml	EKG: lateral ST elevation myocardial infarction cMRI: LVEF = 56%, consistent with myocardial edema (T2 mapping) and myocardial injury (focal LGE) in the basal inferior, mid- to distal lateral/ inferolateral walls	Coronary angiogram: no luminal irregularities
C	36	Male	Gastroesophageal reflux disease	Chest pain 2-day post-2nd vaccine	mRNA-1273 Moderna/NIH	Troponin T = 0.35 ng/ml	EKG: lateral ST elevations Echo: LVEF = 55-60% cMRI: LVEF = 56%, consistent with myocardial edema (T2 mapping) and myocardial injury (focal LGE) in the mid- to distal inferolateral and lateral walls	Coronary angiogram: no luminal irregularities

Another possible mechanism includes impaired development of T cell memory and subsequent exaggerated upregulation of cytokines [9]. Other considerations include a cross-reactivity of existing memory T cells from prior infections with other coronaviruses, which can result in a heterologous T cell memory with resultant exaggerated cytokine release [9].

The smallpox vaccine is linked to myocarditis. In 2002, recommendations were made for smallpox (variola virus) vaccination of enlisted military personnel as well as civilian health care workers. Of 730,580 armed forces personnel vaccinated with live vaccinia vaccine (Dryvax), 86 cases of myopericarditis occurred, at a rate 7.5 times higher than the expected background rate. In a subsequent prospective study of the ACAM2000 vaccine approved in 2007, 7 out of 1307 vaccinated individuals developed myocarditis with no fatalities. However, these vaccines do represent an entirely different model of vaccination as compared to COVID-19 vaccines given their use of live virus to generate an immune response [10].

4. Conclusion

There have been early reports of a presumed link between COVID-19 vaccination and subsequent development of myocarditis, but no causative link has been established. Our cases add to others where a temporal relationship between vaccination and myocarditis has been described. Ultimately, further exploration of this clinical phenomenon is warranted.

Consent

No written consent has been obtained from the patients as there is no patient identifiable data included in this case report/series.

References

[1] F. P. Polack, S. J. Thomas, N. Kitchin et al., "Safety and efficacy of the BNT162b2 mRNA COVID-19 vaccine," *New England Journal of Medicine*, vol. 383, no. 27, pp. 2603–2615, 2020.

[2] J. Montgomery, M. Ryan, R. Engler et al., "Myocarditis following immunization with mRNA COVID-19 vaccines in members of the US military," *JAMA cardiology*, vol. 6, no. 10, p. 1202, 2021.

[3] G. A. Diaz, G. T. Parsons, S. K. Gering, A. R. Meier, I. V. Hutchinson, and A. Robicsek, "Myocarditis and pericarditis after vaccination for COVID-19," *JAMA*, vol. 326, no. 12, p. 1210, 2021.

[4] C. Tschope, E. Ammirati, B. Bozkurt et al., "Myocarditis and inflammatory cardiomyopathy: current evidence and future directions," *Nature Reviews Cardiology*, vol. 18, no. 3, pp. 169–193, 2021.

[5] D. Levin, G. Shimon, M. Fadlon-Derai et al., "Myocarditis following COVID-19 vaccination - a case series," *Vaccine*, vol. 39, no. 42, pp. 6195–6200, 2021.

[6] D. Romero-Alvarez, D. F. Lopez-Cevallos, and I. Torres, "Uninformative and unuseful: why it is necessary to actively challenge COVID-19 antibody testing postvaccination," *Public Health*, vol. 199, pp. 32-33, 2021.

[7] L. McGrath-Cadell, N. K. Bart, L. Lin, S. Ghaly, and C. J. Holloway, "Myocarditis in Crohn's disease: a case report," *Eur Heart J Case Rep.*, vol. 4, no. 4, pp. 1–6, 2020.

[8] A. Lombardi, G. Bozzi, R. Ungaro et al., "Mini review immunological consequences of immunization with COVID-19 mRNA vaccines: preliminary results," *Frontiers in Immunology*, vol. 12, p. 657711, 2021.

[9] N. N. Jarjour, D. Masopust, and S. C. Jameson, "T cell memory: understanding COVID-19," vol. 54, no. 1, pp. 14–18, 2021.

[10] A. Nalca and E. E. Zumbrun, "ACAM2000™: the new smallpox vaccine for United States Strategic National Stockpile," *Drug Design, Development and Therapy*, vol. 4, pp. 71–79, 2010.

12

Blood Cancer and the Heart: Light Chain Cardiomyopathy in Refractory Multiple Myeloma

Abdulbaril Olagunju,[1] **Chandana Shekar**,[2] **Michael Morris**,[3] **Anantharam Kalya**,[2] **Farouk Mookadam**,[2] **and Samuel Unzek**[2]

[1]*Department of Medicine, Creighton University, Phoenix, AZ, USA*
[2]*Heart Center, Banner University Medical Center, University of Arizona College of Medicine-Phoenix, Phoenix, AZ, USA*
[3]*Department of Diagnostic Radiology, Banner University Medical Center, University of Arizona College of Medicine-Phoenix, Phoenix, AZ, USA*

Correspondence should be addressed to Abdulbaril Olagunju; abdulbarilolagunju@creighton.edu
Academic Editor: Gopal Chandra Ghosh

We report a case of a 57-year-old woman with a history of multiple myeloma (MM) and light chain (AL) amyloidosis who presented due to worsening dyspnea on exertion. Her MM has been refractory to multiple chemotherapy regimens and two autologous bone marrow transplantation. Diagnostic evaluations including serum kappa and lambda chains, echocardiogram, pyrophosphate cardiac scan, and cardiac magnetic resonance were indicative of a progression to AL cardiomyopathy. Addition of daratumumab to her regimen appeared to ameliorate the progression of AL cardiomyopathy. However, it was stopped due to adverse effects of pancytopenia and allergic reactions including skin rash and hives. She was hospitalized for heart failure exacerbation and died approximately 2 months following the discontinuation of daratumumab. This case highlights the late presentation of AL cardiomyopathy in refractory MM.

1. Introduction

Multiple myeloma (MM) is a plasma cell malignancy that is responsible for approximately 10% of all hematologic malignancies [1, 2]. As of 2015, about 124,733 were living with MM in the United States; an additional 32,000 new cases were diagnosed in the year 2020, accounting for 1.8% of new cancer diagnosis [1]. Approximately 12-15% of MM patients develop light chain (AL) amyloidosis [2]. In these patients, the progression to AL cardiomyopathy remains a significant cause of morbidity and mortality [3]. Here, we present a case of refractory MM that was complicated by AL cardiomyopathy.

2. Case Presentation

A 57-year-old woman with a history of refractory MM and AL amyloidosis presented to the emergency department with acute exertional dyspnea and palpitations. She denied cough, chest pain, paroxysmal nocturnal dyspnea, fever, chills, and smoking history. Her MM was refractory to multiple combination of treatments including lenalidomide/bortezomib/dexamethasone, carfilzomib/pomalidomide/dexamethasone, high-dose melphalan with autologous bone marrow transplant, pomalidomide/ixazomib/prednisone, cyclophosphamide/bortezomib/dexamethasone (CyBorD), isatuximab/pomalidomide, and a second autologous bone marrow transplant with carfilzomib/lenalidomide/dexamethasone.

Physical exam was notable for jugular venous distention and bilateral lower extremity pitting edema. There were no murmurs, rubs, or gallops. The differential diagnoses included acute systolic heart failure due to cancer-related drug treatments, atrial fibrillation with rapid ventricular response (AFRVR) with acute diastolic heart failure, acute myocardial infarction, and acute pulmonary embolism.

Vital signs were remarkable for heart rate of 101 beats per minute (bpm). Laboratory data were remarkable for hemoglobin 63 g/L (normal range, 135-170 g/L), platelets 54 K/μL (normal range, 130-450 K/microL), white blood cell 3.9×10^9/L (normal range, 4.0-11.0 $\times 10^9$/L), NT-proBNP 4,375 pmol/L (normal range, <14.8 pmol/L), troponin 117 mcg/L (normal range, <14 mcg/L), and serum kappa and lambda chains 1.62 mg/L and 1302 mg/L (normal range, 3.3 to 19.4 mg/L and 5.71 to 26.3 mg/L, respectively). Twelve lead electrocardiogram (ECG) showed sinus tachycardia with low voltage in the limb leads (Figure 1). Computed tomography angiogram of the chest was negative for pulmonary embolism. Echocardiogram revealed left ventricular (LV) ejection fraction of 65%, severely increased LV posterior wall end diastolic thickness (17 mm) (normal: 6 to 9 mm), grade II diastolic dysfunction, mildly enlarged right ventricular (RV) chamber with mildly reduced systolic function, RV systolic pressure of 56 mmHg, and reduced peak average global longitudinal strain with apical sparing of the LV on strain imaging and polar map (Figure 2). Cardiac magnetic resonance (CMR) showed thick myocardial walls with patchy subendocardial late gadolinium enhancement (LGE) prominent along the lateral, inferoseptal walls from the base through the midventricle and papillary muscles (Figure 3). T1 times were very elevated compared to CMR from a year earlier suggesting progressive cardiomyopathy. Basal anteroseptal and inferolateral wall thickness increased from 17-22 mm and 13-19 mm, respectively. No focal regional wall motion abnormality was identified. A pyrophosphate (PYP) cardiac scan compared to a year earlier was positive for scintigraphic evidence of evolving amyloid deposition (Figure 4).

She was transfused with red blood cells with a target hemoglobin of at least 8 g/dL. Diuresis was initiated with intravenous furosemide. This significantly improved her dyspnea and reduced ankle swelling. She was transitioned to torsemide at discharge. Daratumumab (Darzalex) was added to her MM regimen: daratumumab/melflufen/dexamethasone. Due to the refractoriness of her MM, she was not a candidate for heart transplant. At 6-month follow-up, she was asymptomatic, and her cardiac and renal function remained stable. However, a bone marrow biopsy showed stable clonal plasma cells (13%). Furthermore, daratumumab was stopped due to worsening pancytopenia and allergic reactions including skin rash and hives. Her cardiac and renal function remained stable; however, she complained of progressive neuropathy. She was readmitted approximately two months following discontinuation of daratumumab for an acute exacerbation of her heart failure. She suddenly became tachycardic with a heart rate of 140 bpm and was unresponsive and noted to have pulseless electrical activity (PEA). A cardiopulmonary resuscitation was not performed due to her wishes. The cause of her death was thought to be an obstructive shock due to a massive pulmonary embolism.

3. Discussion

Approximately 50% of patients with AL amyloidosis have cardiac involvement [3]. The development of heart failure symptoms portends a poor prognosis with a median survival < 6 months in patients without adequate management of the instigating plasma cell dyscrasia [3].

Echocardiogram in the early stage typically reveals a preserved ejection fraction; however, a reduction in the global longitudinal strain that spares the cardiac apex and manifests in a reduction in stroke volume index indicates significant cardiac dysfunction [4, 5]. In addition, a symmetric biventricular increased wall thickness may be noted on echocardiogram, creating abroad differential for thick-walled cardiomyopathies [4]. CMR is important in the diagnosis of cardiac amyloidosis to assess extent and severity, with tissue biopsy being the gold standard of course [4, 5]. LGE is a significant prognostic factor that correlates with the degree of cardiac infiltration by the light chains [5], with subendocardial LGE in early stages of the disease and transmural LGE seen in in the later stages of the disease [5]. Furthermore, CMR T1 relaxation time is directly proportional to the degree of cardiac light chain infiltration and hence serves a useful method to quantify the progression of cardiac involvement [5]. Unlike transthyretin amyloidosis, PYP scan is positive only in about 40% of AL cardiomyopathy cases [6]. In patients with unconfirmed AL amyloidosis, a tissue biopsy which typically reveals an apple-green birefringence on polarized light microscopy is required [7]. This should be followed by further evaluation to assess for the presence of MM through bone marrow plasma cell quantification, quantification of AL in serum and urine, lytic lesions in skeleton, presence of soft tissue deposits, and other end organ manifestation as described by the International Myeloma Working Group 2014 criteria [8].

The management of heart failure symptoms in patients with AL cardiomyopathy is different from other forms of heart failure [9]. Diuresis with loop diuretics and aldosterone receptor antagonists are important in achieving and maintaining euvolemia [9]. Except in patients with AFRVR, beta-blockers (BB) are generally avoided because they worsen hypotension by suppressing the compensatory sinus tachycardia required to maintain normotension [9]. Angiotensin-converting enzyme inhibitors and angiotensin receptor blockers are also not well tolerated because they aggravate hypotension [9]. Digoxin binds to the amyloid fibrils which increases the risk for digoxin toxicity [9]. Hence, it must be used with caution in patients with AFRVR that cannot tolerate BB due to hypotension [9]. Calcium channel blockers are typically avoided because their negative inotropic effect worsens heart failure symptoms [9].

In addition to relieving heart failure congestion with diuresis, the prognosis of AL cardiomyopathy centers on the treatment of the underlying plasma cell dyscrasia [3]. The available treatment options include hematopoietic stem cell transplantation (HCT) and/or chemotherapy [3]. The combination of high dose melphalan and HCT is associated with a high rate of complete hematologic and organ response and overall survival [3]. However, the significant treatment-related mortality in patients with AL amyloidosis makes the combination available to only 25-30% of patients [3]. These are patients without advanced cardiomyopathy, advanced age, multiple organ involvement, hypotension,

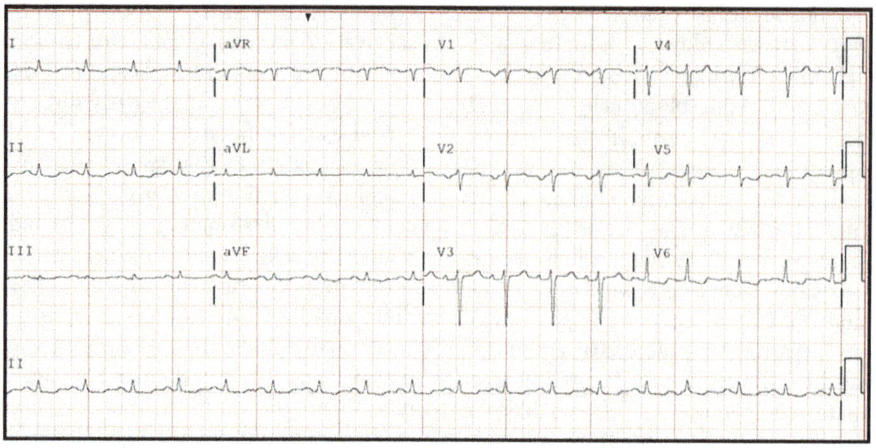

FIGURE 1: ECG showed sinus rhythm with low voltage in the limb leads.

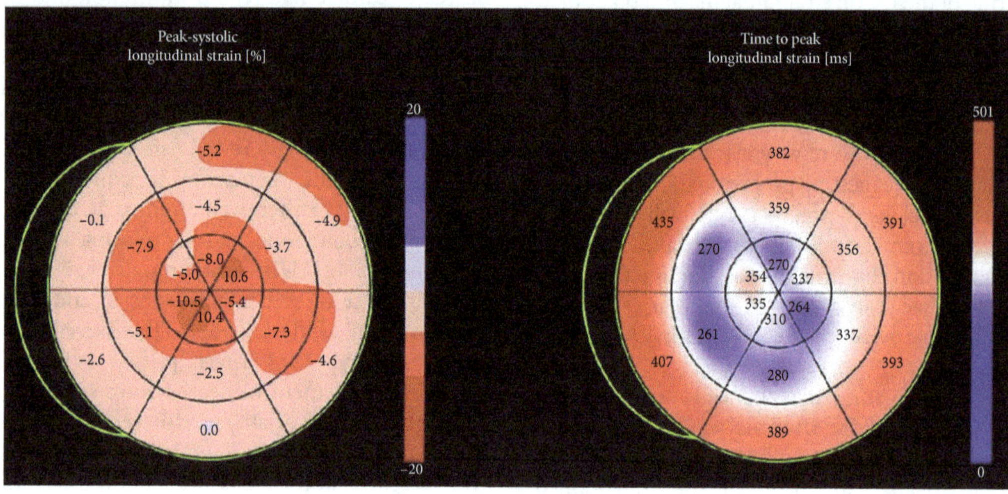

FIGURE 2: Echocardiographic polar map highlighted a decrease in global longitudinal strain.

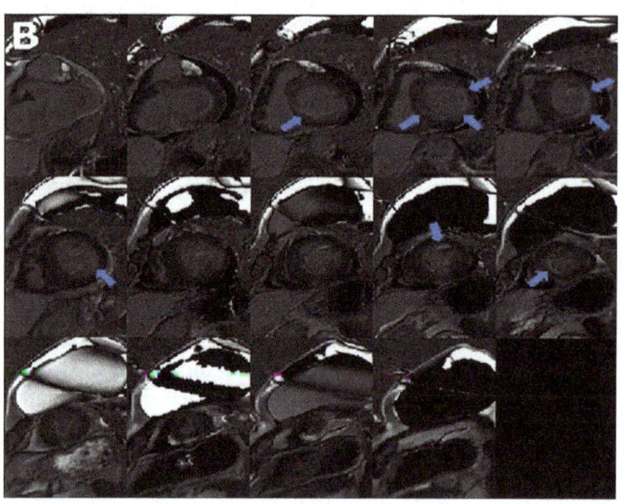

FIGURE 3: CMR revealed patchy midmyocardial and subendocardial LGE.

and low serum albumin levels [8]. The prognosis of AL amyloidosis can be assessed using the European modification of the Mayo 2004 staging [10]. The staging is based on the serum concentration of the NT-proBNP and troponin; the cut-off values are 332 ng/L (normal range, ≤169.4 ng/L) and 0.035 mcg/L (normal range, ≤0.1 mcg/L), respectively [9] (Table 1).

Traditionally, patients who are ineligible for HCT have been treated either with melphalan and dexamethasone or bortezomib-based regimen including bortezomib, melphalan, and dexamethasone or CyBorD [11]. Bortezomib should be used with caution due to its association with worsening heart failure [12]. CyBorD is a more commonly used regimen based on outcomes of trials that demonstrated higher hematologic and organ response compared to BMD [11]. Daratumumab, a monoclonal antibody against the CD38 protein expressed on the clonal plasma cells, was associated with a shorter time to first hematologic and deep response as well as a highly significant improvement in cardiac and renal

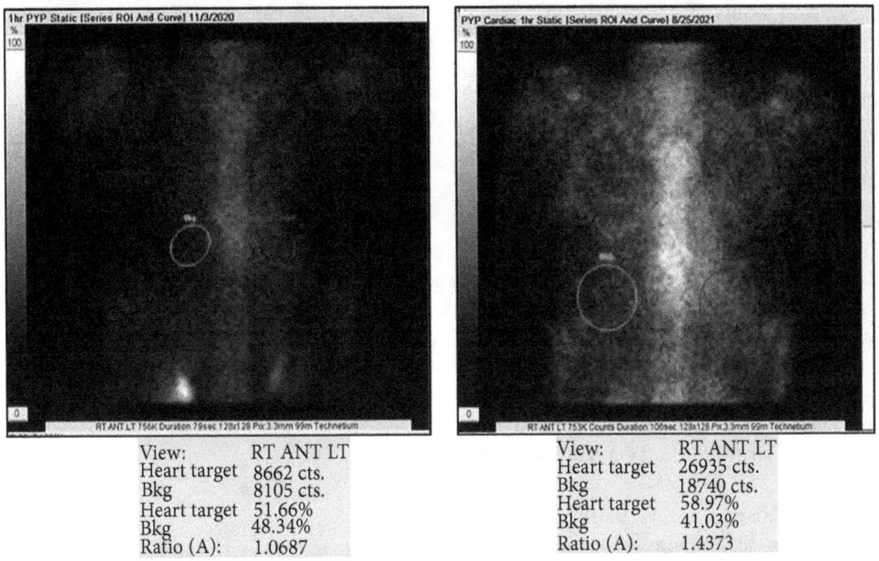

FIGURE 4: Right PYP scan showed increased PYP uptake compared to the left PYP scan done almost a year earlier.

TABLE 1: Cut-off values for NT-proBNP and troponin based on the European modification of the Mayo 2004 staging for prognosticating AL amyloidosis.

Stage	Markers
I	Troponin < 0.035 mcg/L & NT-proBNP < 332 ng/L
II	Troponin ≥ 0.035 mcg/L or NT-proBNP ≥ 332 ng/L
IIIa	Troponin ≥ 0.035 mcg/L & NT-proBNP < 8500 ng/L
IIIb	Troponin ≥ 0.035 mcg/L & NT-proBNP ≥ 8500 ng/L

response in the ANDROMEDA trial either alone or in combination with CyBorD [10–12]. These outcomes were also the highlight of phase II trials that evaluated the impact of daratumumab in patients with refractory and relapsed AL amyloidosis [12]. CD38 plays a role in protecting myeloma cells from immune system destruction [11]. Hence, the level of CD38 expression in AL amyloidosis is proportional to the severity of cardiac involvement and the serum concentration of NT-proBNP [12]. The binding of daratumumab to CD38 results in immune-mediated plasma cell death via multiple mechanisms including apoptosis, complement-dependent cytotoxicity, antibody-dependent cellular cytotoxicity, and antibody-dependent cellular phagocytosis [11]. Besides daratumumab, doxycycline has been associated with a higher rate of organ response and survival in a retrospective study [13]. However, in a recent randomized controlled trial, doxycycline did not prolong survival [14].

Our patient had Mayo stage IIIB AL amyloidosis that remained refractory to multiple chemotherapy regimens and two HCTs, and hence, daratumumab was added with the hope of achieving some cardiac response. It is likely that her readmission for acute exacerbation of heart failure was associated with the discontinuation of daratumumab.

4. Conclusion

We present a case of refractory MM complicated by progressive AL cardiomyopathy in the setting of AL amyloidosis. In general, the prognosis is poor. Daratumumab is a novel immune modulating agent that may help even after a few doses and offers hope for cardiac response. However, our patient discontinued it after 6 months due to worsening pancytopenia and allergic reactions. This was followed by hospitalization for acute heart failure exacerbation during which she developed a PEA and expired.

References

[1] J. Mikhael, N. Ismaila, M. Cheung et al., "Treatment of multiple myeloma: ASCO and CCO joint clinical practice guideline," *Journal of Clinical Oncology*, vol. 37, no. 14, pp. 1228–1263, 2019.

[2] C. Plummer, C. Driessen, Z. Szabo, and M. Mateos, "Management of cardiovascular risk in patients with multiple myeloma," *Cancer Journal*, vol. 9, no. 3, p. 26, 2019.

[3] U. Tahir, G. Doros, J. Kim, L. Connors, D. Seldin, and F. Sam, "Predictors of mortality in light chain cardiac amyloidosis with heart failure," *Scientific Reports*, vol. 9, no. 1, p. 8552, 2019.

[4] M. Maurer, P. Elliott, R. Comenzo, M. Semigran, and C. Rapezzi, "Addressing common questions encountered in the diagnosis and management of cardiac amyloidosis," *Circulation*, vol. 135, no. 14, pp. 1357–1377, 2017.

[5] D. S. Knight, G. Zumbo, W. Barcella et al., "Cardiac structural and functional consequences of amyloid deposition by cardiac magnetic resonance and echocardiography and their prognostic roles," *JACC: Cardiovascular Imaging*, vol. 12, no. 5, pp. 823–833, 2019.

[6] J. Gillmore, M. Maurer, R. Falk et al., "Nonbiopsy diagnosis of cardiac transthyretin amyloidosis," *Circulation*, vol. 133, no. 24, pp. 2404–2412, 2016.

[7] C. Quarta, J. Kruger, and R. Falk, "Cardiac amyloidosis," *Circulation*, vol. 126, no. 12, p. 12, 2012.

[8] S. V. Rajkumar, M. A. Dimopoulos, A. Palumbo et al., "International myeloma working group updated criteria for the diagnosis of multiple myeloma," *The Lancet Oncology*, vol. 15, no. 12, pp. e538–e548, 2014.

[9] R. Falk, K. Alexander, R. Liao, and S. Dorbala, "AL (light-chain) cardiac amyloidosis: a review of diagnosis and therapy," *Journal of the American College of Cardiology*, vol. 68, no. 12, pp. 1323–1341, 2016.

[10] A. Dispenzieri, F. Buadi, S. Kumar et al., "Treatment of immunoglobulin light chain amyloidosis: mayo stratification of myeloma and risk-adapted therapy (mSMART) consensus statement," *Mayo Clinic Proceedings*, vol. 90, no. 8, pp. 1054–1081, 2015.

[11] F. Theodorakakou, M. Dimopoulos, and E. Kastritis, "Daratumumab plus CyBorD for patients with newly diagnosed light chain (AL) amyloidosis," *Therapeutic Advances in Hematology*, vol. 12, article 204062072110583, 2021.

[12] G. Palladini, P. Milani, F. Malavasi, and G. Merlini, "Daratumumab in the treatment of light-chain (AL) amyloidosis," *Cell*, vol. 10, no. 3, p. 545, 2021.

[13] A. Wechalekar and C. Whelan, "Encouraging impact of doxycycline on early mortality in cardiac light chain (AL) amyloidosis," *Blood Cancer Journal*, vol. 7, no. 3, article e546, 2017.

[14] K.-N. Shen, W.-J. Fu, Y. Wu et al., "Doxycycline combined with bortezomib-cyclophosphamide-dexamethasone chemotherapy for newly diagnosed cardiac light-chain amyloidosis: a multicenter randomized controlled trial," *Circulation*, vol. 145, no. 1, pp. 8–17, 2022.

13

Clinical Presentations of Chagas Cardiomyopathy

Malik Shehadeh,[1] **Ana Barac**,[1,2] **and Rachel Marcus**[3]

[1]*Medstar Washington Hospital Center, Washington, D. C, USA*
[2]*Medstar Heart and Vascular Institute, Washington, D. C, USA*
[3]*Medstar Union Memorial Hospital and Latin American Society of Chagas (LASOCHA), USA*

Correspondence should be addressed to Malik Shehadeh; malik.z.shehadeh@medstar.net
Academic Editor: Assad Movahed

Chronic Chagas cardiomyopathy (CCC) is the most common cause of nonischemic cardiomyopathy in endemic Latin American countries. Immigrants to the United States suffer from this disease, but it is underrecognized. We describe the three hallmark clinical presentations: stroke, ventricular arrhythmias, and heart failure, which should prompt suspicion for CCC.

1. Introduction

Chagas disease is a chronic systemic parasitic infection caused by the protozoan Trypanosoma cruzi that is transmitted to humans by triatomine insects in endemic areas of Latin America [1].

CCC typically appears 15-30 years after the initial infection, and 20-30% of infected individuals present with manifestations such as heart failure, stroke, and brady- and tachyarrhythmias [1–3]. Because of lack of awareness of this disease on the part of US-based health care professionals, the diagnosis is underrecognized.

In this case series, we describe the experience of a high-volume referral center with different presentations of Chagas cardiomyopathy, highlighting presentations that should raise suspicion for Trypanosoma cruzi infection.

2. First Presentation: Stroke

A 28-year-old El Salvadorian male was referred to cardiology for palpitations after an electrocardiogram (ECG) showed bifascicular block. A transthoracic echocardiogram (TTE) showed normal biventricular size and function, and a cardiac magnetic resonance imaging (MRI) was suggested because of the ECG abnormalities. This showed a small area of transmural myocardial fibrosis with focal dyskinesis of the true apex, muscular diverticula, and midapical lateral hypokinesis. Because of the myocardial scar, a coronary computed tomography angiography was suggested to evaluate for coronary atherosclerosis, but the patient was lost to follow-up.

2 years later, he presented with new right hemiparesis of indeterminate duration. Brain MRI revealed acute ischemic infarct in the left middle cerebral artery territory (Figure 1). Thrombolytic therapy was not considered given the unknown onset of stroke, and he was admitted to the hospital for further ischemic workup.

Electrocardiogram (ECG) showed normal sinus rhythm with right bundle branch block (RBBB), left anterior fascicular block (LAFB), and secondary T wave changes (Figure 2). TTE with contrast showed normal left ventricular ejection fraction (LVEF), and with echo contrast injection, an apical aneurysm was noted.

Given the patient's country of origin, ECG, and TTE findings, CCC was considered. Commercial Hemagen followed by CDC confirmatory assays were positive for Trypanosoma cruzi infection, which confirmed the diagnosis.

Patient was discharged to a rehabilitation facility and continued to follow up with our clinic. Family screening was discussed as an outpatient.

3. Second Presentation: Ventricular Tachycardia

A 46-year-old El Salvadorian female with a history of alcohol abuse presented to our hospital with hemodynamically unstable ventricular tachycardia requiring cardioversion.

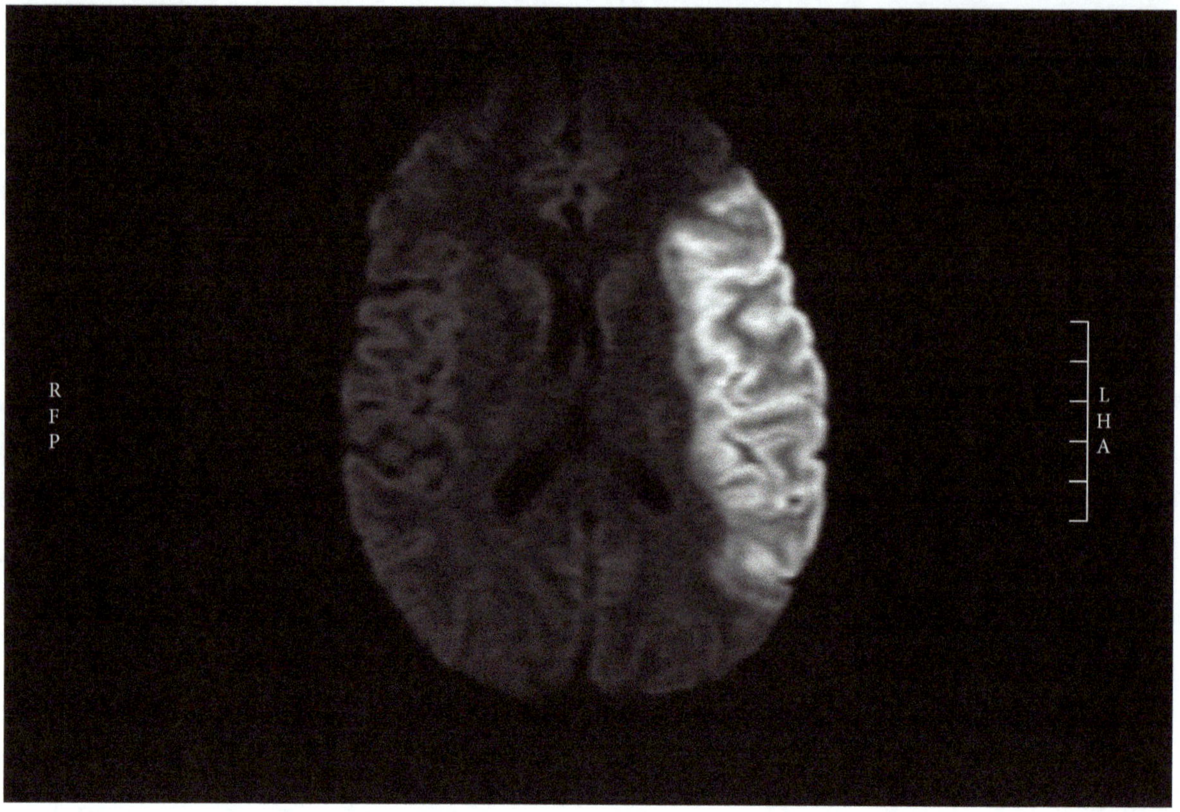

FIGURE 1: Diffusion-weighted brain magnetic resonance imaging (MRI) showing acute stroke in the left middle cerebral artery territory.

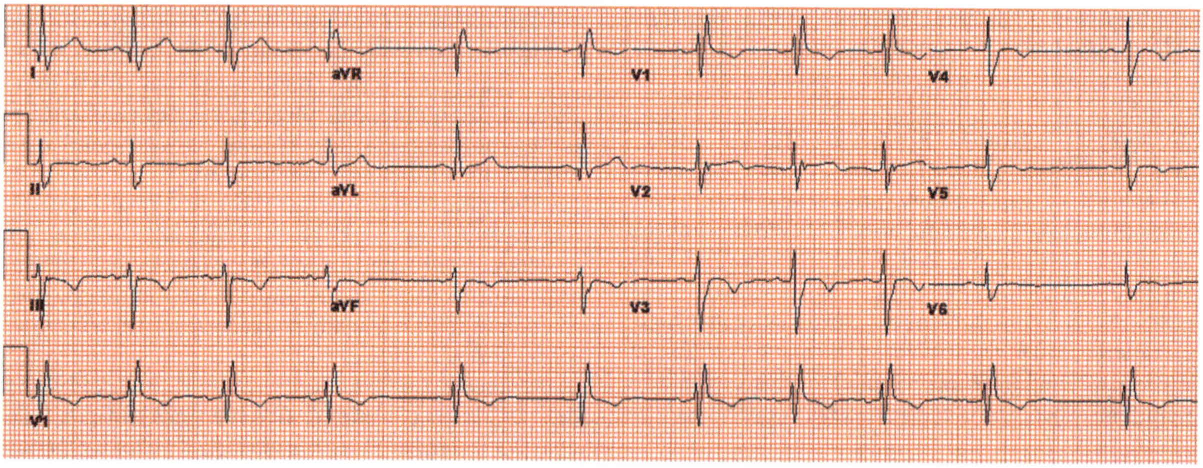

FIGURE 2: Electrocardiogram showing normal sinus rhythm with right bundle branch block, left anterior fascicular block, and secondary T wave changes.

She presented with chest tightness and dizziness of 2-hour duration and was found to be in monomorphic ventricular tachycardia requiring cardioversion. Laboratory investigations showed low potassium and magnesium levels which were repleted. Thyroid function was normal. Troponin I was 0.581 ng/ml (reference range < 0.045 ng/ml). ECG after cardioversion showed normal sinus rhythm with RBBB and LAFB (Figure 3).

Coronary angiography showed no coronary artery disease. TTE showed normal biventricular function without regional wall motion abnormalities. Cardiac MRI showed extensive transmural basal lateral wall gadolinium enhancement suggestive of fibrosis (Figure 4). Commercial Trypanosoma cruzi enzyme-linked immunosorbent assay (ELISA) followed by CDC serologic testing confirmed the diagnosis of CCC.

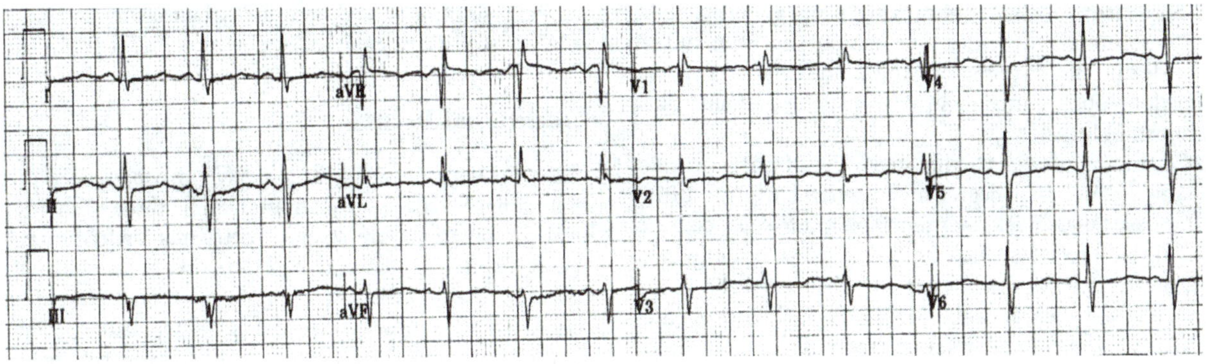

FIGURE 3: Electrocardiogram showing normal sinus rhythm with bifascicular block (right bundle branch block and left anterior fascicular block).

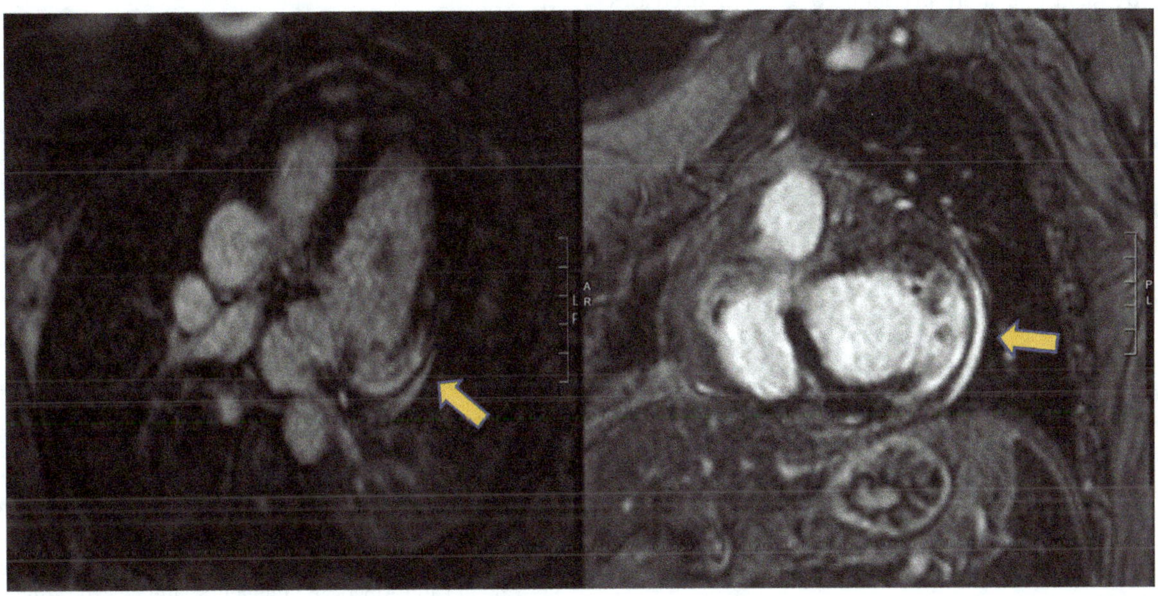

FIGURE 4: Cardiac magnetic resonance imaging (MRI) showing transmural late gadolinium enhancement in the basal lateral wall (yellow arrows) which is highly concerning of Chagas cardiomyopathy.

The patient received a single-chamber implantable cardioverter defibrillator for secondary prevention. Family screening was discussed as an outpatient; the patient was made aware that all children of an infected mother must receive testing to evaluate for congenital transmission.

4. Third Presentation: Heart Failure

A 43-year-old El Salvadorian male with heart failure from CCC required left ventricular assist device (LVAD) implantation and subsequently orthotopic heart transplantation.

The patient presented at the age of 22 with a syncopal event for which a dual-chamber pacemaker was placed. After developing symptoms of heart failure in his early 30's, he was found by TTE to have severe systolic dysfunction with an ejection fraction of 10%. Coronary angiography showed no obstructive coronary artery disease. Nonischemic lab analysis was unrevealing.

He underwent right heart catheterization with biopsy which showed multifocal chronic inflammation with fibrosis and myocardial necrosis. Given his country of origin, there was high suspicion of Chagas disease as the precipitating cause of his nonischemic cardiomyopathy. Trypanosoma cruzi serologic assays were obtained and were positive.

Despite guideline-directed medical therapy, he required inotropic support and subsequently a HeartWare LVAD was placed. Two years later, the patient received a heart transplant and within 2 weeks of transplant was diagnosed with acute reactivation of Chagas by polymerase chain reaction assay. He responded well to benznidazole therapy.

5. Discussion

Chagas Cardiomyopathy is the most important clinical presentation of Chagas disease. While only 20-30% of infected patients will develop cardiomyopathy [3], those who do will have a spectrum of findings ranging from abnormal ECG alone to severe biventricular dysfunction and even sudden cardiac death. The three major clinical presentations of Chagas cardiomyopathy include arrhythmias, heart failure, and thromboembolism [1, 3].

ECG findings that are highly suggestive of Chagas cardiomyopathy include first-degree atrioventricular block, RBBB, LAFB, bifascicular block, or premature ventricular contractions [3]. Nevertheless, the absence of these findings does not mean the diagnosis is not present. Hallmark echocardiographic features include regional wall motion abnormalities, particularly of the basal inferolateral wall, and an apical aneurysm/thrombus that can be difficult to image without contrast or cardiac MRI, especially when the remainder of the left ventricle is normal [4]. Gadolinium uptake on cardiac MRI is frequent and more pronounced as LVEF decreases. Studies demonstrate that gadolinium uptake correlates well with the risk of arrhythmias [4].

Patients with Chagas cardiomyopathy with preserved or mildly depressed ejection fraction are still at risk for lethal ventricular arrhythmias as well as strokes, and strong consideration should be given to risk to stratify those patients with cardiac imaging [3, 4].

All children of seropositive women and any additional family members of an infected individual should be screened for the disease because of the risk of maternal-fetal transmission and the higher rates of Chagas disease in immediate family members [2, 6].

Most importantly, physicians in the United States who work with Latin American immigrants should be aware that this disease in not uncommon in patients presenting with unexplained cardiac symptoms and/or suspicious electrocardiographic features. Seroprevalence studies have shown high rates of Chagas disease in Latin American immigrants from Chagas-endemic countries to the U.S.: at the Olive View Medical Center in Los Angeles County, 5% of patients with conduction abnormalities [7], 7.5% of patients with pacemakers [9], 18% of patients with bifascicular block [7], and 19% of patients with nonischemic cardiomyopathy were found to have Chagas disease [8], and at Elmhurst hospital in the Bronx, 13% of nonischemic cardiomyopathy patients were found to have Chagas disease [5].

6. Conclusion

Chagas disease should be strongly suspected in Latin American immigrant patients from endemic countries who present with stroke, ventricular arrhythmias, or heart failure.

Abbreviations

CCC: Chronic Chagas cardiomyopathy
ECG: Electrocardiogram
TTE: Transthoracic echocardiogram
MRI: Magnetic resonance imaging
RBBB: Right bundle branch block
LAFB: Left anterior fascicular block
LVEF: Left ventricular ejection fraction
CDC: Centers for Disease Control and Prevention
ELISA: Enzyme-linked immunosorbent assay
LVAD: Left ventricular assist device.

Additional Points

Learning Objectives. (1) Chagas cardiomyopathy can present with different clinical presentations. The three hallmark clinical presentations are stroke, ventricular arrhythmias, and heart failure. (2) Chagas cardiomyopathy should be suspected in Latin American immigrant patients from endemic countries who present with unexplained cardiac symptoms and/or suspicious ECG features. (3) Chagas cardiomyopathy can have serious manifestations even in the presence of normal LVEF.

References

[1] A. Rassi Jr., A. Rassi, and J. A. Marin-Neto, "Chagas disease," *The Lancet*, vol. 375, no. 9723, pp. 1388–1402, 2010.

[2] C. Bern, L. A. Messenger, J. D. Whitman, and J. H. Maguire, "Chagas disease in the United States: a public health approach," *Clinical Microbiology Reviews*, vol. 33, no. 1, pp. 1–42, 2019.

[3] M. C. P. Nunes, A. Beaton, H. Acquatella et al., "Chagas cardiomyopathy: an update of current clinical knowledge and management: a scientific statement from the American Heart Association," *Circulation*, vol. 138, no. 12, pp. e169–e209, 2018.

[4] H. Acquatella, F. M. Asch, M. M. Barbosa et al., "Recommendations for multimodality cardiac imaging in patients with Chagas disease; a report from the American Society of Echocardiography in collaboration with the InterAmerican Association of Echocardiography (ECOSIAC) and the Cardiovascular Imaging Department of the Brazilian Society of Cardiology (DIC-SBC)," *Journal of the American Society of Echocardiography*, vol. 18, pp. 3–25, 2018.

[5] L. Kapelusznik, D. Varela, S. P. Montgomery et al., "Chagas disease in Latin American immigrants with dilated cardiomyopathy in New York City," *Clinical Infectious Diseases*, vol. 57, no. 1, pp. e7–e7, 2013.

[6] S. Hernandez, C. J. Forsyth, C. A. Flores, and S. K. Meymandi, "Prevalence of Chagas disease among family members of previously diagnosed patients in Los Angeles, California," *Clinical Infectious Diseases*, vol. 69, no. 7, pp. 1226–1228, 2019.

[7] M. I. Traina, S. Hernandez, D. R. Sanchez et al., "Prevalence of Chagas disease in a U.S. population of Latin American immigrants with conduction abnormalities on electrocardiogram," *PLOS Neglected Tropical Diseases*, A. Debrabant, Ed., vol. 11, no. 1, p. e0005244, 2017.

[8] M. I. Traina, D. R. Sanchez, S. Hernandez et al., "Prevalence and impact of Chagas disease among Latin American immigrants with nonischemic cardiomyopathy in Los Angeles, California," *Circulation: Heart Failure*, vol. 8, no. 5, pp. 938–943, 2015.

[9] S. Park, S. K. Meymandi, J. S. Bradfield et al., "The prevalence of Chagas disease among Latin American immigrants with pacemakers in Los Angeles, California," *The American Journal of Tropical Medicine and Hygiene*, vol. 96, no. 5, pp. 1139–1142, 2017.

14

Hypertrophic Cardiomyopathy and Wolff-Parkinson-White Syndrome in a Young African Soldier with Recurrent Syncope

Mohammed Abdullahi Talle,[1,2] Faruk Buba,[1,2] Aimé Bonny,[3] and Musa Mohammed Baba[1,4]

[1]*Department of Medicine, College of Medical Sciences, University of Maiduguri, Nigeria*
[2]*Cardiology Unit, Department of Medicine, University of Maiduguri Teaching Hospital, Maiduguri, Nigeria*
[3]*University of Douala, Cameroon*
[4]*Cardiology Unit, Department of Medicine, College of Medical Sciences, Gombe State University, Gombe, Nigeria*

Correspondence should be addressed to Mohammed Abdullahi Talle; abdultalle@yahoo.com
Academic Editor: Kathleen Ngu

Syncope is a common manifestation of both hypertrophic cardiomyopathy (HCM) and Wolff-Parkinson-White (WPW) syndrome. The most common arrhythmia in HCM is ventricular tachycardia (VT) and atrial fibrillation (AF). While preexcitation provides the substrate for reentry and supraventricular tachycardia (SVT), AF is more common in patients with preexcitation than the general population. Concurrence of HCM and WPW has been reported in many cases, but whether the prognosis or severity of arrhythmia is different compared to the individual disorders remains unsettled. We report a case of HCM and Wolff-Parkinson-White (WPW) syndrome in a 28-year-old male Nigerian soldier presenting with recurrent syncope and lichen planus.

1. Introduction

Inherited cardiac arrhythmogenic disorders are less reported in Africa, and their burden as causes of sudden cardiac death (SCD) in Africa is unknown [1]. The lack of the often-needed expensive state-of-the-art diagnostic equipment compounds the challenges that hinder establishing the epidemiology of cardiac arrhythmias in sub-Saharan African (SSA) countries [2]. This makes the reporting of every single case of clinical arrhythmia (symptomatic or otherwise) imperative, to aid in better understanding of the burden of arrhythmic cardiac disorders in SSA.

Concurrence of HCM and WPW has been variously reported. In a consecutive series of patients presenting with preexcitation, 7.62% were found to have HCM [3]. Of the many phenocopies of HCM, cardiac hypertrophy and preexcitation are typically caused by a mutation of the gamma 2 subunit of the adenosine monophosphate-activated protein kinase (PRKAG2) [4]. Although both HCM and WPW are independently associated with various forms of arrhythmias and SCD, whether their concurrence will result in more frequent and severe arrhythmias or fatalities remains conjectural, and to our knowledge, this has not been reported in SSA. We present a case of HCM with WPW in a young African soldier presenting with recurrent syncope.

2. Case Presentation

A 28-year-old male African soldier from Nigeria was referred to the cardiology clinic of the University of Maiduguri Teaching Hospital in November 2017 for evaluation of recurrent syncope. He complained of paroxysmal palpitations, dizziness, and shortness of breath followed by presyncope and syncope. He has had subtle and infrequent palpitation and shortness of breath since childhood. He experienced his first syncope about 2 years ago which became more frequent three months prior to his referral and has had about 10 episodes of syncope. The last episode was in November 2017, during which a heart rate of 184 beats per minute and blood pressure of 90/50 mmHg with cold clammy extremities were documented by the attending medical officer at a peripheral hospital.

However, ECG was not done due to nonavailability of ECG machine. There was no family history of similar symptoms or SCD. He developed pruritic skin lesions involving all parts of the body but mainly over the extensor surfaces a month prior to presentation. He joined the military 4 years ago after undergoing the rigorous recruit training program and has been actively involved in military operations until recently when his disabling symptoms precluded active participation.

The resting pulse was regular at 78 bpm, and all peripheral pulses were present and normal. He had a comparable blood pressure of 120/76 mmHg on the right and left upper limbs, and jugular venous pressure was normal. Apex was in the fifth left intercostal space at the midclavicular line and was heaving with double apical impulse. The heart sounds were S_4, S_1, and S_2 with a crescendo-decrescendo systolic murmur loudest midway between the apex and the left lower sternal edge, but there was no diastolic murmur. Chest was clear, and no abnormality was detected on abdominal examination. Nervous and musculoskeletal systems were essentially normal. There were widespread silvery scaly skin lesions interspersed with hyperpigmented plaques all over his body but mainly on the extensor surfaces of the upper limb (Figure 1).

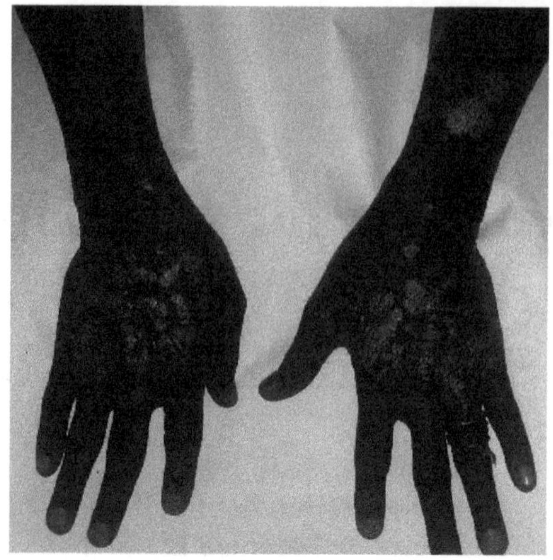

FIGURE 1: Silvery scaly lesions and plaques on the extensor surfaces of the hands and forearm.

Resting ECG (Figure 2) revealed a regular sinus rhythm at the rate of 78 cycles per minute with a QRS axis of +90°. The PR interval was about 100 msec, and there was a delta wave with broad QRS complex; findings are consistent with ventricular preexcitation. The QRS complexes showed positive concordance across precordial leads, with discordant ST segments and T waves. Corrected QT interval (adjusted for the broad QSR complexes) was prolonged at 461 msec.

Two-dimensional transthoracic echocardiography revealed a maximum septal thickness of 27 mm at the basal anterior septum with a corresponding posterior wall thickness of 13 mm (Figures 3(a) and 3(b)). Left ventricular outflow peak gradient was 36 mmHg, with a late peaking of velocity (Figure 4). There was no systolic anterior motion of the mitral valve or mitral regurgitation. The left ventricular end-diastolic dimension and ejection fraction were 21 mm and 80%, respectively. Exercise stress test was aborted within the first 2 minutes due to dizziness. Stress echo, cardiac MRI, cardiac CT, catheterization, ambulatory ECG, and electrophysiology (EP) study were not available.

A diagnosis of HCM with WPW was made, and he was placed on 100 mg of atenolol daily. A medical report was given to his division advising against strenuous activities and the need for further evaluation with ambulatory ECG and EP study. His regular follow-ups were uneventful, and he was recently transferred to the southern part of Nigeria where he will continue his treatment. His skin lesion was reviewed by a dermatologist, and a clinical diagnosis of lichen planus was made and confirmed by histology at another hospital. The third author (AB) offered to sponsor the subsequent evaluation and management of the patient in France or Algeria, but the patient declined the offer.

3. Discussion

This to the best of our knowledge is the first case of concurrence of HCM and WPW being reported from SSA. Both HCM and WPW can independently result in the constellation of symptoms our patient presented with. Hypertrophic cardiomyopathy has a protean manifestation, being generally asymptomatic or minimally symptomatic with a relatively benign course and annual mortality of less than 1% in the adult population. Clinical symptoms include progressive shortness of breath, chest pain, palpitations, light-headedness, syncope, and less commonly SCD. Palpitation in HCM results from supraventricular arrhythmias, commonly AF, and nonsustained ventricular tachycardia [5, 6]. The actual cause of recurrent palpitation and syncope in the index case was not determined because he did present to us while the symptomatic and ambulatory ECG and EP study was not done.

Wolff-Parkinson-White syndrome is an accessory pathway-mediated tachycardia occurring in patients with ventricular preexcitation and is the second most common cause of SVT [7]. Symptoms commonly include palpitations, shortness of breath, presyncope, syncope, and SCD. Thirty percent of people with WPW have AF, and this is associated with increased risk of SCD [8]. The patient reported 10 episodes of syncope in the preceding two years, and all were associated with palpitation. Although none of the episodes was captured on ECG, the last episode of witnessed event with regular pulse of 184 beats per minute before his referral is suggestive of SVT rather than AF. Rapid AF can be swiftly conducted to the ventricle via the accessory pathway resulting in 1 : 1 conduction and ventricular fibrillation with circulatory collapse. Whether the patient's syncopal episodes were associated with AF remains undetermined.

The association of WPW and other primary cardiac disorders has been variously documented. Mutation of PRKAG2 results in familial WPW with HCM [4]. Our patient and his kindred were not subjected to genetic studies due to nonavailability. However, there was no history suggesting familial occurrence of WPW and/or HCM, and the nervous and musculoskeletal disorders as well as conduction system

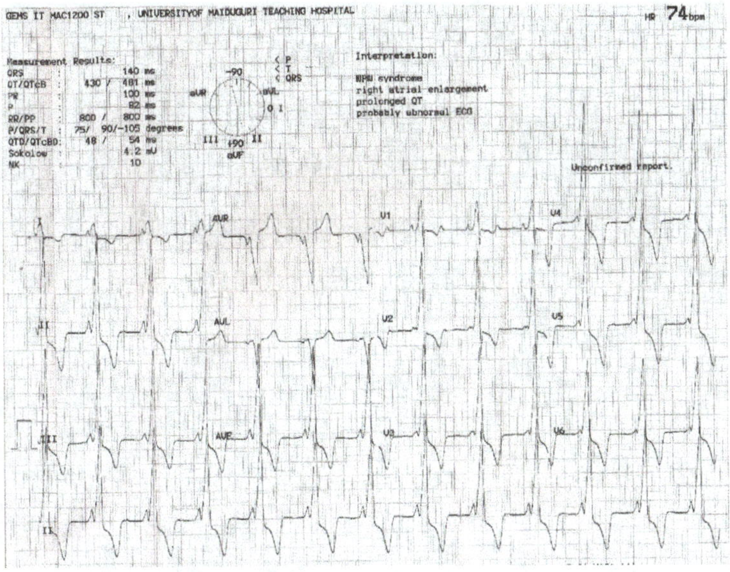

FIGURE 2: Resting 12-lead ECG obtained at presentation showing short PR interval, positive delta wave in V1 (type A Wolff-Parkinson-White pattern), and broad QRS complex.

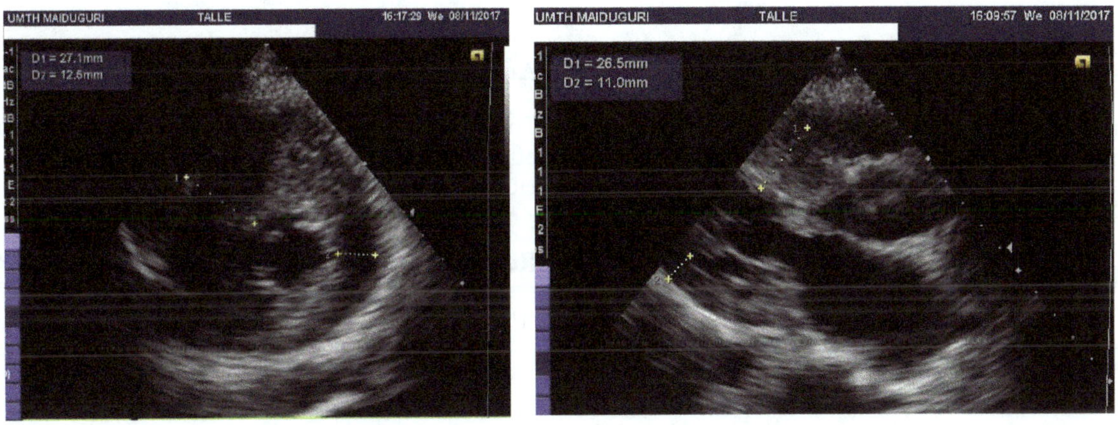

(a) (b)

FIGURE 3: Parasternal short axis (a) and long axis (b) views showing asymmetric septal hypertrophy.

disorders prevalent in this mutation were not documented in this patient.

Resting 12-lead ECG showed features of preexcitation, which along with recurrent palpitations and syncope defines WPW syndrome. The positive delta wave in V1 (type A WPW) and positively concordant QRS complexes across precordial leads are suggestive of the left lateral accessory pathway. However, EP study is required to confirm location and culpability of the pathway in cardiac arrhythmias but was not done due to nonavailability. Although the amplitude of the QRS complexes is in keeping with left ventricular hypertrophy (LVH), voltage criteria for ECG diagnosis of LVH may not be applicable in the setting of preexcitation, especially in persons younger than 40 years. The discordance of ST segments and T wave to the dominant deflection of QRS complexes in this context is more in keeping with ventricular preexcitation than LVH.

The diagnostic hallmark for HCM on echocardiography is asymmetric septal hypertrophy with a septum to posterior wall thickness ratio of greater than 1.5 or 1.3 in people with a family history of HCM. Our patient had asymmetric septal hypertrophy with a septum to posterior wall ratio of 2.5 and resting LVOT gradient of 36 mmHg. The military background of the patient makes physiologic LVH (athleticism) a pertinent consideration. However, the septal thickness of 27 mm is well out of the "grey zone" of 13 to 15 mm that commonly results in such diagnostic challenges. Similarly, the presence of restrictive LV filling pattern on spectral Doppler suggesting diastolic dysfunction and limited left ventricular end-diastolic dimension favours HCM.

Whether this patient's recurrent syncope was a consequence of arrhythmias related to either WPW or HCM was not established with certainty. Notwithstanding, recurrence of syncope in this context puts the patient at a very high risk and requires further evaluation and implementation of definitive treatment strategies to avert SCD. Determining the culprit for the recurrent syncope between WPW and HCM presents a real diagnostic conundrum.

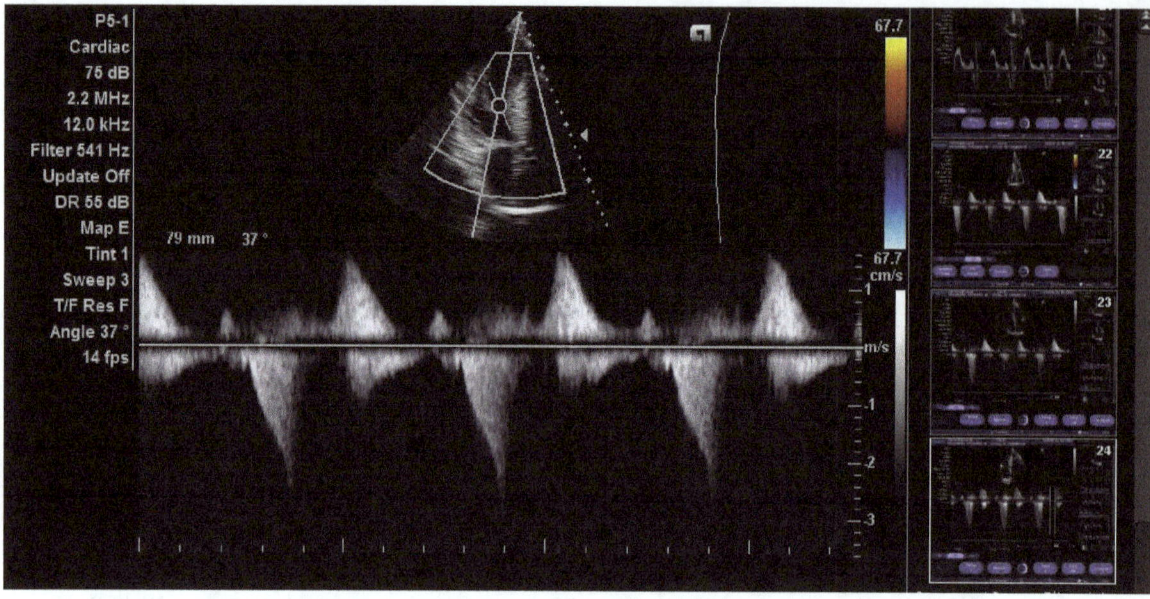

FIGURE 4: Late peaking of flow (dagger shape) across the left ventricular outflow tract.

Ambulatory ECG and EP study would have provided insights. The frequency of syncope remarkably improved on 100 mg of atenolol, and the patient had only one episode in four months.

The diagnosis of lichen planus may add another layer of intrigue to the case. An association has been established between dermatologic disorders (e.g., psoriasis) and cardiovascular diseases, reflecting the role of inflammation as a common denominator. However, no such link has been established between Lichen planus and WPW and/or HCM. Hypertrophic cardiomyopathy was reported in a 59-year-old woman with lichen planus and rheumatoid arthritis receiving etanercept and methotrexate [9]. Similarly, adalimumab (Humira), a tumour necrosis factor blocker used in the treatment of psoriatic arthritis, has been associated with HCM [10]. Skin manifestation is an integral part of Fabry's disease, a storage disorder having identical phenotype with HCM, but the appearance is different from the lesions in this patient.

The evaluation and management of this patient was limited by lack of facilities and the requisite expertise. Ambulatory ECG, EP study, cardiac MRI, and genetic testing would have undoubtedly provided pertinent information that will fine-tune the management but were not available. Consequently, decisions regarding ablation therapy and/or implantable cardioverter-defibrillator could not be accomplished. This case exemplifies the prevailing practices in many countries of sub-Saharan Africa, especially in management of cardiac arrhythmias.

Consent

Informed consent was duly obtained from the patient for publishing this case report.

Acknowledgments

The authors wish to acknowledge the contribution of the staff of cardiology lab of the University of Maiduguri Teaching Hospital during the evaluation of this patient.

References

[1] A. Bonny, K. Tibazarwa, S. Mbouh et al., "Epidemiology of sudden cardiac death in Cameroon: the first population-based cohort survey in sub-Saharan Africa," *International Journal of Epidemiology*, vol. 46, no. 4, pp. 1230–1238, 2017.

[2] M. A. Talle, A. Bonny, W. Scholtz et al., "Status of cardiac arrhythmia services in Africa in 2018: a PASCAR Sudden Cardiac Death Task Force report," *Cardiovascular Journal of Africa*, vol. 29, no. 2, pp. 115–121, 2018.

[3] A. M. Perosio, L. D. Suarez, A. M. Bunster et al., "Pre-excitation syndrome and hypertrophic cardiomyopathy," *Journal of Electrocardiology*, vol. 16, no. 1, pp. 29–39, 1983.

[4] M. H. Gollob, M. S. Green, A. S. Tang, and R. Roberts, "PRKAG2 cardiac syndrome: familial ventricular preexcitation, conduction system disease, and cardiac hypertrophy," *Current Opinion in Cardiology*, vol. 17, no. 3, pp. 229–234, 2002.

[5] I. Olivotto, F. Cecchi, S. A. Casey, A. Dolara, J. H. Traverse, and B. J. Maron, "Impact of atrial fibrillation on the clinical course of hypertrophic cardiomyopathy," *Circulation*, vol. 104, no. 21, pp. 2517–2524, 2001.

[6] L. Monserrat, P. M. Elliott, J. R. Gimeno, S. Sharma, M. Penas-Lado, and W. J. McKenna, "Nonsustained ventricular tachycardia in hypertrophic cardiomyopathy: an independent marker of sudden death risk in young patients," *Journal of the American College of Cardiology*, vol. 42, no. 5, pp. 873–879, 2003.

[7] H. J. Vidaillet Jr., J. C. Pressley, E. Henke, F. E. Harrell Jr., and L. D. German, "Familial occurrence of accessory atrioventric-

ular pathways (preexcitation syndrome)," *The New England Journal of Medicine*, vol. 317, no. 2, pp. 65–69, 1987.

[8] C. Blomström-Lundqvist, M. M. Scheinman, E. M. Aliot et al., "ACC/AHA/ESC guidelines for the management of patients with supraventricular arrhythmias— executive summary: a Report of the American College of Cardiology/American HeartAssociation Task Force on Practice Guidelines and the European Society of Cardiology Committee for Practice Guidelines (Writing Committee to Develop Guidelines for the Management of Patients With Supraventricular Arrhythmias) Developed in collaboration with NASPE–Heart Rhythm Society," *European Heart Journal*, vol. 24, no. 20, pp. 1857–1897, 2003.

[9] A. N. Chiriac, L. I. Foia, A. E. Chiriac et al., "Lichen planus secondary complications associated with the use of biologic therapy for rheumatoid arthritis," *Romanian Journal of Morphology and Embryology*, vol. 54, 3 Suppl, pp. 829–831, 2013.

[10] *Humira and Hypertrophic Cardiomyopathy-From FDA Reports*, April 2018, https://www.ehealthme.com/ds/humira/hypertrophic-cardiomyopathy/.

15

Multivessel Coronary Artery Vasospasm-Induced Takotsubo Cardiomyopathy

Vishal I. Patel[1,2] **and Serap Sobnosky**[1,2,3]

[1]*St. Mary Medical Center, Department of Internal Medicine, USA*
[2]*UCLA David Geffen School of Medicine, USA*
[3]*St. Mary Medical Center, Department of Cardiology, USA*

Correspondence should be addressed to Vishal I. Patel; vishal.ishwar.patel@gmail.com

Academic Editor: Antonio de Padua Mansur

Takotsubo cardiomyopathy is associated with a constellation of cardiac findings including reversible left ventricular dysfunction and an acute triggering stressor. Epicardial coronary vasospasm is a rarely reported etiology for takotsubo cardiomyopathy, and its pathophysiologic mechanisms still remain incompletely understood. We present the case of a 54-year-old female with chest pain and ST-elevation myocardial infarction who was found to have takotsubo cardiomyopathy due to diffuse multivessel coronary artery vasospasm in the absence of obstructive coronary artery disease. To our knowledge, this is the first angiographically confirmed case of this rare phenomenon to be reported, as most literature involves focal, segmental, or single coronary artery involvement. Moreover, we review current literature and develop a discussion on the targeted treatment of vasospastic disease as part of the multimodal approach to the management of takotsubo syndrome.

1. Introduction

Takotsubo cardiomyopathy, or takotsubo syndrome (TTS), is characterized by transient left ventricular dysfunction with apical dyskinesia, typically in the setting of a physical or emotional stressor. Initially thought to be a benign finding, further study over the past decade has revealed that TTS may be associated with severe complications including heart failure and sudden death, leading to intensification of understanding the underlying pathophysiological basis [1]. Of the several proposed mechanisms, multivessel epicardial coronary artery vasospasm is a rare and unique finding that is not yet well understood as most reported cases involve single arteries or focal vasospasm. Here, we present a case of TTS due to diffuse multivessel vasospasm of the right coronary artery (RCA), left anterior descending (LAD) artery, and left circumflex artery (LCx), managed with targeted vasodilatory and antianginal therapies.

2. Case Presentation

A 54-year-old female was brought to the emergency department with nonexertional chest pain worsening for the past several hours. She reported profound psychosocial stress due to the recent sudden and tragic death of a grandchild. On examination, blood pressure was 188/112 mmHg with an otherwise unremarkable cardiopulmonary and vascular examination. Medical history was notable for hypertension, chronic obstructive pulmonary disease, tobacco dependence with a 30 pack-year history, peptic ulcer disease, and morbid obesity. Laboratory studies were notable for a troponin of 0.003 ng/mL and brain natriuretic peptide of 13 pg/mL. Electrocardiogram (ECG) revealed sinus bradycardia, first-degree atrioventricular block, and concave 2 mm ST-segment elevation in leads II, III, and aVF, with reciprocal depression in aVL (Figure 1(a)). Chest radiography demonstrated an enlarged cardiac silhouette but otherwise no acute

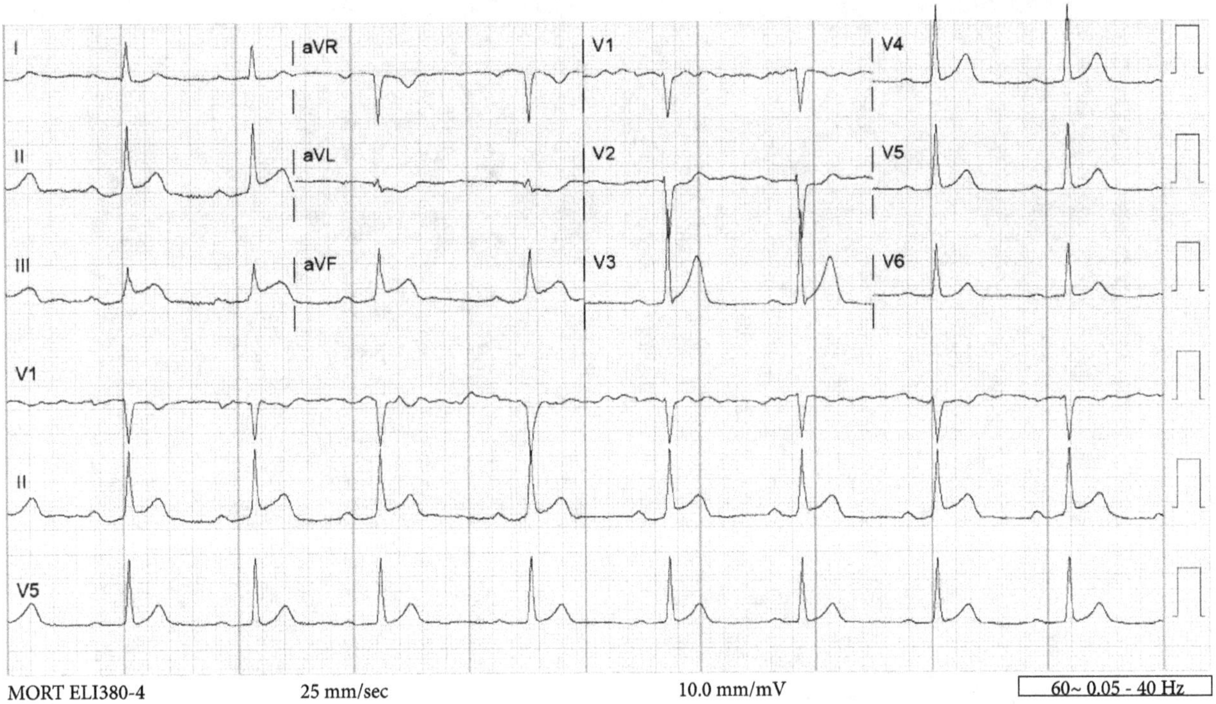

(a)

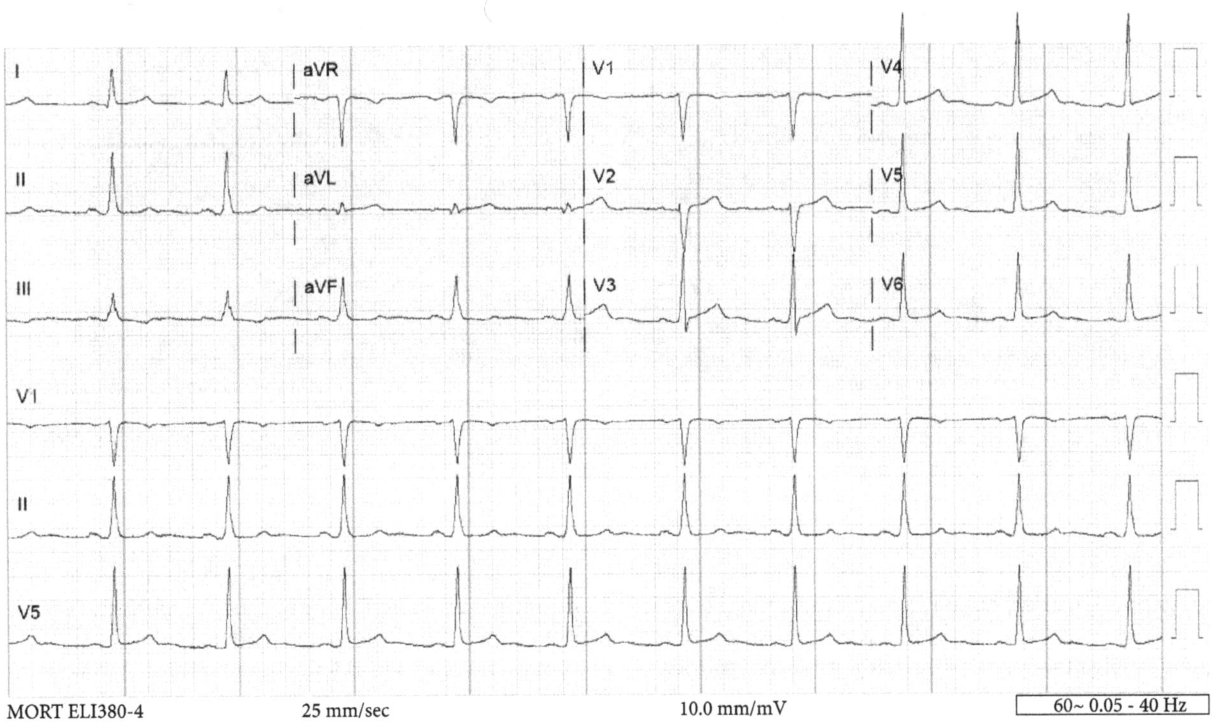

(b)

FIGURE 1: 12-lead electrocardiogram. At presentation to the emergency department (a), showing sinus bradycardia (HR 51 bpm); 2 mm ST-segment elevations in leads II, III, and aVF with reciprocal depression in aVL; and first-degree AV block (PR 200 ms). Approximately one hour later (b), there is resolution of ST-segment changes in leads II, III, and aVF as well as resolution of first-degree AV block (PR 179 ms).

pulmonary process. A computed tomography angiography of the chest was negative for aortic dissection. The patient was taken emergently to the cardiac catheterization laboratory for coronary angiography. A repeat ECG just prior to transport demonstrated sinus rhythm with essentially resolved ST-segment abnormalities seen on presentation (Figure 1(b)); however, the patient still had significant chest pain. Review of medical records, including coronary angiography three years

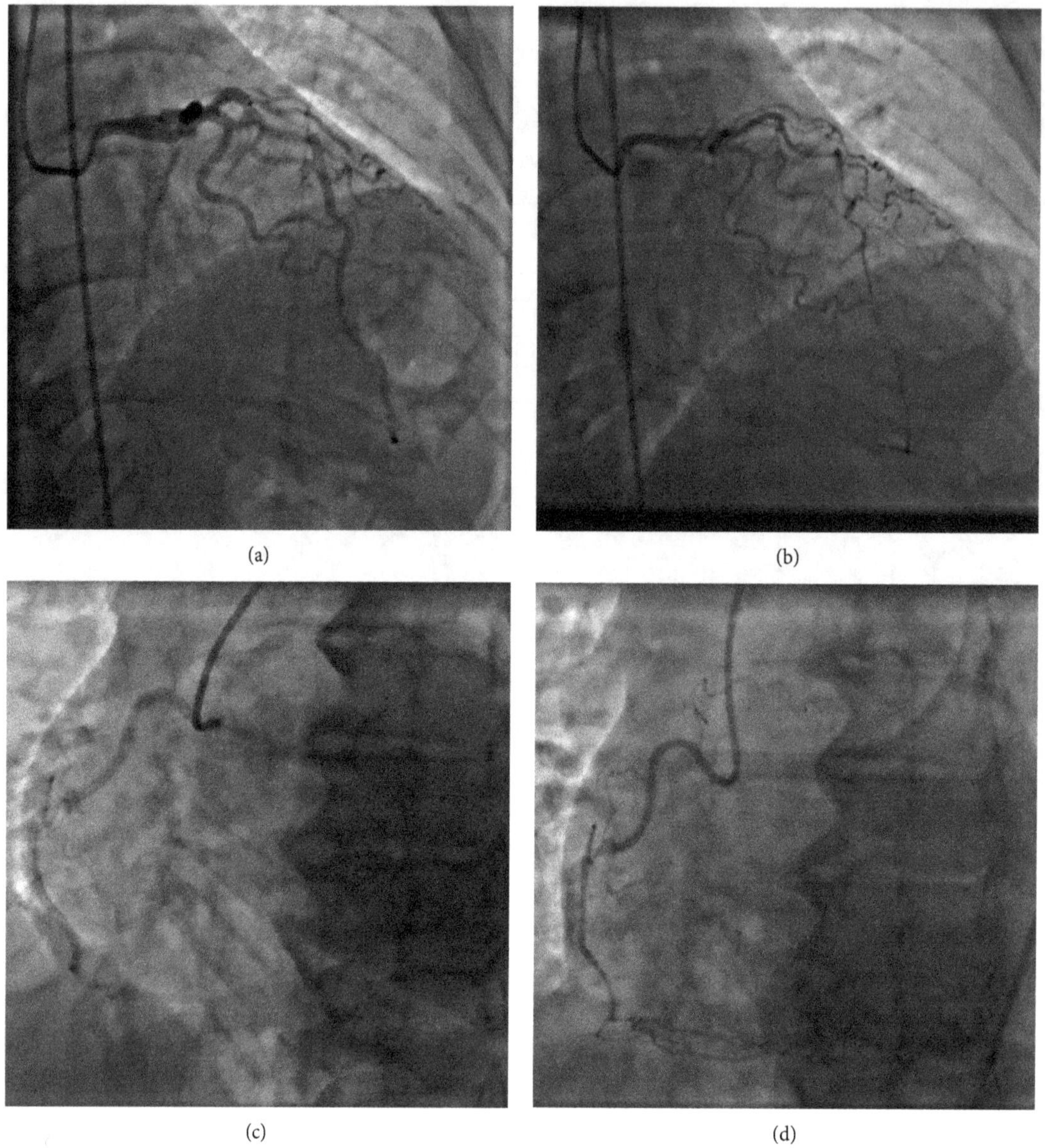

FIGURE 2: Coronary angiography demonstrates (a) normal left coronary artery system three years prior, (b) diffuse severe LAD and LCx vasospasm, (c) normal right coronary artery system three years prior, and (d) mild RCA vasospasm.

prior, was notable for myocardial bridging of the left anterior descending (LAD) artery but no significant stenosis of the coronary arteries (Figures 2(a) and 2(c)). A transthoracic echocardiogram (TTE) three years prior had normal left ventricular (LV) contractility (Figure 3(a)).

In the cardiac catheterization laboratory, coronary angiography demonstrated diffuse vasospasm of the LAD which caused narrowing of the vessel diameter to 0.5 mm and reduced flow to thrombolysis in myocardial infarction (TIMI) 2 (Figure 2(b)). There was also vasospasm of the LCx as well as the smaller nondominant RCA (Figure 2(d)). There was no significant flow-limiting focal stenoses of the coronary arteries. A left ventriculogram also demonstrated apical ballooning; however, the images could not be retrieved due to a software error. The patient was given sublingual nitroglycerin 0.4 mg twice which resulted in rapid improvement in her chest pain and vasospasm. Further provocation testing was deemed unnecessary due to demonstrative real-time angiographic findings. A TTE with contrast revealed a moderately impaired LV systolic function with apical ballooning, associated with a depressed LV ejection fraction of 40% (Figure 3(b)) (Video 1). The clinical picture was consistent with takotsubo cardiomyopathy. She was initiated on medical management for vasospastic anginal disease with an oral calcium-channel blocker, long-acting nitrate, and low-dose beta-blocker. The final duration of these medications was to be determined on follow-up visits, with expected titration as symptoms improved. The patient's symptoms resolved, and she was discharged home in a stable condition. A repeat TTE was done 4 weeks later with resolution of apical ballooning and recovery of ventricular function, confirming the diagnosis (Video 2).

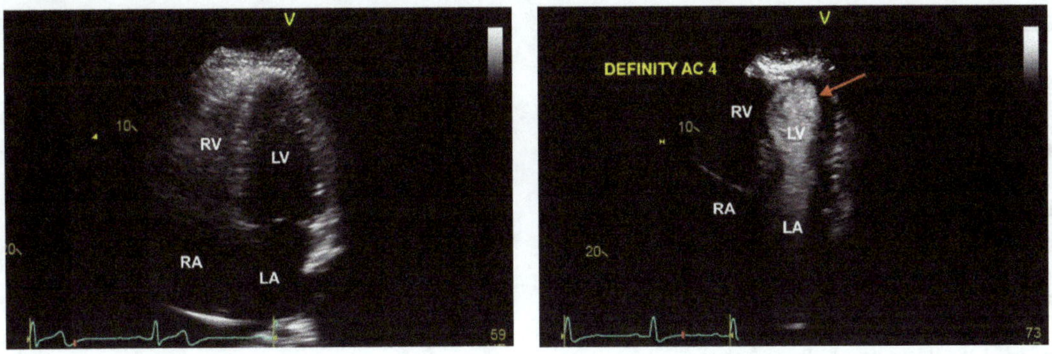

(a) (b)

Figure 3: Transthoracic echocardiogram, apical 4-chamber view, demonstrates (a) normal LV contractility three years prior and (b) contrasted study with LV dysfunction with apical dyskinesia (red arrow), consistent with takotsubo cardiomyopathy.

3. Discussion

Although described as early as the 1980s, the term "takotsubo cardiomyopathy" is credited to the work of Dote and Sato in the early 1990s based on their report of the characteristic LV appearance reminiscent of an "octopus trap" or "octopus pot." Since then, the term "takotsubo syndrome" (TTS) has become the nomenclature recommended by expert consensus as it is more comprehensive; however, it is still commonly known as stress, ampulla, or takotsubo cardiomyopathy, broken-heart syndrome, or apical ballooning syndrome [1]. Based on recently revised diagnostic criteria, TTS is defined as a transient LV dysfunction in the absence of obstructive coronary artery disease (CAD), associated with new ECG changes or elevated cardiac biomarkers, and typically triggered by an emotional or physical stressor. TTS typically affects postmenopausal women, most commonly in the sixth decade of life [2]. Several pathophysiological mechanisms have been proposed, including myocardial ischemia, LV outflow tract obstruction, catecholamine cardiotoxicity, and autonomic nervous system modulation [3]. Many of these theories result from understanding the triggers or clinical settings in which TTS is diagnosed, including among others, sudden loss of a loved one, financial loss, surgery, trauma, drug intoxication, or intensive physical demands [2, 4]. Clinical presentation therefore can often be indistinguishable from acute coronary syndrome (ACS) [1, 2, 5]. As the incidence of TTS continues to uptrend annually, characterizing the underlying pathophysiology and targeting management remain key to impacting worldwide morbidity and mortality [3, 6].

Within the realm of myocardial ischemia as an etiological basis for TTS, data on epicardial coronary artery vasospasm remains rather sparse. Fairly few cases of angiographically confirmed vasospasm have been reported, and all have focal or single coronary artery involvement. Diffuse multivessel coronary artery vasospasm has not yet been reported at the time of our review of literature. Plausibility of the vasospastic theory has been studied through provocative testing to induce coronary vasospasm. Tsuchihashi et al. reported a retrospective analysis with 10 of 48 (21%) patients with TTS demonstrating positive provocative vasospasm, 5 of whom had both right and left coronary artery involvement [7]. Angelini reported a series of four cases of TTS in which provocative vasospasm could reproduce TTS echocardiographic findings or suggestive symptoms [8].

Given the rarity of coronary vasospasm in TTS, management typically defers to a case-by-case evaluation of clinical symptoms and management of potential triggers. Pharmacologic therapy of vasospastic disease is often the first step in intervention, with initiation of calcium-channel blockers, beta-blockers (in certain cases), and long-acting nitrates [4, 9, 10]. Further studies are needed to definitively characterize coronary vasospasm and the role of provocative testing in TTS, as well as optimization of medical therapies for the development of robust guidelines. We hypothesize that there may be a role for prophylactic intervention in high-risk scenarios to prevent vasospasm-induced myocardial injury. This case uniquely captured vasospastic disease in real-time linked to TTS in the appropriate clinicopathological setting, with demonstrated normal cardiac function and coronary angiography prior, as well as demonstrated resolution of LV dysfunction.

In conclusion, we presented the first angiographically confirmed case of diffuse multivessel epicardial coronary artery vasospasm-induced TTS in the setting of a known psychosocial stressor. This case highlights vasospastic disease as a culprit process and utilizes a targeted management plan to encourage further development of robust prevention and treatment strategies.

Abbreviations

ACS: Acute coronary syndrome
CAD: Coronary artery disease
ECG: Electrocardiogram
LAD: Left anterior descending artery
LCx: Left circumflex artery
LV: Left ventricular
RCA: Right coronary artery
TIMI: Thrombolysis in myocardial infarction
TTE: Transthoracic echocardiogram
TTS: Takotsubo syndrome.

Supplementary Materials

Video 1: Transthoracic echocardiogram, apical 4-chamber view, with contrast, showing ventricular dysfunction with apical dyskinesia, consistent with takotsubo cardiomyopathy. Video 2: Transthoracic echocardiogram, apical 4-chamber view, showing complete recovery of ventricular function about 4 weeks later. *(Supplementary Materials)*

References

[1] J. R. Ghadri, I. S. Wittstein, A. Prasad et al., "International expert consensus document on takotsubo syndrome (part I): clinical characteristics, diagnostic criteria, and pathophysiology," *European Heart Journal*, vol. 39, no. 22, pp. 2032–2046, 2018.

[2] N. Khalid, S. A. Ahmad, E. Shlofmitz, and L. Chhabra, *Pathophysiology of takotsubo syndrome*, StatPearls, 2021, https://www.ncbi.nlm.nih.gov/books/NBK538160/.

[3] S. Y. Hassan and P. Tornvall, "Epidemiology, pathogenesis, and management of takotsubo syndrome," *Clinical Autonomic Research*, vol. 28, no. 1, pp. 53–65, 2018.

[4] M. R. Summers and A. Prasad, "Takotsubo cardiomyopathy: definition and clinical profile," *Heart Failure Clinics*, vol. 9, no. 2, pp. 111–122, 2013.

[5] F. Pelliccia, J. C. Kaski, F. Crea, and P. G. Camici, "Pathophysiology of Takotsubo syndrome," *Circulation*, vol. 135, no. 24, pp. 2426–2441, 2017.

[6] Y. J. Akashi, H. M. Nef, and A. R. Lyon, "Epidemiology and pathophysiology of Takotsubo syndrome," *Nature Reviews. Cardiology*, vol. 12, no. 7, pp. 387–397, 2015.

[7] K. Tsuchihashi, K. Ueshima, T. Uchida et al., "Transient left ventricular apical ballooning without coronary artery stenosis: a novel heart syndrome mimicking acute myocardial infarction," *Journal of the American College of Cardiology*, vol. 38, no. 1, pp. 11–18, 2001.

[8] P. Angelini, "Transient left ventricular apical ballooning: a unifying pathophysiologic theory at the edge of Prinzmetal angina," *Catheterization and Cardiovascular Interventions*, vol. 71, no. 3, pp. 342–352, 2008.

[9] M. Lombardi, R. Vergallo, G. Liuzzo, and F. Crea, "A case report of coronary artery spasm and takotsubo syndrome: exploring the hidden side of the moon," *European Heart Journal - Case Reports*, vol. 5, no. 1, p. ytaa477, 2021.

[10] S. Giusca, T. Eisele, P. Nunninger, B. Münz, and G. Korosoglou, "Aborted sudden cardiac death in a female patient presenting with takotsubo- like cardiomyopathy due to epicardial coronary vasospasm," *Case Reports in Cardiology*, vol. 2017, Article ID 7875240, 4 pages, 2017.

16

A Volume Challenge Reveals the Diagnosis of Pediatric Restrictive Cardiomyopathy

Elyssa Cohen,[1,2] Conor P. O'Halloran,[1,2] Philip T. Thrush,[1,2] T. Marsha Ma,[3] and Paul Tannous[1,2]

[1]*Ann & Robert H. Lurie Children's Hospital of Chicago, Chicago, IL, USA*
[2]*Northwestern University Feinberg School of Medicine, Chicago, IL, USA*
[3]*Loyola University Medical Center, Chicago, IL, USA*

Correspondence should be addressed to Elyssa Cohen; elycohen@luriechildrens.org

Academic Editor: Anca Daniela Farcaş

A healthy 11-year-old girl presented with exercise intolerance of unclear etiology, and her physical exam was notable for a 3/6 systolic ejection murmur at the left upper sternal border with radiation to the back. Extensive noninvasive workup consisted of ECG, transthoracic echocardiogram, and cardiac MRI/MRA, which were all nondiagnostic. She was ultimately referred for cardiac catheterization. Baseline invasive hemodynamics demonstrated a normal cardiac index and pulmonary vascular resistance but was notable for mildly elevated right and left end-diastolic pressures. A diagnosis remained elusive, so a 500 mL volume challenge was performed, which unmasked right and left ventricular waveform transformations to reveal the pathognomonic "square root sign" of restrictive cardiomyopathy with concordant RV/LV respirophasic variation. These findings and her clinical history allowed for the rare pediatric diagnosis of restrictive cardiomyopathy early in her clinical course, prior to the development of overt signs of pathologic myocardial remodeling, such as pulmonary hypertension and biatrial enlargement.

1. Case Report

An 11-year-old healthy female presented to her pediatrician for a well-child check with the new complaint of not being able to keep up with her peers during soccer due to shortness of breath and pain characterized as a shooting sensation down both legs. Physical exam was notable for a 3/6 systolic ejection murmur at the left upper sternal border with radiation to the back, mildly diminished lower extremity pulses, and normal four extremity blood pressures.

An electrocardiogram was performed and demonstrated normal sinus rhythm, no atrial enlargement, no right or left ventricular hypertrophy, and no evidence of right or left ventricle strain. Transthoracic echocardiogram documented flow acceleration across the aortic arch with a peak velocity of 4 m/sec, normal systolic function with an ejection fraction of 70%, normal atrial and ventricular size, and no evidence to suggest decreased compliance. Cardiac MRI/MRA was ordered to further delineate anatomy, and it showed a crenellated aortic arch with mild hypoplasia of the proximal descending thoracic aorta (z-score of -2.88) with a peak velocity of 2.1 m/s, but no discrete coarctation (Figure 1(a)). There were no abdominal aortic lesions or evidence of endocardial fibroelastosis. Given the equivocal nature of data thus far collected and no clear etiology for her exertional symptoms, a cardiac catheterization was performed. Baseline hemodynamics revealed a normal cardiac index of 4.6 L/min/m^2, normal PVR of 1.7 iWU, no arch gradient (Figure 1(b)), mildly elevated RVEDp (12 mmHg) and LVEDp (16 mmHg) with normal diastolic waveforms (Figure 1(c)). Collectively, these data did not provide a unifying diagnosis and the etiology for her exercise intolerance remained uncertain.

To further investigate the significance of her elevated end-diastolic pressures, a 500 mL normal saline bolus was administered, acutely increasing the RVEDp and LVEDp

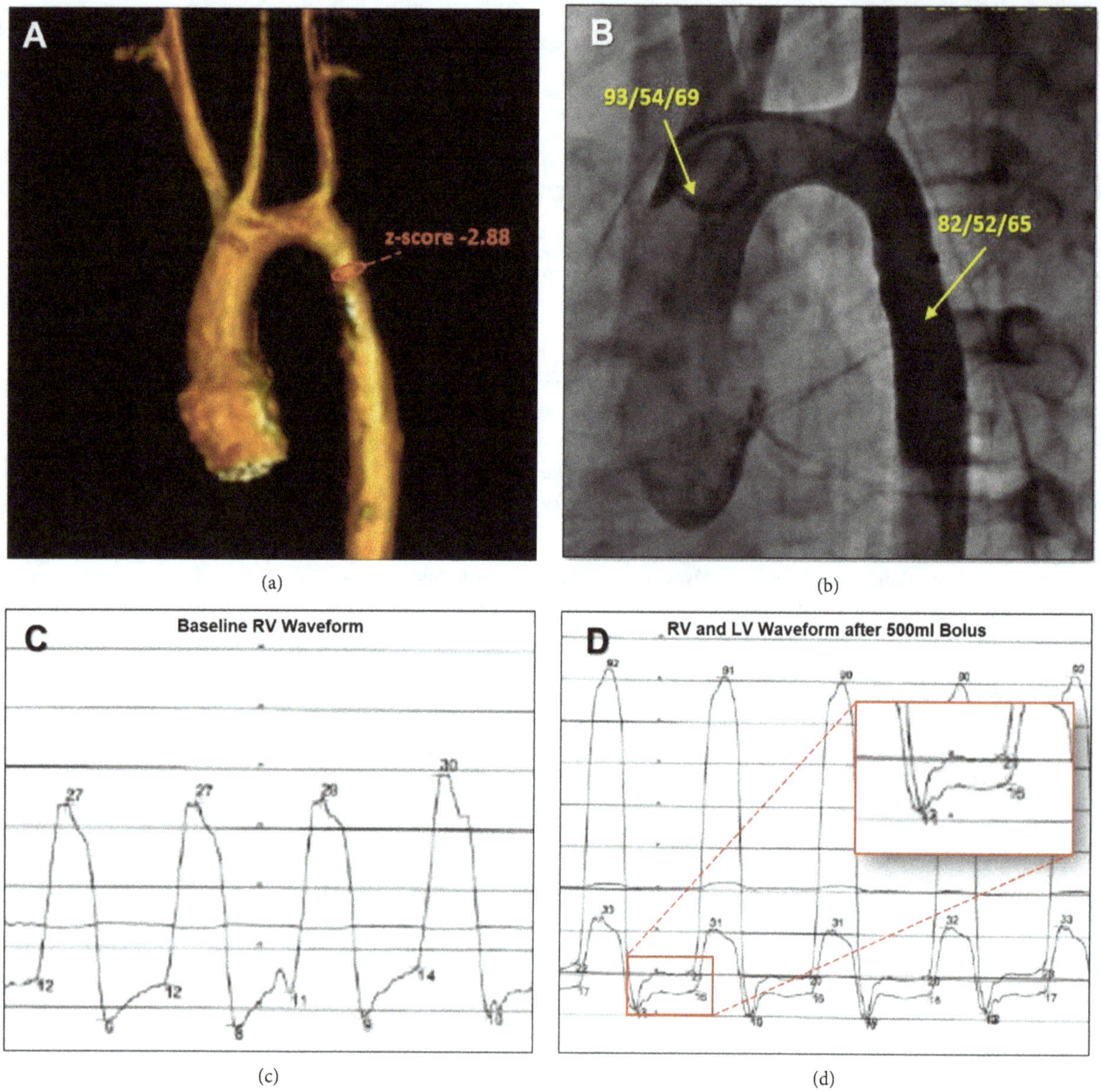

FIGURE 1: Cardiac MRA, aortic arch angiography, and hemodynamic waveforms before and after volume challenge. (a) Cardiac MRA showed a crenellated arch with hypoplasia of the proximal descending thoracic aorta (z-score of −2.88), but no discrete coarctation. (b) Catheterization was performed and confirmed no arch gradient. (c) Pressure tracings document an elevated RVEDp (12 mmHg) and LVEDp (16 mmHg) but with grossly normal diastolic waveforms at the start of the case. (d) After a 500 mL bolus, RVEDp and LVEDp increased to 16 and 20 mmHg, respectively, and dramatic change in the diastolic waveforms was observed with unmasking of a "classic" square root sign and concordant RV/LV respirophasic variation.

to 16 and 20 mmHg, respectively. In addition to the rise in end-diastolic pressure, we observed a dramatic change in the diastolic waveform with unmasking of a "classic" square root sign and concordant RV/LV respirophasic variation (Figure 1(d)). Four-chamber end-diastolic pressures did not equalize as would be seen in constrictive pericardial disease. Collectively, these findings and her clinical history were most consistent with a diagnosis of restrictive cardiomyopathy (RCM). Arch intervention was not indicated, and she was referred to heart failure clinic for medical management.

As an outpatient at heart failure clinic, she was started on 10 mg of Lasix daily for symptom prevention. She had an unremarkable Holter monitor and exercise stress test. Genetic testing has not identified any known cardiomyopathy-associated genes to explain her restrictive phenotype.

Now two years following diagnosis, she is asymptomatic on a daily diuretic. Interval hemodynamic evaluations and echocardiograms demonstrate preserved systolic function and no evidence of pulmonary hypertension. She continues to enjoy being active and participating on her soccer team at a competitive level.

2. Discussion

Restrictive cardiomyopathy is a rare diagnosis in the pediatric population with an incidence of 0.03-0.04 cases per

100,000 children [1, 2]. Patients often present with a history of chronic and subtle progression of symptoms. Diagnosis is typically made later in the disease course than it was for this patient, usually when there are overt signs of pathologic myocardial remodeling such as biatrial enlargement, hepatomegaly, pulmonary hypertension, and pathognomonic changes in intracardiac pressure waveforms [3–5].

This patient presented early with exertional symptoms, and it was her nonspecific physical exam findings that led to the investigation for a cardiac etiology. Prior to cardiac catheterization, she had undergone an extensive workup with an echocardiogram and cardiac MRI/MRA, which were only significant for a mildly hypoplastic distal thoracic aortic arch—insufficient in explaining her symptoms. During her hemodynamic evaluation in the catheterization lab, her end-diastolic ventricular pressures were observed to be mildly elevated; however, the ventricular diastolic waveforms were not consistent with restrictive physiology or constrictive pericarditis. Considering the patient's NPO status and possibility that she was presenting with mild hypovolemia, a 500 mL bolus was administered to replete her volume status. Immediately, the RVEDp and LVEDp increased, the RV and LV diastolic waveforms transformed to reveal the "square root sign," and the ventricular pressures demonstrated concordant respirophasic variation, findings consistent with restrictive cardiomyopathy [6–8]. Thus, her symptoms are most likely secondary to left atrial hypertension exacerbated by peak exercise.

In conclusion, cardiac etiologies should be considered in patients with unexplained exercise intolerance, particularly in the setting of abnormal cardiovascular examination. Dehydration caused by routine fasting before cardiac catheterization may mask the characteristic hemodynamic findings of RCM. Careful fluid administration can unmask these findings, yielding a definitive diagnosis in otherwise unclear cases.

References

[1] S. E. Lipshultz, L. A. Sleeper, J. A. Towbin et al., "The incidence of pediatric cardiomyopathy in two regions of the United States," *The New England Journal of Medicine*, vol. 348, no. 17, pp. 1647–1655, 2003.

[2] A. W. Nugent, P. E. Daubeney, P. Chondros et al., "The epidemiology of childhood cardiomyopathy in Australia," *The New England Journal of Medicine*, vol. 348, no. 17, pp. 1639–1646, 2003.

[3] T. M. Lee, D. T. Hsu, P. Kantor et al., "Pediatric cardiomyopathies," *Circulation Research*, vol. 121, no. 7, pp. 855–873, 2017.

[4] S. G. Wittekind, T. D. Ryan, Z. Gao et al., "Contemporary outcomes of pediatric restrictive cardiomyopathy: a single-center experience," *Pediatric Cardiology*, vol. 40, no. 4, pp. 694–704, 2019.

[5] S. W. Denfield and S. A. Webber, "Restrictive cardiomyopathy in childhood," *Heart Failure Clinics*, vol. 6, no. 4, pp. 445–452, 2010.

[6] J. B. Geske, N. S. Anavekar, R. A. Nishimura, J. K. Oh, and B. J. Gersh, "Differentiation of constriction and restriction: complex cardiovascular hemodynamics," *Journal of the American College of Cardiology*, vol. 68, no. 21, pp. 2329–2347, 2016.

[7] R. Ditaranto, A. G. Caponetti, V. Ferrara et al., "Pediatric restrictive cardiomyopathies," *Frontiers in Pediatrics*, vol. 9, article 745365, 2022.

[8] M. J. Garcia, "Constrictive pericarditis versus restrictive cardiomyopathy?," *Journal of the American College of Cardiology*, vol. 67, no. 17, pp. 2061–2076, 2016.

17

Recurrent Stress Cardiomyopathy: A Rare Variant in a Young Patient with Undiagnosed Pheochromocytoma

Robert Lembo, Paul Wesley, and Joe B. Calkins

Department of Cardiovascular Medicine, Medical College of Georgia, 1120 15th Street, Augusta, GA 30912, USA

Correspondence should be addressed to Robert Lembo; rlembo@augusta.edu

Academic Editor: Christopher S. Snyder

Biventricular stress cardiomyopathy is one of several known anatomical variants of reversible cardiomyopathies to occur. We present a case of a young patient with recurrent stress cardiomyopathy complicated by cardiogenic shock in the perioperative period. The cardiomyopathy observed was in a patient with neurofibromatosis type I and undiagnosed pheochromocytoma who presented for intervention of hydrocephalus. This case demonstrates the importance of vigilance in the young patient who develops shock in the perioperative period.

1. Introduction

Stress cardiomyopathy can often be encountered in the perioperative setting. Shock with rapid hemodynamic collapse in a young patient should raise concern for stress cardiomyopathy.

2. Case Report

A 28-year-old woman with a previous diagnosis of neurofibromatosis type I (NF I) presented to the hospital with dizziness, nausea, emesis, and anorexia. Magnetic resonance imaging of her head demonstrated a left thalamic mass and obstructive hydrocephalus. Seven years prior, the patient underwent ablation of atrioventricular nodal reentry tachycardia. Electrophysiology study at that time demonstrated dual AV nodal physiology, and she underwent successful cryoablation of her slow pathway without further history of palpitations. The ablation was complicated by biventricular failure requiring inotropic infusion for 12 hours. Rapid resolution occurred, and the patient was discharged without further event.

The patient underwent a biopsy of the left thalamic mass and drain placement to relieve obstruction. During anesthesia induction supraventricular tachycardia (SVT) occurred and was terminated with cardioversion. The procedure was aborted, and the patient was returned to the intensive care unit. A postoperative echocardiogram demonstrated severe left and right ventricular function and hypokinetic basal left ventricular segments, with akinesis of all other segments. The EF was less than 10% (see echocardiogram in Figures 1(a)–3(a)). Inotropic support with milrinone was initiated. Three days later, limited echocardiogram demonstrated normal left ventricular size with hyperdynamic systolic function and an EF greater than 70% (see echocardiogram in Figures 1(b)–3(b)). Metoprolol tartrate was initiated to prevent recurrence of SVT. The patient returned to the operating room and underwent successful external ventricular drain placement. Induction of anesthesia was uneventful. The patient was discharged without further cardiac event.

The patient again presented for symptoms with worsening hydrocephalus requiring further intervention. Upon anesthesia induction, the patient again developed SVT requiring cardioversion. Profound hypertension surrounded this arrhythmia with systolic blood pressure greater than 220 mmHg. Given the recurrent intraoperative hemodynamic events, testing of urinary and serum metanephrines was pursued which demonstrated elevated metanephrines and catecholamines. CT scan demonstrated a heterogeneous enhancing mass of the left adrenal gland and dotatate scan demonstrated increased uptake in the left adrenal gland suggestive of pheochromocytoma. Prazosin was initiated prior

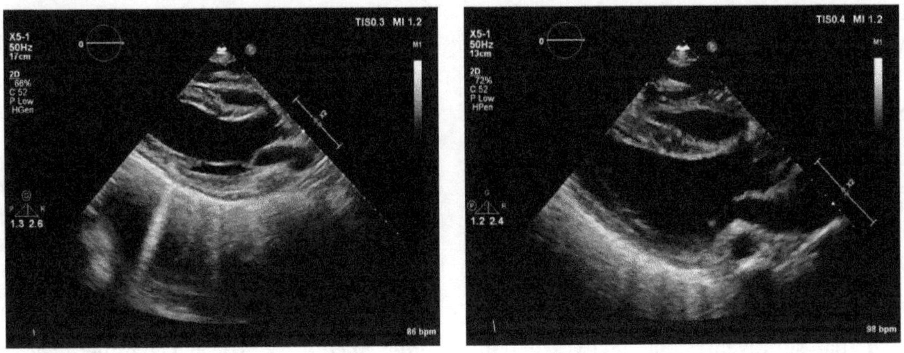

(a) (b)

FIGURE 1: (a–b) Transthoracic echocardiogram demonstrating parasternal long axis view demonstrating hypokinesis of basal left ventricle and akinesis in all other segments (see supplementary material for video of echocardiogram clips in Figures 1–3). (b) Parasternal long axis view demonstrating recovery.

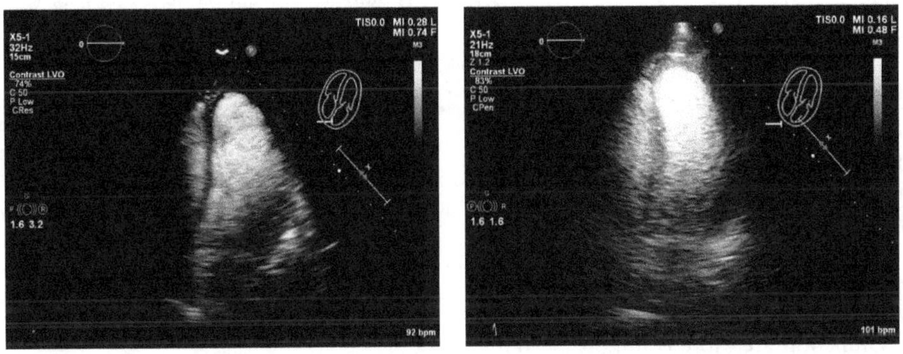

(a) (b)

FIGURE 2: (a–b) Apical 4 chamber view with ultrasound-enhancing agent demonstrating hypokinesis of basal left ventricle and akinesis of all other segments. (b) Apical 4 chamber view with ultrasound-enhancing agent demonstrating recovery.

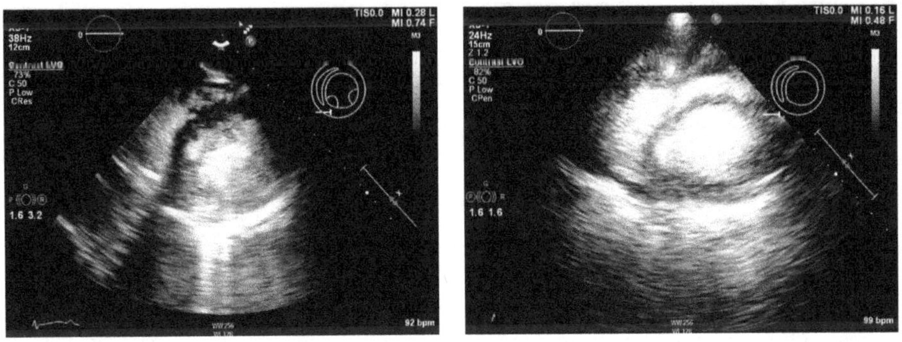

(a) (b)

FIGURE 3: (a–b) Short axis view with ultrasound-enhancing agent demonstrating profound biventricular hypokinesis. (b) Short axis view with ultrasound-enhancing agent demonstrating recovery.

to definitive treatment of the hydrocephalus and pheochromocytoma. She underwent robotic-assisted laparoscopic left adrenalectomy in addition to left ventriculoperitoneal shunt placement. Pathology confirmed pheochromocytoma. The patient was discharged without further event and with normal left ventricular function.

3. Discussion

Pheochromocytoma and NF1 are rarely observed in the same patient and occur with an incidence of about 1% of individuals affected with NF1 [1]. Common presenting symptoms of pheochromocytoma are paroxysms of hypertension, headache, palpitations, and diaphoresis which occur in 50% of the cases. However, 10% of the patients remain normotensive and asymptomatic thereby limiting diagnosis [2]. It is common for pheochromocytoma to be first detected during anesthetic induction [3]. Uncontrolled catecholamine release can occur in the periinduction period causing cardiovascular complications including cardiogenic shock, takotsubo cardiomyopathy, myocardial infarction, and aortic dissection [4]. Furthermore, young patients without prior history who suffer from acute cardiac decompensation intraoperatively must be considered for entities such as pheochromocytoma. It has been suggested that supraventricular tachycardia in the presence of pheochromocytoma has led to acute depression in ventricular function, despite cardioversion of the arrhythmia [5].

As in this patient, the diagnosis of pheochromocytoma was considered after labile hemodynamics and rhythm abnormalities were encountered during two anesthetic inductions. Reversible biventricular dysfunction occurred after initial cryoablation seven years earlier, likely due to the same process; however, clinical details are limited. An atypical stress cardiomyopathy with biventricular dysfunction with hypokinesis at the base and subsequent akinesis in all other segments occurred in this patient.

Five anatomical variants of stress cardiomyopathy have been reported in the literature with apical ballooning (typical) occurring with a prevalence of 75-80% [6]. This biventricular anatomic variant that was observed in our patient occurs with a prevalence of less than 0.5%. Atypical patterns of left ventricular dysfunction are more common in young individuals and are associated with the development of shock. In the absence of LVOT obstruction, supportive care with inotropic use is indicated. Patients may require mechanical support in the form of an intraaortic balloon pump or percutaneous left ventricular assist devices until ventricular function recovers [5]. Kumar et al. report that a perioperative catecholamine surge may be attenuated with pretreatment with IV benzodiazepine, although this has not been extensively studied [3]. Recovery of left ventricular function from stress cardiomyopathy will vary from days to weeks as observed in the International Takotsubo Registry. Clinical factors unfavorable with ventricular recovery include male sex, baseline LVEF < 45%, and acute neurologic events associated with the cardiomyopathy [7].

This case demonstrates the importance of vigilance in the young patient who develops acute cardiomyopathy with biventricular involvement in the perioperative setting. Pheochromocytoma should be investigated in these instances. The biventricular variant of stress cardiomyopathy may be related to pheochromocytoma and appears to be reversible. Supportive care with inotropic therapy and serial echocardiographic evaluation is indicated and evaluation of possible pheochromocytoma is paramount.

Additional Points

Learning Objectives. (i) Shock in the perioperative setting in young patients should raise the possibility of stress cardiomyopathy. (ii) Supportive care with inotropic therapy and serial reevaluation with echocardiography is paramount. (iii) Biventricular variant stress cardiomyopathy may be related to pheochromocytoma and appears to be reversible.

Supplementary Materials

Supplementary 1. Transthoracic echocardiogram demonstrating parasternal long axis view (a) with hypokinesis of basal left ventricle and akinesis in all other segments with subsequent recovery (b).

Supplementary 2. Apical 4 chamber view (a) with ultrasound-enhancing agent demonstrating hypokinesis of basal left ventricle and akinesis of all other segments with subsequent recovery (b).

Supplementary 3. Short axis view (a) with ultrasound-enhancing agent demonstrating profound biventricular hypokinesis and subsequent recovery (b).

References

[1] V. Kantorovich and K. Pacak, "Pheochromocytoma and paraganglioma," *Progress in Brain Research*, vol. 182, pp. 343–373, 2010.

[2] E. L. Bravo and R. W. Gifford, "Pheochromocytoma: diagnosis, localization and management," *The New England Journal of Medicine*, vol. 311, no. 20, pp. 1298–1303, 1984.

[3] V. Kumar, J. Spivey, M. Arthur, and M. Castresana, "Pheochromocytoma detected during anesthesia induction," *Journal of Cardiothoracic and Vascular Anesthesia*, vol. 25, no. 5, pp. e43–e44, 2011.

[4] M. S. Lord and J. G. T. Augoustides, "Perioperative Management of Pheochromocytoma: Focus on Magnesium, Clevidipine, and Vasopressin," *Journal of Cardiothoracic and Vascular Anesthesia*, vol. 26, no. 3, pp. 526–531, 2012.

[5] H. Shawa, M. Bajaj, and G. R. Cunningham, "Pheochromocytoma-induced atrial tachycardia leading to cardiogenic shock and cardiac arrest: resolution with atrioventricular node ablation and pacemaker placement," *Texas Heart Institute Journal*, vol. 41, no. 6, pp. 660–663, 2014.

[6] H. M. de Chazal, M. G. Del Buono, L. Keyser-Marcus et al., "Stress Cardiomyopathy Diagnosis and Treatment:," *Journal of the American College of Cardiology*, vol. 72, no. 16, pp. 1955–1971, 2018.

[7] S. Jurisic, S. Gili, V. L. Cammann et al., "Clinical predictors and prognostic impact of recovery of wall motion abnormalities in Takotsubo syndrome: results from the International Takotsubo Registry," *Journal of the American Heart Association*, vol. 8, no. 21, article e011194, 2019.

18

Defects in Very Long-Chain Fatty Acid Oxidation Presenting as Different Types of Cardiomyopathy

Fariba Alaei[1] **Marjan Shakiba**[2] **Hedyeh Saneifard**[2] **Kourosh Vahidshahi**[3] **and Mastaneh Alaei**[4]

[1]*Pediatric Cardiology Department, Mofid Children's Hospital, Faculty of Medicine, Shahid Beheshti University of Medical Sciences, Tehran, Iran*
[2]*Pediatric Endocrinology and Metabolism Department, Mofid Children's Hospital, Faculty of Medicine, Shahid Beheshti University of Medical Sciences, Tehran, Iran*
[3]*Pediatric Cardiology, Shahid Modarres Hospital, Faculty of Medicine, Shahid Beheshti University of Medical Sciences, Tehran, Iran*
[4]*Blood Transfusion Research Center, High Institute for Research and Education in Transfusion Medicine, Tehran, Iran*

Correspondence should be addressed to Hedyeh Saneifard; h.saneifard@sbmu.ac.ir

Academic Editor: Yigit Canga

Cardiac involvement may accompany various inborn errors of metabolism (IEM) including fatty acid oxidation (FAO) disorders, presenting as rhythm disturbances, conduction abnormalities, cardiomyopathies, pericardial effusion, and sudden cardiac death. FAO disorders are rare mitochondrial diseases with variable organ involvements and clinical presentations. Very long-chain acyl-CoA dehydrogenase deficiency (VLCADD) is a FAO disorder with diverse clinical presentations. We report two VLCADD patients with cardiac involvement and diverse presentations. The first patient represents with cardiogenic shock and dilated cardiomyopathy (DCM) at childhood. The second patient represents with suspicious sepsis at early infancy and hypertrophic cardiomyopathy (HCM) at further evaluation. IEM should be thought of in every individual case with suspicious sepsis or cardiac failure regardless of age or previous history.

1. Introduction

Very long-chain acyl-CoA dehydrogenase deficiency (VLCADD) is an autosomal recessive fatty acid beta-oxidation disorder of mitochondrial origin. It involves the initial step of beta oxidation in mitochondrial matrix [1]. Disease is caused by mutations in the *ACADVL* gene (17p13.1) and has an incidence of 1 : 50000-1 : 100000 in newborns [2]. It has different presentations and three phenotypes. Early onset type, usually presents within the first months of life, with hypoglycemia, liver disease, cardiomyopathy (CMP), arrhythmias, and pericardial effusion. Infantile/childhood onset type with a later onset usually presents with hypoglycemia and rarely CMP. Late-onset type detected in older children and young adults usually present with isolated skeletal muscle involvement, myalgia, rhabdomyolysis, and myoglobinuria [3].

Diagnosis is made by tandem mass spectrometry in which blood acylcarnitine profile demonstrates increased C14-C18 (C16:1, C14:2, C14:1, and C18:1). Confirmation is performed by VLCAD activity measurement in the fibroblast or lymphocyte culture or by genetic evaluation revealing two pathogenic mutations in the ACADVL gene [4].

The major cardiac manifestations include arrhythmia, conduction abnormalities, CMP with or without pericardial effusion, and sudden death mainly initiated by fasting, exercise, sickness, and fever [2].

Long-chain fatty acids and carnitine need to be transported across the sarcolemma, as fatty acids are the major source of energy for myocardial cells. Any disturbance in energy production in this disorder results in low availability of glucose (hypoglycemia) and formation of ketone bodies, especially during periods of fasting and sickness. On the other hand, accumulation of toxic metabolites (long-chain fatty acids (LCAD)) is cardiotoxic and can explain CMP following toxic metabolite accumulation [2].

In this study, we report 2 cases of VLCADD with CMP, one presenting at early infancy with hypertrophic CMP and the other presenting at childhood with dilated type. No written consent has been obtained from the patients as there is no patient identifiable data included in this case report.

2. Case Report

2.1. Patient 1. A 4-year and 3-month baby girl was admitted in the ICU with GI symptoms and decreased level of consciousness. She had suffered from abdominal pain, headache, nausea, vomiting, and decreased appetite since 10 days ago. At the time of admission, she was afebrile and hemodynamically unstable with blood pressure of 72/35 mmHg, heart rate of 145/min, weak pulses, and increased capillary refill time. Physical examination revealed grade 3 heart murmurs at left sternal border and apical regions, diffuse expiratory wheezing across the chest, and hepatomegaly. Examination of the abdomen showed no tenderness or guarding. Lab tests demonstrated normal leukocyte count and differential for her age. Acute phase reactants were within normal range. Blood chemistry tests were normal but liver function tests were disrupted (aspartate aminotransferase (AST) = 293 IU/l, alanine aminotransferase (ALT) = 612 IU/L, total bilirubin = 3.48 mg/dl, and direct bilirubin = 1.44 mg/dl). Chest X-ray revealed increased cardiothoracic ratio and pulmonary vascular marking with no significant consolidation. Sinus tachycardia appeared on electrocardiography. Echocardiography showed all chambers dilation, severe mitral, tricuspid and pulmonary regurgitation, reduced ejection fraction (DCM), and mild pulmonary hypertension (Figure 1). She was treated with inotropes and diuretics. Metabolic and rheumatologic evaluation was implemented for evaluation of secondary CMP. Rheumatologic studies were normal. Metabolic work-up revealed normal serum and urine amino acid chromatography as well as normal urine organic acid profile, but increased C14-C14.1-C14.2-C16-C16.1-C18-C18.1 and C18.2 was detected at acylcarnitine profile. Thus, medium chain triglyceride (MCT) oil, low-fat and high-carbohydrate diet was started with the diagnosis of VLCADD.

2.2. Patient 2. A 35-day baby girl was admitted with vomiting, poor feeding, poor weight gain, lethargy, and suspicious sepsis. She was the first child of a consanguineous couple, born through an uneventful pregnancy. Anthropometric indices were normal at birth (weight: 2880 g, height: 50 cm, and head circumference: 34 cm). Physical examination revealed heart rate of 185/min and blood pressure of 65/40 mmHg, severe failure to thrive ($W = 2900$ g, height = 50 cm, and head circumference = 34 cm), hypotonia, and hepatomegaly.

During admission, she experienced recurrent episodes of hypoglycemia, so was evaluated for IEM. She appeared normoglycemic when receiving glucose infusion, but hypoglycemia and deterioration of clinical condition recurred repeatedly following restarting of breast feeding and minimizing glucose infusion. Chest radiography demonstrated increased cardiothoracic ratio and echocardiographic evaluation revealed a small ASD with increased left ventricular thickness and normal systolic function in favor of HCM.

Lab tests demonstrated normal complete blood count and electrolytes for age. Uric acid, cholesterol, triglyceride, and creatine kinase (CK) were also within normal limits. Minimal blood glucose level was 30 mg/dl during hypoglycemic episodes, and urine ketone bodies were negative. AST, ALT, and gamma glutamyl transferase (GGT) levels were 146 IU/L, 172 IU/L, and 204 IU/L, respectively. Arterial blood gas exam demonstrated mild metabolic acidosis to normal results during hospitalization. Plasma amino acids profile, serum ammonia and lactate levels, urine carbohydrate chromatography, and galactose 1-phosphate uridyl transferase activity were within normal limits.

Acyl carnitine profile showed specific feature compatible with VLCAD or carnitine palmitoyl transferase 2 deficiency (CPT-2) (C12: 0.64 μmol/l (<0.55), C14: 2.72 μmol/l (<0.5), C14:1: 2.23 μmol/l (<0.25), C14:2: 0.24 μmol/l (<0.2), C16: 16.48 μmol/l (<7) C18: 4.97 μmol/l (<2.5), C18:1: 6.33 μmol/l (<3), and C18:2: 0.73 μmol/l (<0.7)); thus, MCT-based formula was started. This resulted in a dramatic response. Glucose infusion was tapered, and the patient was discharged. During follow-up, she had gained weight, and her height and head circumference had reached normal values. Further cultured fibroblast enzyme activity demonstrated decreased VLCAD activity (CPT2 = 8 (8.5-17.3), VLCAD < 0.18 (1.48-5.2), and Sanger sequencing revealed splicing defect mutation c1269+1G>A in VLFAD gene, both tests confirming VLCADD.

3. Discussion

CMPs are primary disorders of myocardium with structural remodeling and resultant ventricular dysfunction. In this regard, a variety of disease classifications has been developed according to the clinical presentation, genetics, and natural history. The main CMP categories include dilated, hypertrophic, restrictive, arrhythmogenic right ventricular, left ventricular noncompaction, and unclassified. CMPs may be primary or secondary to other disorders such as infectious, genetic, toxic, metabolic, endocrine, hematologic, neoplastic, nutritional, neuromuscular, and inflammatory conditions [5, 6].

IEM are consequences of absence or abnormal levels of specific enzymes or enzyme cofactors, resulting in accumulation or deficiency of particular metabolites, mostly inherited as autosomal recessive traits. CMPs may be seen in various IEM and are typically related to energy metabolism impairment or substance storage due to conditions such as glycogen storage diseases, mucopolysaccharidoses, FAO disorders, organic acidemias, and mitochondrial disorders. Newborn screening was offered in all states of United State of America, specific parts of Europe, Australia, and Canada to identify treatable inborn error of metabolism including FAO. Not many developing countries in Asia and Middle East have newborn screening. Japan and China are Asian countries with long experience in newborn screening. Qatar and Saudi Arabia are Middle East countries which started newborn screening during recent years. Newborn screening was started in Iran since 2019. Newborn screening was

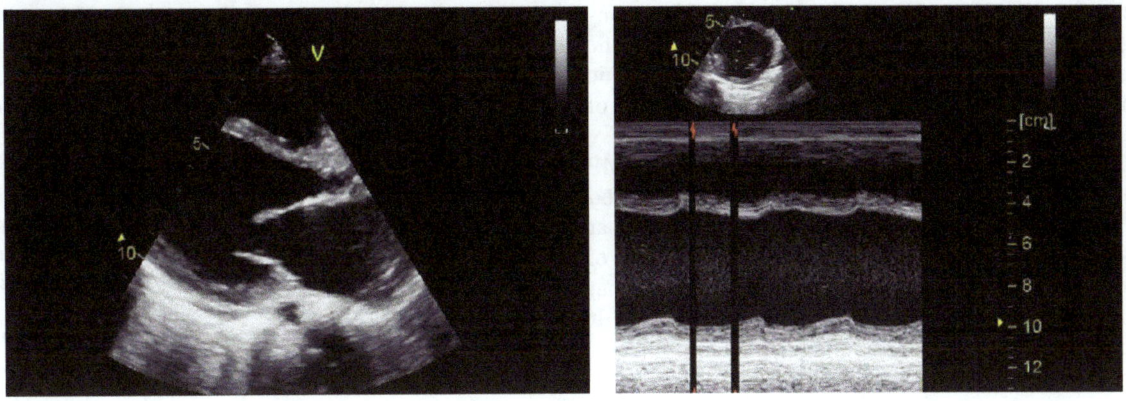

(a) (b)

Figure 1: Echocardiographic evaluation at parasternal Log axis (a) and short axis (b) views shows left ventricular dilatation and decreased contractility.

Table 1: VLCADD patients' natural history.

Study	Age at presentation	Clinical manifestation	Cardiac presentation	Diagnosis	Outcome
Dereddy NR	2 months	Respiratory distress, failure to thrive, hepatomegaly, hypotonia	Left ventricular hypertrophy and dilatation, reduced systolic function and pericardial effusion	Skin fibroblasts enzyme activity	Normal cardiac function after 8 years follow-up
	4 months	Metabolic acidosis, cardiogenic shock	Left ventricular dilatation with reduced systolic function	Gene mutation	Acceptable cardiac size and function after 4 years follow-up
Katz S	2 days	Lethargy, increased CK and liver transaminases	First: small ASD After 6 months: Massive pericardial effusion, left ventricular hypertrophy and systolic dysfunction requiring ECMO	Plasma acyl carnitine profile, gene mutation	Death
Mathur A*	1day to 22 months	a variety of presentations	Dilated and hypertrophic cardiomyopathy	Gene mutation	Normal systolic function in 6
Sharef SW	Immediate neonatal period	Neonatal hypoglycemia, positive family history	Dilated and hypertrophic left ventricle, reduced ejection fraction, pericardial effusion	Acylcarnitine profile, skin fibroblast enzyme activity	Normal cardiac function after 4 years follow-up

*This study consisted of 18 genetically documented VLCADD cases.

initiated in a limited area of Iran and is going to cover all parts of the country.

FAO disorders including defects of beta-oxidation enzymes, carnitine deficiency syndromes, and fatty acid transport defects are rare causes of CMP in children. In these disorders, free fatty acids are not metabolized and are stored in the cytoplasm as triglycerides, resulting in myopathy, CMP, and fatty liver [7].

Treatment should include energy supplying to prevent catabolic state, avoiding fasting, and regulating nutritional fat, restricting LCAD consumption and providing MCT supplementation to minimize production of abnormal fatty acid metabolites, by-pass the enzymatic block in β-oxidation, and providing ketone bodies as appropriate sources of energy [8].

Therefore, it is important to consider curable genetic conditions, including FAO disorders such as VLCADD, as potential causes of infantile or delayed onset CMPs. VLCADD encompasses a continuum of severity, including minimal symptoms to life-threatening conditions in different age groups, resulting in a very heterogeneous clinical outcome.

There are some case reports discussing cardiac involvement in VLCADD with variety of manifestations presenting in Table 1 [9–11].

Mathur and colleagues studied 37 patients suspicious of FAO disorders and identified 18 genetically documented VLCADD. Among them, 12 (67%) presented with CMP (11 DCM and 1 HCM), in infancy. Finally, 8 survived and 6 gained normal systolic function [12].

Tucci and colleagues performed cardiac function evaluation in VLCADD mice applying magnetic resonance imaging (MRI) and magnetic resonance spectroscopy (MRS). Cardiac dysfunction and dilatation developed during 1-

year follow-up despite MCT supplementation. They concluded that cardiac function deterioration was due to specific MCT regimen and as the result of its induced ketogenic state, inhibition of glucose oxidation and transforming of MCT into long-chain fatty acids (LCT) [13].

There are few reports of VLCADD presenting with CMP in the literature. Most cases have presented at neonatal period or early infancy. Our first case demonstrated the disorder at age of 4 years with dilated CMP and no previous history of myopathy or cardiac disorder. The second case presented at early infancy with hypoglycemia and hypertrophic CMP. It seems that early detection and prompt treatment implementation may be lifesaving in this group of patients.

References

[1] L. D. Pena, S. C. van Calcar, J. Hansen et al., "Outcomes and genotype-phenotype correlations in 52 individuals with VLCAD deficiency diagnosed by NBS and enrolled in the IBEM-IS database," *Molecular genetics and metabolism.*, vol. 118, no. 4, pp. 272–281, 2016.

[2] C. Cecatto, A. U. Amaral, J. C. da Silva et al., "Metabolite accumulation in VLCAD deficiency markedly disrupts mitochondrial bioenergetics and Ca2+ homeostasis in the heart," *The FEBS journal.*, vol. 285, no. 8, pp. 1437–1455, 2018.

[3] U. Spiekerkoetter, T. Tenenbaum, A. Heusch, and U. Wendel, "Cardiomyopathy and pericardial effusion in infancy point to a fatty acid b-oxidation defect after exclusion of an underlying infection," *Pediatric Cardiology*, vol. 24, no. 3, pp. 295–297, 2003.

[4] S. J. Knottnerus, J. C. Bleeker, R. C. I. Wüst et al., "Disorders of mitochondrial long-chain fatty acid oxidation and the carnitine shuttle," *Reviews in Endocrine & Metabolic Disorders*, vol. 19, no. 1, pp. 93–106, 2018.

[5] R. M. Kliegman and J. S. Geme, *Nelson Textbook of Pediatrics E-Book*, Elsevier Health Sciences, 2019.

[6] H. D. Allen, R. E. Shaddy, D. J. Penny, T. F. Feltes, and F. Cetta, *Moss and Adams' Heart Disease in Infants, Children, and Adolescents: Including the Fetus and Young Adult*, Wolters Kluwer, 2016.

[7] J. M. Saudubray, M. R. Baumgartner, and J. H. Walter, *Inborn Metabolic Diseases: Diagnosis and Treatment*, Springer, Berlin Heidelberg, 2016.

[8] S. C. Van Calcar, M. Sowa, F. Rohr et al., "Nutrition management guideline for very-long chain acyl-CoA dehydrogenase deficiency (VLCAD): an evidence- and consensus-based approach," *Molecular Genetics and Metabolism*, vol. 131, no. 1-2, pp. 23–37, 2020.

[9] S. W. Sharef, K. Al-Senaidi, and S. N. Joshi, "Successful treatment of cardiomyopathy due to very long-chain acyl-CoA dehydrogenase deficiency: first case report from Oman with literature review," *Oman Medical Journal*, vol. 28, no. 5, pp. 354–356, 2013.

[10] N. R. Dereddy, D. Kronn, and U. Krishnan, "Defects in long chain fatty acid oxidation presenting as severe cardiomyopathy and cardiogenic shock in infancy," *Cardiology in the Young*, vol. 19, no. 5, pp. 540–542, 2009.

[11] S. Katz, Y. Landau, B. Pode-Shakked et al., "Cardiac failure in very long chain acyl-CoA dehydrogenase deficiency requiring extracorporeal membrane oxygenation (ECMO) treatment: a case report and review of the literature," *Molecular Genetics and Metabolism Reports*, vol. 10, pp. 5–7, 2017.

[12] A. Mathur, H. F. Sims, D. Gopalakrishnan et al., "Molecular heterogeneity in very-long-chain acyl-CoA dehydrogenase deficiency causing pediatric cardiomyopathy and sudden death," *Circulation*, vol. 99, no. 10, pp. 1337–1343, 1999.

[13] S. Tucci, U. Flögel, S. Hermann, M. Sturm, M. Schäfers, and U. Spiekerkoetter, "Development and pathomechanisms of cardiomyopathy in very long-chain acyl-CoA dehydrogenase deficient (VLCAD$^{-/-}$) mice," *Biochimica et Biophysica Acta*, vol. 1842, no. 5, pp. 677–685, 2014.

19

Left Ventricular Noncompaction: A Rare Case of Nonischemic Cardiomyopathy

Julia Tian,[1] Asif Uddin,[1] and Philippe Akhrass[2]

[1]*Department of Medicine, Northwell Health at Staten Island University Hospital, Staten Island, NY 10305, USA*
[2]*Department of Electrophysiology, Northwell Health at Staten Island University Hospital, Staten Island, NY 10305, USA*

Correspondence should be addressed to Asif Uddin; asif1uddin@gmail.com
Academic Editor: Magnus Baumhäkel

Isolated left ventricular noncompaction (LVNC) is a rare form of cardiomyopathy that is characterized by deep intertrabecular recesses and abnormal trabeculations that can be observed on transthoracic echocardiogram (TTE) or cardiac MRI (CMR) studies. Our case describes a 41-year-old male who presented with exertional chest pain and was discovered to have significantly reduced left ventricular ejection fraction (LVEF) which was nonischemic in etiology as confirmed by cardiac catheterization. Subsequent evaluation with CMR imaging revealed noncompaction of the left ventricle. The patient received defibrillation and lifelong anticoagulation given his elevated risk of sudden cardiac death (SCD). This case highlights the importance of considering unconventional etiologies of cardiomyopathy when investigating new-onset heart failure as well as the necessity of life-saving measures such as anticoagulation and defibrillator implantation in view of arrhythmogenic structural heart diseases.

1. Introduction

Left ventricular noncompaction (LVNC) is an uncommon cardiomyopathy estimated to occur between 0.014 and 1.3 percent in the general population. It is characterized by deep intertrabecular recesses and abnormal trabeculations popularly believed to result from a failure of a phase of cardiac development during which the normal myocardium compacts inward. However, it can also involve abnormalities during ventricular wall formation or remodeling which can be transient or permanent [1, 2].

Clinical manifestations vary widely and can range from asymptomatic disease to symptoms of heart failure, left ventricular systolic dysfunction, thromboembolism, Wolff-Parkinson-White (WPW) syndrome, atrial and ventricular arrhythmias, bundle branch blocks, and sudden cardiac death. The most common manifestations are heart failure and ventricular systolic dysfunction.

There is currently no universally-accepted criteria for classifying and diagnosing LVNC. Depending on the organization, it may be classified as a genetic cardiomyopathy or as an unclassified cardiomyopathy [3, 4]. Diagnosis of LVNC can be made using imaging studies such as echocardiography, computed tomography, or CMR. Similar to the clinical criteria, no standard imaging criteria currently exist. The Jenni, Chin, and Stollberger criteria emphasize different components of the echocardiogram [5, 6]. A summary of all three would involve evidence of a two-layered structure (thin compacted epicardial layer and thick endocardial layer) with a noncompacted to compacted ratio of greater than 2 (greater than 2.3 on CMR), an epicardial-to-trabeculation trough to epicardial-to-trabeculation peak ratio of less than 0.5, and more than three trabeculations from the ventricular wall (not sensitive for CMR) [7, 8].

2. Case Presentation

The patient was a 41-year-old male with a past medical history of unspecified congenital heart disease, hypothyroidism, and hypogonadism (taking intramuscular testosterone injections twice weekly), who presented with a chief complaint of chest pain during exertion of 1-month duration. The pain

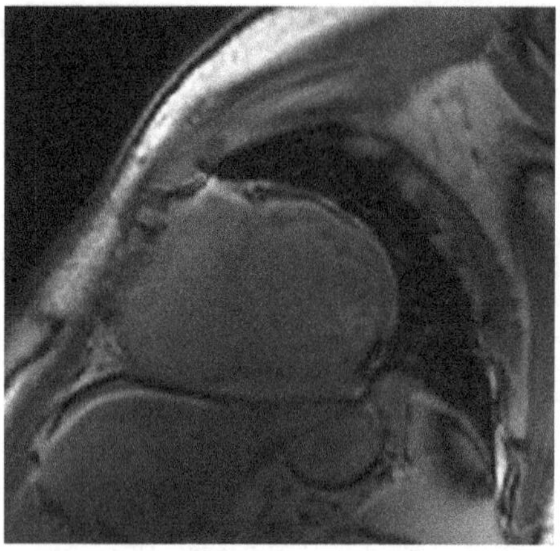

FIGURE 1: Short axis view of cardiac magnetic resonance (CMR) reveals a noncompact-to-compact myocardium ratio of greater than 2.3.

was described as 10 out of 10 in intensity, burning with a band-like tightness in nature, and located in the epigastric area with radiation toward the substernal region. His initial cardiac enzymes were significant for a troponin level of 0.62 ng/mL. His B-type natriuretic peptide (BNP) level was 1,190. An electrocardiogram (ECG) revealed a sinus rhythm with right superior axis deviation, biatrial enlargement, and right ventricular hypertrophy. Further evaluation with a TTE revealed that the patient had a LVEF of 20-29% with a markedly dilated left atrium and left ventricle. Subsequently, a cardiac catheterization did not reveal evidence of obstructive coronary artery disease. Given the trivial history of congenital heart disease and nonischemic cardiomyopathy, a cardiac MRI was then conducted and revealed a noncompacted to compacted myocardium ratio of greater than 2.3 in the left ventricle, global hypokinesis with severely depressed left and right ventricle ejection fractions of 27% and 26%, biatrial enlargement, and no evidence of a left ventricular thrombus (Figures 1 and 2). His hospital course was complicated by an episode of nonsustained ventricular tachycardia, which given his LVNC and low ejection fraction, placed him at an elevated risk for SCD. The patient subsequently received an internal cardiac defibrillator (ICD) and was discharged home with aspirin, beta blocker, angiotensin-receptor blocker, and anticoagulation therapy with warfarin.

3. Case Discussion

In summary, LVNC is an uncommon and controversial cause of cardiomyopathy. It is becoming a popular topic in the field of cardiology due to its multiple possible etiologies, pathogenesis, diagnostic criteria, and clinical course. Due to its highly variable manifestations, the management of this condition should be individualized. Patients with evidence of heart failure should receive guideline-directed medical therapy (GDMT). Some literature supports the use of anticoagulation in patients with LVEF less than 40%, a history of atrial fibrillation, or a prior cardioembolic event

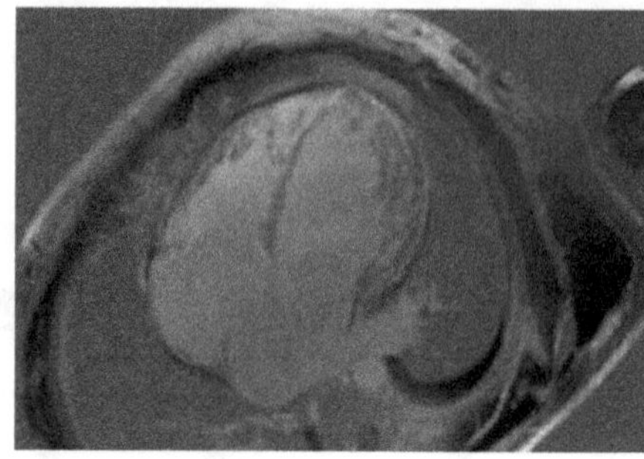

FIGURE 2: Four-chamber view of cardiac magnetic resonance (CMR) reveals dilation of all chambers of the heart.

[9]. All patients should also receive family and genetic counseling. As an uncommon disease with a multitude of life-threatening complications, it is imperative to perform a thorough cardiac evaluation in cases of new-onset heart failure with or without arrhythmia. In addition, further research and collaboration from major organizations are necessary to create a standardized criteria for the diagnosis and management of this disorder.

References

[1] H. Chen, W. Zhang, D. Li, T. M. Cordes, R. Mark Payne, and W. Shou, "Analysis of ventricular hypertrabeculation and noncompaction using genetically engineered mouse models," *Pediatric Cardiology*, vol. 30, no. 5, pp. 626–634, 2009.

[2] E. Arbustini, F. Weidemann, and J. L. Hall, "Left ventricular noncompaction: a distinct cardiomyopathy or a trait shared by different cardiac diseases?," *Journal of the American College of Cardiology*, vol. 64, no. 17, pp. 1840–1850, 2014.

[3] B. J. Maron, J. A. Towbin, G. Thiene et al., "Contemporary definitions and classification of the cardiomyopathies: an American Heart Association scientific statement from the Council on Clinical Cardiology, Heart Failure and Transplantation Committee; Quality of Care and Outcomes Research and Functional Genomics and Translational Biology Interdisciplinary Working Groups; and Council on Epidemiology and Prevention," *Circulation*, vol. 113, no. 14, pp. 1807–1816, 2006.

[4] P. Elliott, B. Andersson, E. Arbustini et al., "Classification of the cardiomyopathies: a position statement from the European Society of Cardiology Working Group on Myocardial and Pericardial Diseases," *European Heart Journal*, vol. 29, no. 2, pp. 270–276, 2008.

[5] B. S. Frischknecht, C. H. Attenhofer Jost, E. N. Oechslin et al., "Validation of noncompaction criteria in dilated cardiomyopathy, and valvular and hypertensive heart disease," *Journal of the American Society of Echocardiography*, vol. 18, no. 8, pp. 865–872, 2005.

[6] T. K. Chin, J. K. Perloff, R. G. Williams, K. Jue, and R. Mohrmann, "Isolated noncompaction of left ventricular myocardium. A study of eight cases," *Circulation*, vol. 82, no. 2, pp. 507–513, 1990.

[7] G. Fazio, G. Novo, L. D'angelo et al., "Magnetic resonance in isolated noncompaction of the ventricular myocardium," *International Journal of Cardiology*, vol. 140, no. 3, pp. 367–369, 2010.

[8] C. Stöllberger, W. Kopsa, R. Tscherney, and J. Finsterer, "Diagnosing left ventricular noncompaction by echocardiography and cardiac magnetic resonance imaging and its dependency on neuromuscular disorders," *Clinical Cardiology*, vol. 31, no. 8, pp. 383–387, 2008.

[9] K. Kido and M. Guglin, "Anticoagulation Therapy in Specific Cardiomyopathies: Isolated Left Ventricular Noncompaction and Peripartum Cardiomyopathy," *Journal of Cardiovascular Pharmacology and Therapeutics*, vol. 24, no. 1, pp. 31–36, 2019.

20

Permanent Pacemaker Implantation in a Patient with Takotsubo Cardiomyopathy and Complete Atrioventricular Block

Toshihiro Terui,[1,2,3] **Masumi Iwai-Takano**,[4,5,6] **and Tomoyuki Watanabe**[1]

[1]*Division of Internal Medicine, Health Co-op, Watari Hospital, Fukushima, Japan*
[2]*International Community Health, Graduate School of Medicine, Fukushima Medical University, Fukushima, Japan*
[3]*Department of Neuropsychiatry, Fukushima Medical University, Fukushima, Japan*
[4]*Department of Epidemiology, Fukushima Medical University, Fukushima, Japan*
[5]*Division of Cardiovascular Surgery, Fukushima Medical University, Fukushima, Japan*
[6]*Fukushima Prefectural General Hygiene Institute, Fukushima, Japan*

Correspondence should be addressed to Masumi Iwai-Takano; masumi@fmu.ac.jp
Academic Editor: Christopher S. Snyder

This case report presents a patient with Takotsubo cardiomyopathy (TCM) and complete atrioventricular (AV) block who was treated with permanent pacemaker implantation. A 78-year-old woman with a history of hypertension presented with a 6-month history of palpitations. On initial evaluation, her heart rate was 40 beats/minute. Electrocardiography revealed a complete AV block and T-wave inversion in these leads: I, II, aVL, aVF, and V3–6. Echocardiography showed akinesis from the midventricle to the apex and hyperkinesis on the basal segments. The patient was diagnosed with TCM and complete AV block. Because improvement of TCM may subsequently improve the AV node dysfunction associated with TCM, the patient was admitted for treatment of heart failure without pacemaker implantation. The left ventricular (LV) abnormal wall motion improved gradually; however, the AV block persisted intermittently. On hospital day 14, a pause of 5–6 seconds without LV contraction was observed, and permanent pacemaker implantation was performed. On day 92, echocardiography revealed normal LV wall motion. However, electrocardiography revealed that the pacemaker rhythm with atrial sensing and ventricular pacing remained. Although specific degree of damage that may result from AV block associated with TCM is unknown, some of these patients require pacemaker implantation, despite improvement of abnormality in LV wall motion.

1. Introduction

Takotsubo cardiomyopathy (TCM) is known as stress-induced heart disease that occurs with transient acute left ventricle (LV) apical ballooning without coronary artery stenosis. Various pathogeneses of TCM are presumed, and strong emotional or physical stress has been reported to be triggers [1]. Various types of arrhythmias can complicate acute phase TCM, such as ventricular tachycardia, ventricular fibrillation, Torsades de pointes, atrial fibrillation, sinus node dysfunction, and atrioventricular (AV) block [1–3]. Contrary to the reversible, transient pathophysiology of TCM alone, some cases of arrhythmia-complicated TCM developed into more life-threatening conditions, such as intermittent asystole or sudden cardiac death [2]. However, only a few reports have described TCM patients with AV block who underwent pacemaker implantation. Among those reports, AV node dysfunction remained even after LV contraction was improved [4–6]. However, AV node conduction normalized for some patients over a long-term follow-up period [7]. Because the specific degree of damage that occurs in AV conduction in the setting of TCM is unknown, the best method for the management of advanced AV block associated with TCM remains unclear [8]. This case report presents a patient with persistent AV block-complicated TCM, the treatment of which was permanent pacemaker implantation in the process of improving LV dysfunction.

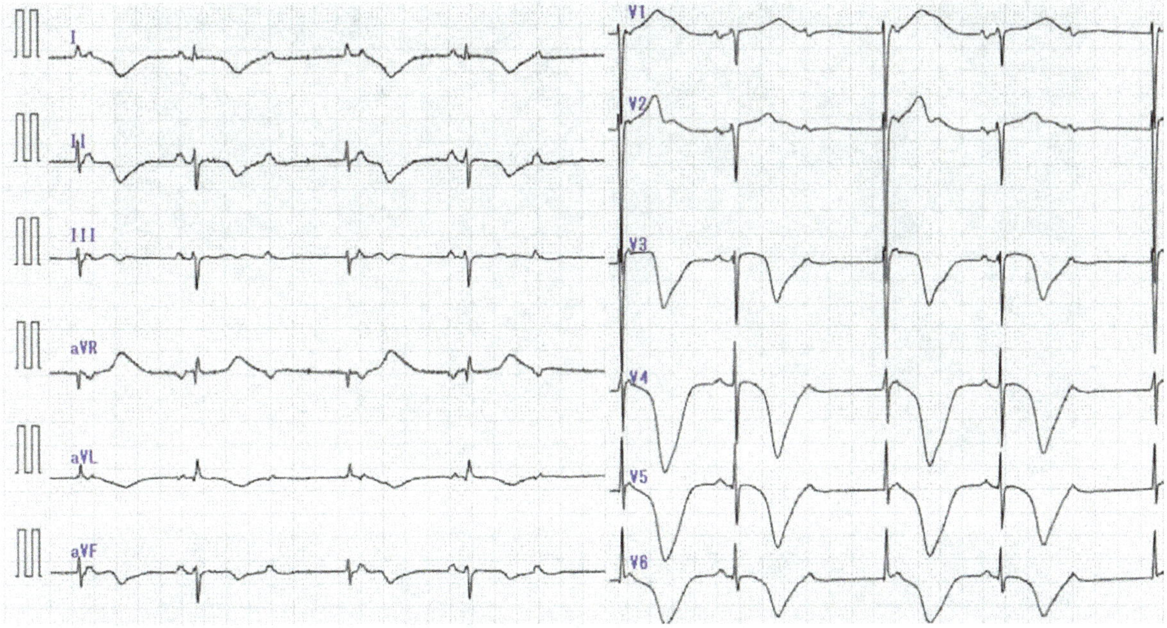

FIGURE 1: The initial electrocardiogram in the emergency department shows complete atrioventricular block with a heart rate of 40 beats/minute and T-wave inversion in the I, II, aVL, aVF, and V3–6 leads.

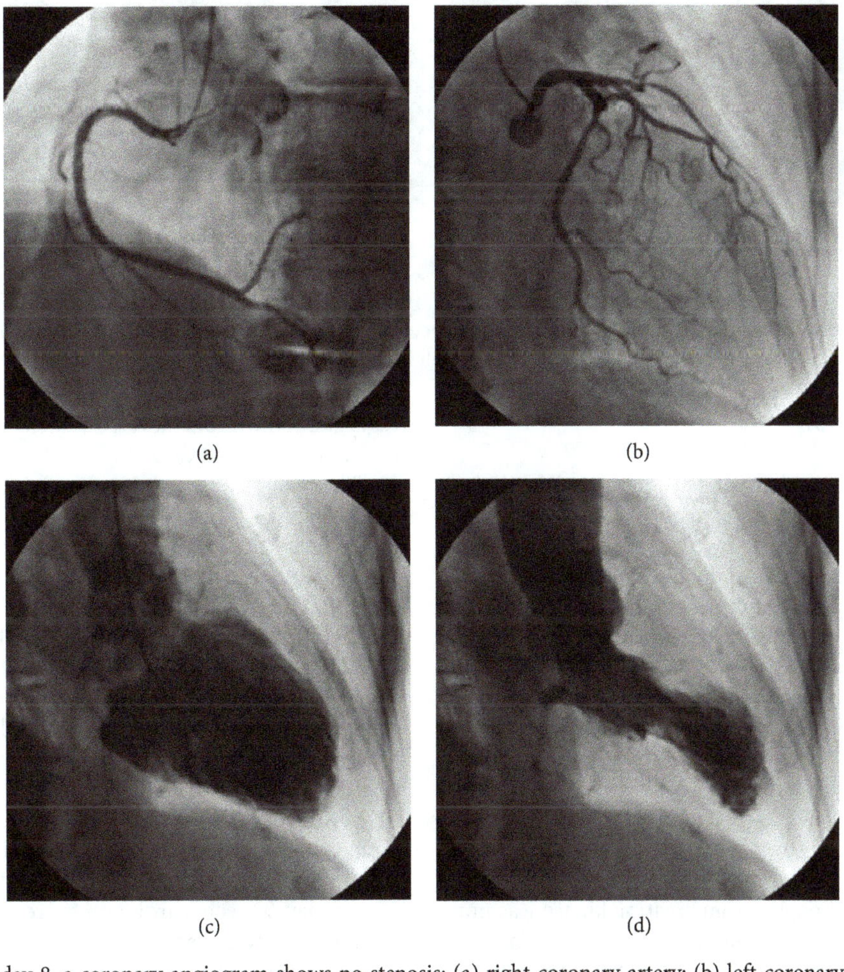

FIGURE 2: On hospital day 8, a coronary angiogram shows no stenosis: (a) right coronary artery; (b) left coronary artery. Left ventricular angiography shows hypokinesis from the midventricle to the apex and hyperkinesis in the basal segments: (c) end-diastole; (d) end-systole.

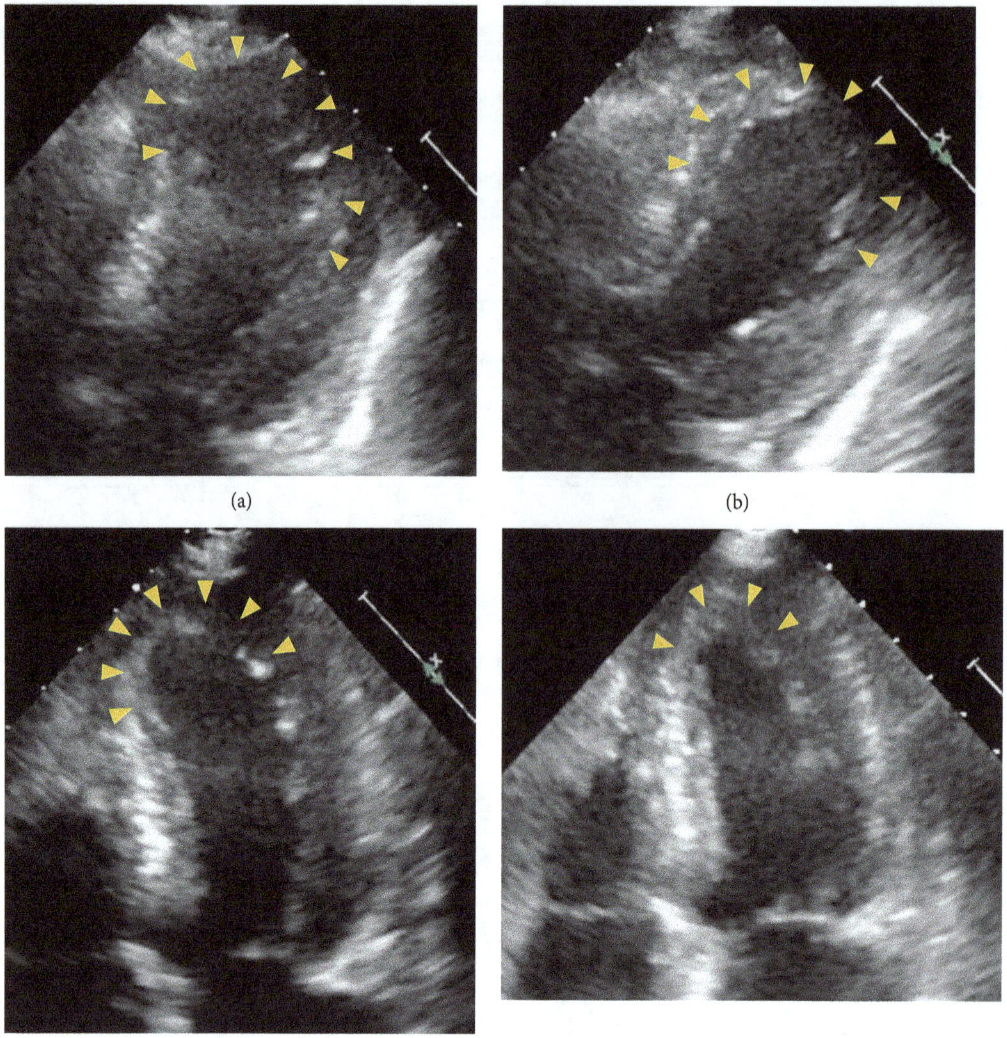

(a) (b) (c) (d)

FIGURE 3: Echocardiogram shows gradual improvement of left ventricular systolic dysfunction: (a) admission (day 0), (b) hospital day 2, (c) day 5, and (d) day 9. Yellow arrow indicates an area of abnormal wall motion in end-systole.

2. Case Presentation

A 78-year-old woman with hypertension complained a 6-month history of palpitations and presented to her local clinic, where physical examination showed bradycardia. She was then referred to the authors' hospital for further evaluation.

On physical examination, blood pressure was 153/78 mmHg, heart rate was 46 beats/minute, and peripheral capillary oxygen saturation was 96% on room air. Chest radiography showed enlargement of the cardiothoracic ratio and blunting of the right costophrenic angle. Initial electrocardiography revealed complete AV block with a junctional escape rate of 40 beats/minute, and T-wave inversion in these leads: I, II, aVL, aVF, and V3–6 (Figure 1). Laboratory data showed elevations of troponin T 184 ng/L (normal, <50 ng/L) and brain natriuretic peptide 287.5 pg/mL (normal, <18.4 pg/mL), although serum creatine kinase was normal. Echocardiography showed akinesis from the midventricle to the apex of the LV and hyperkinesis on the basal segments. Mild mitral regurgitation and mild tricuspid regurgitation without elevated velocity of tricuspid regurgitation were also observed.

The patient was diagnosed with TCM and complete AV block. Because AV node dysfunction associated with TCM may be recovered after improvement of TCM, she was conservatively treated for heart failure without pacemaker implantation. On hospital day 8, coronary angiography showed no significant stenosis, and left ventriculography revealed apical ballooning (Figure 2).

Echocardiography showed improvement of LV abnormal wall motion gradually over admission through hospital day 9 (Figure 3); however, AV block persisted intermittently (Figure 4(a)). On day 14, a pause of 5–6 seconds without LV contraction was observed (Figure 4(b)), and the patient underwent temporary pacemaker implantation. On day 15, a permanent pacemaker was implanted.

On day 92, echocardiography revealed normal LV wall motion. However, electrocardiography showed that the pacemaker rhythm (DDD mode, AV delay 180 msec) with atrial sensing and ventricular pacing remained.

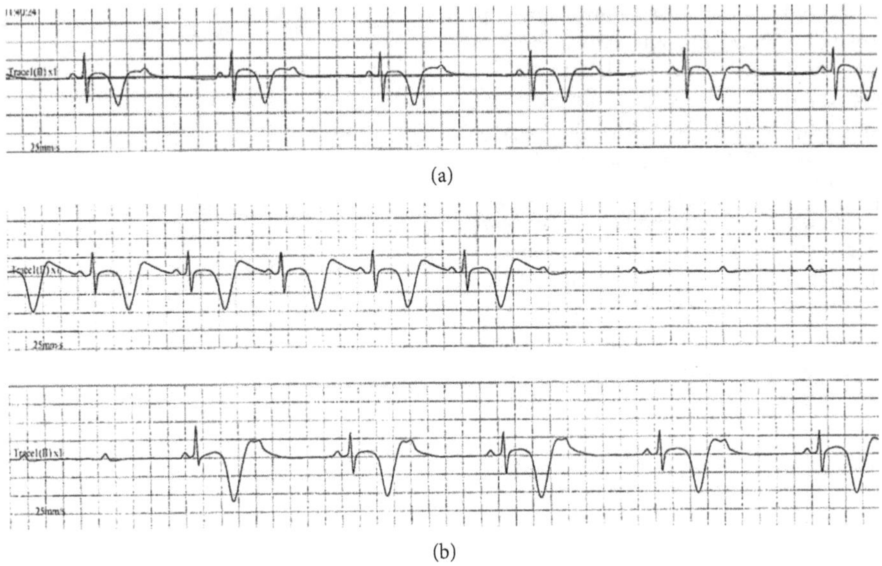

FIGURE 4: Electrocardiogram shows transient advanced atrioventricular block on hospital day 2 (a) and day 14 (b).

3. Discussion

The occurrence of AV block is rarely associated with TCM, with a prevalence of about 2.9% [2]. Previous AV block and its intervention, such as temporary or permanent pacemaker implantation, can be triggers of myocardial dyskinesis [9, 10]. Subsequently, myocardial abnormalities such as fibrosis or edema have the pathologic potential to create ventricular electrical stimuli. However, the definitive demonstration of a cause/effect relationship between myocardial edema and electrical abnormalities, not only in TCM but also in other conditions of reversible ventricular dysfunction, is still lacking [11]. Thus, it remains unknown whether TCM causes AV block or AV node dysfunction as complications or conversely whether AV block as a physical stressor causes TCM.

Patient's age may be a contributor to AV dysfunction, and AV block may be more common in older adult women. [12]. In the current case, a 78-year-old woman experienced palpitations before developing TCM. It was expected that the AV block would recover along with improvement of LV systolic dysfunction; however, the AV block remained despite improvement of the abnormality in LV wall motion. Thus, the hypothesis was that previous AV node dysfunction, which progressed with aging, induced the TCM in this patient. Moreover, 3 months after permanent pacemaker implantation, echocardiography showed normal LV wall motion, but the patient's AV block persisted.

It remains unclear whether permanent pacemaker implantation in patients with AV block complicated by TCM is an appropriate treatment, and it is not possible to predict proper implantation in the acute phase of TCM. Some reports describe patients who underwent permanent pacemaker implantation for AV block-complicated TCM on day 1 to day 18 [8–10, 12–14]. However, AV block has been reported to improve in the acute phase of TCM (on day 3) in some cases [7], and the recovery of AV node dysfunction 3 months after permanent pacemaker implantation in a patient with TCM has also been reported [15]. In contrast, AV block remained in several reported patients after improved LV wall motion abnormality in the chronic phase of TCM [8, 14]. Several investigators have suggested that permanent pacemaker implantation in the acute phase of TCM is required in these patients with AV block because of the persistence of AV block in this setting and the prognosis [16, 17].

Because the specific degree of damage of AV conduction in TCM is unknown, the treatment strategy for AV block in TCM patients remains unclear. However, some cases require permanent pacemaker implantation for advanced AV block despite improvement of LV wall motion abnormality.

4. Conclusion

Permanent pacemaker implantation was performed in a patient with AV block-complicated TCM. Some cases require permanent pacemaker implantation for advanced AV block, despite improvement of LV wall motion abnormality.

Authors' Contributions

Toshihiro Terui and Masumi Iwai-Takano contributed equally to this work.

References

[1] S. M. Said, E. Saygili, O. R. Rana et al., "Takotsubo cardiomyopathy: what we have learned in the last 25 years? (a comparative literature review)," *Current Cardiology Reviews*, vol. 12, no. 4, pp. 297–303, 2016.

[2] F. F. Syed, S. J. Asirvatham, and J. Francis, "Arrhythmia occurrence with takotsubo cardiomyopathy: a literature review," *Europace*, vol. 13, no. 6, pp. 780–788, 2011.

[3] K. H. Brown, R. G. Trohman, and C. Madias, "Arrhythmias in takotsubo cardiomyopathy," *Cardiac Electrophysiology Clinics*, vol. 7, no. 2, pp. 331–340, 2015.

[4] P. Korantzopoulos, D. N. Nikas, K. Letsas et al., "High-grade

atrioventricular block and takotsubo cardiomyopathy: case report and review of the literature," *International Cardiovascular Research Journal*, vol. 9, no. 2, pp. 119–124, 2015.

[5] D. T. Gamble, K. J. Shuttleworth, C. Scally, and S. J. Leslie, "Takotsubo cardiomyopathy with severe bradyarrhythmia following epidural insertion," *BMJ Case Reports*, vol. 2016, p. bcr2016216946, 2016.

[6] B. Morawiec, S. Degrauwe, J. F. Iglesias, and O. Muller, "First report on biventricular stress cardiomyopathy with concomitant atrio-ventricular high-grade conduction disorder," *Cardiology Journal*, vol. 24, no. 1, pp. 98–100, 2017.

[7] T. Sugiura, Y. Dohi, S. Yamashita et al., "Midventricular ballooning Takotsubo cardiomyopathy complicated by transient complete atrioventricular block," *Internal Medicine*, vol. 52, no. 17, pp. 1919–1921, 2013.

[8] M. Inoue, H. Kanaya, T. Matsubara, Y. Uno, T. Yasuda, and K. Miwa, "Complete atrioventricular block associated with Takotsubo cardiomyopathy," *Circulation Journal*, vol. 73, no. 3, pp. 589–592, 2009.

[9] Z. H. Wei, Q. Dai, H. Wu, J. Song, L. Wang, and B. Xu, "Takotsubo cardiomyopathy after pacemaker implantation," *Journal of Geriatric Cardiology*, vol. 15, no. 3, pp. 246–248, 2018.

[10] N. D. Brunetti, R. Ieva, M. Correale et al., "Combined exogenous and endogenous catecholamine release associated with Tako-Tsubo like syndrome in a patient with atrio-ventricular block undergoing pace-maker implantation," *Acute Cardiac Care*, vol. 13, no. 2, pp. 112–114, 2011.

[11] F. Migliore, A. Zorzi, M. Perazzolo Marra, S. Iliceto, and D. Corrado, "Myocardial edema as a substrate of electrocardiographic abnormalities and life-threatening arrhythmias in reversible ventricular dysfunction of takotsubo cardiomyopathy: imaging evidence, presumed mechanisms, and implications for therapy," *Heart Rhythm*, vol. 12, no. 8, pp. 1867–1877, 2015.

[12] E. H. Cativo, R. Valvani, T. O. Mene-Afejuku, D. P. Cativo, and S. Mushiyev, "A rare association of Takotsubo cardiomyopathy with high-degree atrioventricular block," *Case Reports in Cardiology*, vol. 2017, Article ID 6989438, 4 pages, 2017.

[13] R. Shanmugasundaram, K. Tamilarasu, G. Rajendiran, and A. Murali, "An uncommon presentation of a rare disease - high-degree AV block with takotsubo cardiomyopathy," *Indian Heart Journal*, vol. 64, no. 5, pp. 511–514, 2012.

[14] S. Kurisu and Y. Kihara, "Clinical management of Takotsubo cardiomyopathy," *Circulation Journal*, vol. 78, no. 7, pp. 1559–1566, 2014.

[15] H. M. Nef, H. Möllmann, J. Sperzel et al., "Temporary third-degree atrioventricular block in a case of apical ballooning syndrome," *International Journal of Cardiology*, vol. 113, no. 2, pp. e33–e35, 2006.

[16] T. Stiermaier, K. P. Rommel, C. Eitel et al., "Management of arrhythmias in patients with Takotsubo cardiomyopathy: is the implantation of permanent devices necessary?," *Heart Rhythm*, vol. 13, no. 10, pp. 1979–1986, 2016.

[17] M. T. Le, C. Grimard, O. Varenne, R. Jakamy, and J. Rosencher, "Tako-Tsubo cardiomyopathy and high-degree atrio-ventricular block: do we need to wait left ventricular function recovery to implant a pacemaker?," *International Journal of Cardiology*, vol. 176, no. 2, pp. e56–e59, 2014.

21

Frequently Recurrent Takotsubo Syndrome in COPD

Juan Vaz, [1] **Rikard Berggren**, [2] **and Berne Eriksson** [1,3]

[1] *Department of Medicine, Halmstad Hospital, Halmstad, Sweden*
[2] *Department of Cardiology, Halmstad Hospital, Halmstad, Sweden*
[3] *Krefting Research Centre, Institute of Medicine, University of Gothenburg, Gothenburg, Sweden*

Correspondence should be addressed to Juan Vaz; juan.vazleonidas@regionhalland.se

Academic Editor: Hajime Kataoka

Cardiovascular disease is common among patients with chronic obstructive pulmonary disease (COPD). Takotsubo syndrome (TTS) is a transient cardiac disorder that, in its typical form, involves left ventricular dysfunction with apical ballooning and mimics acute coronary syndrome (ACS). "Bronchogenic TTS" has been proposed as a specific form of TTS (during severe acute dyspnea in asthma or COPD) with atypical presentation. Recurrent TTS in COPD seems to be exceptionally rare since only a handful of clinical cases have previously been reported in the literature. Here, we present a unique case of a frequently recurrent TTS during COPD exacerbation in a 70-year-old woman, with at least 4 different episodes of TTS within 5 years. This case report exemplifies the difficulties of the diagnosis of TTS at the onset of acute COPD exacerbation. Potential pathophysiological mechanisms and therapeutic strategies are also briefly discussed.

1. Introduction

Cardiovascular disease is common among patients with chronic obstructive pulmonary disease (COPD). More than 3.2 million COPD patients die annually, and in approximately 30% of the cases, cardiovascular disease and its complications are the main causes of death [1, 2]. Despite formerly being referred to as "stress cardiomyopathy," Takotsubo syndrome (TTS) is a complex transient cardiac disorder that, in its typical form, involves left ventricular dysfunction with apical ballooning, and mimics acute coronary syndrome (ACS) [3, 4]. The prevalence of TTS is unknown, but it is estimated to be 2-3% of all patients with diagnosed ACS [5]. Cumulative incidence of recurrence in TTS has been reported to be approximately 5% at 6 years, and the annual rate of recurrence is only 1-2% [3, 6]. TTS has also been related to severe dyspnea during respiratory disease [7, 8], but the pathophysiological mechanisms remain mostly unknown [9]. "Bronchogenic TTS" has been proposed as a specific form of TTS that occurs during severe acute dyspnea in asthma or COPD, with atypical presentation [10–12]. Recurrent TTS in COPD seems to be exceptionally rare since only a handful of clinical cases have previously been reported in the literature [13, 14]. Here, we present a unique case of frequently recurrent TTS during COPD exacerbation with at least 4 different episodes of TTS.

2. Case Presentation

At first medical contact (FMC), a 70-year-old Caucasian woman who admitted to be a heavy smoker and was slightly overweight, presented to the emergency room (ER) with severe dyspnea. Her past medical history, medications, and background information are summarized in Table 1.

Hypoxia with pulse oxygen saturation < 85%, tachypnea, tachycardia, and hypertension were present. Signs of infection, cyanosis, and peripheral edema were absent. Clinical examination revealed expiratory wheezes and prolonged expiration. Chest pain and electrocardiogram (ECG) abnormalities were absent. Chest radiography exhibited bilateral flattening of the diaphragm but no pulmonary infiltrates or pneumothorax. White blood cell count (WBC) and C-reactive protein (CRP) were mainly normal, but troponin T (TPNT) level was elevated (53 ng/L: normal level, <15 ng/L). The patient was admitted to the hospital, and standard treatment for acute exacerbation of COPD was initiated.

Table 1: Characteristics of a 70-year-old woman presenting with severe dyspnea.

	Diagnosis	Medications	Timeline
Psychiatric history	Bipolar disorder	Lithium Lamotrigine Escitalopram Zopiclone	35 years before FMC Regular contact with psychiatrist
Medical history	Previous ischemic stroke with remaining minute weakness of the right leg	Aspirin Simvastatin	12 years before FMC
	Lithium-induced hypothyroidism	Levothyroxine	20 years before FMC
	Fibromyalgia	Paracetamol	5 years before FMC
Surgical history	Endometrial cancer	Curative hysterectomy with bilateral salpingo-oophorectomy Adjuvant radiochemotherapy	15 years before FMC
Allergies		None	
Family history		Endometrial and colon cancer	
Alcohol use		None	
Nicotine use		Heavy smoker. 35-Pack-year history	

FMC: first contact with the emergency room due to severe dyspnea.

Soon after admission, increased dyspnea and vague chest discomfort were observed despite normal pulse oxygen saturation. ECG revealed T-wave inversion in several leads, normal QT interval (Figure 1, FMC), and an increased TPNT level of 108 ng/L. Pulmonary embolism and aortic dissection were outruled via computed tomography (CT). Echocardiography (ECHO) revealed a normal left ventricular ejection factor (LVEF) without dyskinesia, at the time (see under Discussion). Dual antiplatelet therapy (DAPT), in concordance with the existing guidelines of the European Society of Cardiology (ESC) for ACS, was initiated, and coronary angiography was performed. The latter showed no signs of significant stenosis or other pathologies that could explain the patient's symptoms. During the following days, no other episodes of dyspnea or chest pain were registered, ECG and TPNT level returned to normal, and the patient was discharged from the hospital with prescriptions for standard treatment for COPD. Upon the initially assumed absence of pathology in ECHO, the patient was diagnosed with myocarditis and followed up 3 months after FMC with a new ECHO, which was without abnormalities. During the follow-up period, the patient managed to quit smoking.

Almost 32 months after FMC, the patient was again admitted to the hospital. This time she was suffering from exhaustion, dyspnea, and leg swelling for 2 weeks. Bilateral crackles and pitting edema of legs were present. ECG revealed T-wave inversions on several leads without QT interval prolongation (Figure 1). TPNT level was elevated (58 ng/L). Likewise, NT-probrain natriuretic peptide (NT-pro-BNP) level was also abnormal (2088; normal age-adjusted level, <450 pg/mL). CT scan showed no signs of pulmonary embolism, aortic dissection, or pleural effusion. ECHO, at the time, revealed severe left ventricular hypokinesia, most prominent in the inferolateral wall and the septum. LVEF was approximately 30%. Subsequent analysis revealed severe midventricular hypokinesia instead of inferolateral (see under Discussion). DAPT and heparin were given and acute coronary angiography was performed. Once again, no significant pathology was found despite the patient's severe acute heart failure. Also, as during FMC and upon treatment with diuretics and standard COPD medications, dyspnea and chest pain disappeared, ECG returned to normal, and crackles and pitting edema were gone. TPNT levels decreased as well (Table 2). The patient was then diagnosed with non-Q-wave myocardial infarction, and she was prescribed metoprolol, ramipril, and eplerenone. Cardiac magnetic resonance imaging (CMR) was performed 3 weeks after discharge from the hospital. Oddly, no signs of previous myocardial infarction or myocarditis were found, LVEF was calculated to be 55%, and hypokinesia was absent. Subsequent follow-ups confirmed that the patient was feeling well without symptoms of heart failure or angina pectoris. Moreover, NT-pro-BNP level was normal and a new ECHO was completely normal. Treatment with eplerenone was discontinued due to adverse side effects, and after some months, follow-ups were discontinued on the patient's initiative.

Eight months after the second episode (4 months after the last follow-up), the patient was once again hospitalized due to acute COPD exacerbation. Chest pain was denied, but a burning feeling over the back was present. Clinical examination was concomitant with previous episodes, but pitting edema and crackles were absent. The initial ECG at ER was normal except for sinus tachycardia, and cardiac troponin, NT-pro-BNP, CRP, and WBC levels were normal.

During the first hours after admission, severe dyspnea was observed and TPNT levels increased to 244 ng/L. ECG now revealed T-wave inversions similar to those found at previous hospitalizations (Figure 1). A small quantity of pleural effusion was found at CT scan, but pulmonary embolism and aortic dissection were absent. ECHO showed severe left ventricular hypokinesia, most manifest in the apical and midventricular segments. LVEF was estimated at 20%. NT-pro-BNP level increased from the previous normal level to 1000 pg/mL. As chest pain was still absent,

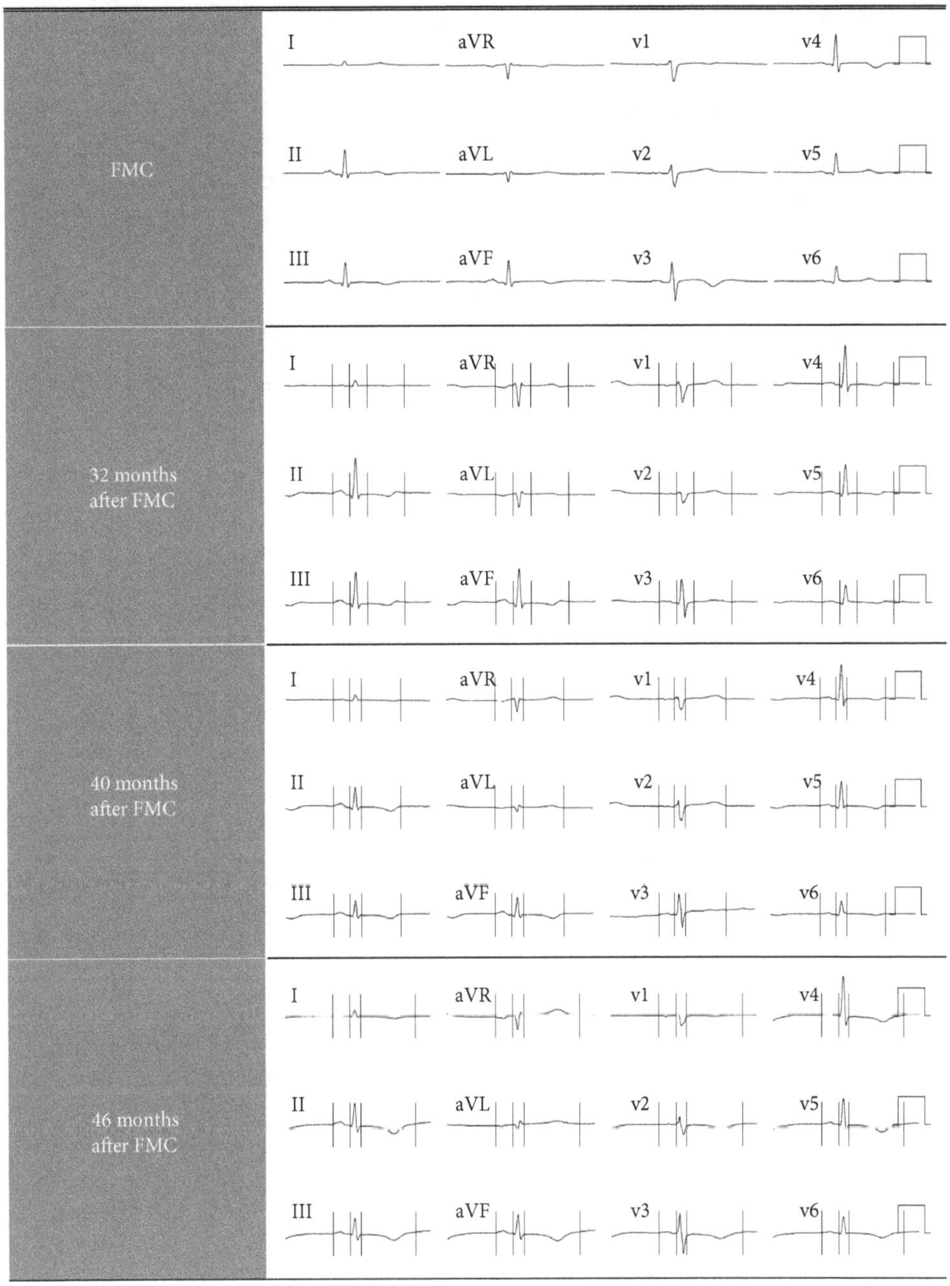

FIGURE 1: ECG abnormalities in a 70-year-old female COPD patient with recurrent TTS.

treatment with intravenous diuretics was started; the patient's status improved rapidly, but the TPNT level remained unchanged. On day 4, severe chest pain started and the TPNT level increased to 300 ng/L. ECG was still abnormal with unspecific T-wave inversions. DAPT was given, and coronary angiography was once again normal. Astonishingly, soon after coronary angiography, chest pain ceased, ECG and NT-pro-BNP were normal, TPNT levels decreased considerably, and ECHO revealed an LVEF of 50-60% without hypokinesia. She was again diagnosed with myocarditis, and furosemide was prescribed. A follow-up within a month was planned.

Almost 2 weeks after being sent home, the patient returned to the ER with dyspnea and acute chest pain. Crackles were present, but chest radiography was normal. Pitting edema was absent. TPNT level was 107 pg/mL. The patient was again admitted to the hospital, and ECHO performed on the next day was evaluated as normal. At this point, the patient was completely recovered and stated that she had had a rough week with high stress levels. The TPNT level decreased, and since a follow-up was previously planned, she was discharged without new prescriptions. She was diagnosed with unspecific chest pain.

During the succeeding follow-ups, a grade 3 COPD was confirmed via spirometry (FEV1/FVC0.39, FEV1 39% of normal) and her COPD treatment was adjusted. Treatment with metoprolol was substituted with amlodipine, and a new ECHO was normal with an LVEF of 60%.

Table 2: Clinical presentation of a 70-year-old female COPD patient with recurrent TTS.

	FMC	32 months after FMC	40 months after FMC	40.5 months after FMC	46 months after FMC	48 months after FMC
Symptoms	Severe dyspnea	Dyspnea, exhaustion	Severe dyspnea, cough	Dyspnea, chest pain	Severe dyspnea	Dyspnea
ECG (Figure 1)	T-wave inversion	T-wave inversion	T-wave inversion	Mainly normal	T-wave inversion	Mainly normal
TPNT (ng/L)	53-108-54-14	58-288-285-88	19-200-300-240-54	107-112-52	31-431-521-574-51	42-74-107
NT-pro-BNP (pg/mL)	Normal	2088	1000	Normal	Normal	Normal
CT scan or CR	Normal	Normal	Bilateral pleural effusion	Normal	Normal	Normal
Coronary angiography	Normal	Normal	Normal	None	None	None
ECHO	Normal LVEF 60%	Hypokinesia in the septum and inferolateral wall. LVEF 30%	Global hypokinesia (partially preserved function in the basal wall). LVEF 20%	Normal	Midventricular akinesia but less affected function in apical and basal segments LVEF < 20%	None
ECHO (reviewed images)	Discrete apical hypokinesia	Severe hypokinesia, most prominent midventricular	Severe hypokinesia, most prominent midventricular and apical	Further analysis not possible due poor image quality	As above	None
Days at hospital	7	4	16	5	7	1
Initial diagnose	Myocarditis	Non-Q-wave MI	Myocarditis	Chest pain (UNS)	Midventricular TTC	Dyspnea (UNS)
Diagnose (after review)	Possible TTC	Midventricular TTC	Midventricular TTC	Unclear	Midventricular TTC	Unclear
Follow-up	ECHO: normal	CMR: normal ECHO: normal	ECHO: normal	ECHO: normal	ECHO: normal LVEF Minor basal hypokinesia	CCTA: no significant stenosis

CCTA: cardiac computed tomography angiography; CMR: cardiac magnetic resonance imaging; COPD: chronic obstructive pulmonary disease; CR: chest radiography; ECG: electrocardiogram; ECHO: echocardiography; FMC: first medical contact; LVEF: left ventricular ejection fraction; MI: myocardial infarction; NT-pro-BNP: NT-probrain natriuretic peptide; TPNT: troponin T; TTS: Takotsubo syndrome; UNS: unspecified.

Six months after past hospitalization (4 months after the last follow-up), the patient was again admitted to the hospital due to severe dyspnea. Chest pain was negated, ECG showed T-wave inversion on leads AVL and I, and TPNT was slightly elevated. ECHO at ER revealed severe generalized left ventricular hypokinesia with midventricular akinesia, but the basal and apical segments were less affected. LVEF was estimated to be less than 20%. On day 2, TPNT level increased to 431 ng/L, NT-pro-BNP level was normal, and T-wave inversions on several leads were observed (Figure 1). During the following days, the patient recovered, ECG returned to normal, and TPNT level decreased considerably. Importantly, chest pain was never observed. ECHO previous to discharging from the hospital showed normal global function with an LVEF of 50% with remaining left basal hypokinesia. Treatment with carvedilol was started since the patient did not tolerated amlodipine, and verapamil was considered contraindicated due to a potential interaction with lithium (see Table 1). During this hospitalization, the patient was given the diagnosis of TTS for the first time. Additionally, a comprehensive review of the patient's previous medical history and saved ECHO images exposed several episodes of TTS (see under Discussion).

Finally, 2 months after her first diagnosed TTS, she was again admitted to the hospital due to dyspnea and elevated TPNT (107 ng/L). ECG was mainly normal. For unknown reasons, an ECHO wasn't performed and the patient was discharged on the first day. Cardiac computed tomography angiography (CCTA) was performed after two months, and no significant stenosis was observed. A previously planned ECHO showed normal LVEF and minor left basal hypokinesia. To date, no new TTS episodes have been observed and concurrently, no new acute COPD exacerbations have been noted.

3. Discussion

A case of recurrent TTS with different wall motion patterns in the same patient has previously been reported [15]. "Bronchogenic TTS" has been defined as an atypical form of TTS [10–12], and acute respiratory failure has also been associated to atypical TTS [8]. Our review of our patient's preceding medical data uncovered four probable episodes of atypical TTS. In three of them, our ECHO expert established the presence of midventricular hypokinesia, and in one case, akinesia was established; no signs of right ventricular strain and/or pulmonary hypertension were found (Table 2). Midventricular TTS is a rare form of TTS, found in only 14.6% of the cases [3, 4]. Likewise, in FMC, our ECHO expert found signs of apical hypokinesia but not apical ballooning that might be similar to those found in focal type TTS [3]. In one of the episodes, the quality of the data was insufficient for analysis of ECHO images, and in the last episode, no ECHO was performed. In summary, based on the recently published International Takotsubo Diagnostic Criteria (InterTAK Diagnostic Criteria) [4], International Takotsubo Diagnostic Score (InterTAK Diagnostic Score), and diagnostic algorithm of Takotsubo syndrome [16], we advocate that our patient had had 4 different episodes of atypical TTS (1 focal type TTS and 3 midventricular TTS), the last 3 occurring with high frequency (Table 2). This postulation is supported by the occurrence of new ECG abnormalities (T-wave inversions) combined with transient elevation of cardiac troponins, confirmed transient echocardiographic hypokinesia compatible with TTS, and no evidence of infection, myocarditis (even if the patient was previously diagnosed with myocarditis, there is enough clinical data to dismiss this diagnosis since there is no sign of myocarditis on CMR), or significant coronary artery spasms (coronary angiography and CCTA).

TTS is a puzzling and complex medical condition with a largely unknown pathophysiology, and a comprehensive review of it is beyond the scope of this article. Nevertheless, since TTS is frequently elicited by emotional or physical stressors, sympathetic stimulation has long been proposed as a key factor in TTS [4, 17]. Among others, oxidative stress, infective agents, genetic predisposition, transient coronary artery spasm, and estrogen deficiency appear to be involved in the development of TTS [4, 18, 19].

There are several factors in this case that may have contributed to the high recurrence of TTS observed. Female sex, emotional and physical stresses, no ST-segment depression, and psychiatric disorders are the main risk factors in this case, according to the InterTAK Diagnostic Score [16].

3.1. Female Sex and Hormonal Factors. Approximately 90% of TTS patients are postmenopausal women [3], which might support estrogen-deficiency theories [20]. In our patient, bilateral salpingo-oophorectomy was performed approximately 15 years before FMC and she had had no estrogen supplementation (Table 1). Estrogen supplementation might attenuate glucocorticoid and catecholamine responses to mental stress in perimenopausal women [21]. However, there is no evidence of similar responses in postmenopausal women and clear associations between estrogen levels and the development of TTS have not been reported yet. Hypothyroidism might predispose to TTS since 35% of the patients in a single center retrospective study (predominantly elderly female) had a history of hypothyroidism and the use of levothyroxine did not have protective effects [22, 23]. Still, the role of hypothyroidism in TTS is unknown and multicentric prospective studies are lacking.

3.2. ECG Changes. The InterTAK Registry reports a 41% T-wave inversion frequency in TTS [3]. Moreover, initial T-wave inversion has been described in atypical TTS due to acute respiratory failure [8] and even in "bronchogenic TTS" [10]. Our patient's initial ECG showed unspecific T-wave inversions in all TTS episodes (Figure 1, Table 2). However, no QT interval prolongation was observed, which otherwise is found in up to 50% of TTS patients at admission [3] and might cause life-threatening ventricular arrhythmias during the subacute phase [16]. Interestingly, in a recent study, no ECG differences were found on admission among patients with TTS due to emotional stress compared to patients with TTS secondary to neurological diseases, physical activities, and medical conditions or procedures, respectively [24].

3.3. COPD. In 3 of the episodes (including FMC), the development of TTS was observed during the first hours after hospitalization and after successful respiratory therapy with inhaled drugs. Normally, COPD patients are given high doses of a beta agonist (such as terbutaline or salbutamol) combined with ipratropium. As elevated catecholamine levels seem to play a key role in TTS [4], the additional stimulation of cardiac beta-2-adrenergic receptors might potentiate the development of TTS in patients under extreme stress, such as under hypoxia and acidosis. It has been suggested that epinephrine has a stunning effect on myocardial tissue in TTS due to the induction of beta-2 receptors, which in turn were more frequently found in the cardiac apex during TTS [25]. Thus, the use of a high dose of a beta-2 agonist at the ER might have been important for our patient's TTS development. In one occasion, the patient presented to the ER with manifest heart failure (Table 2). The medical records reveal that the patient had been inhaling high doses of salbutamol and ipratropium prior to hospitalization. Remarkably, ipratropium has also been proposed as an inducer in "bronchogenic TTS" [26]. Still, the use of ipratropium may mainly have favorable effects in "bronchogenic TTS" since it may reduce the need of beta-2-agonist administration. Even if hypothetically promising, the use of beta blockers in TTS is controversial and, at 1 year, there is no evidence of survival benefit for the use of beta blockers [3]. Glucocorticoids, such as prednisolone or betamethasone, are often administrated in high doses during acute COPD exacerbation. There is no known relationship between the use of systemic steroids and TTS. Despite being a stressor, high-dose corticosteroids may have had favorable effects in our patient since (as with ipratropium) this obviously reduced the need for beta-2-agonist administration during the subacute phase. Moreover, the anti-inflammatory effects of cortisone might have relieved the patient's chronic muscle pain, decreasing the underlying stress levels and possibly even the level of catecholamines.

3.4. Chronic Pain and Psychiatric Illness. Chronic pain diseases, such as fibromyalgia, may be related to nocturnal "sympathetic overdrive," and in animal models, increased plasma cortisol and epinephrine levels have been noticed upon long-lasting stress due to chronic pain [27].

Up to 42% of TTS patients suffer from psychiatric illness, and half of those had previously been diagnosed with an affective disorder [3]. Elevated sympathetic activity and reduced catecholamine uptake might be responsible for persistent cardiac sympathetic stimulation, increasing the risk for TTS in these patients, when exposed to stressful situations [28, 29]. Furthermore, the use of selective serotonin reuptake inhibitors (SSRIs) has been associated with a lower survival rate in TTS [30]. In animal models, lithium appears to stimulate catecholamine release from the adrenal gland and increase catecholamine concentration in the plasma [31]. However, lithium seems to reduce plasma epinephrine response upon insulin stimulation in humans [32]. Thus, it is unclear if a long-standing medication with SSRIs and/or lithium plays a role in the development of TTS.

A strong connection between the central nervous system (CNS) and the heart in TTS is highly probable as sympathetic overactivity seems to be an important factor in the development of TTS [17, 33]. Moreover, substantial anatomical alterations in the limbic system have been reported in TTS patients [34]. Decreased cortical thickness in the limbic system might result in less efficient emotional control, predisposing then for TTS. However, this hypothesis need to be confirmed in longitudinal studies [34]. Interestingly, similar brain alterations in the limbic system were found in major depression and bipolar disease when compared that in to healthy controls [35, 36]. These alterations have also been coupled to emotional dysregulation in bipolar disease [36].

Previous to FMC, the patient had a long history of bipolar disorder with several episodes of mania or severe depression. Her last hospitalization due to severe psychiatric illness was registered two years before FMC. There is no data indicating that the patient's background psychiatric illness was acutely aggravated prior to her hospitalizations due to dyspnea. During the 48 months between FMC and the last contact with the ER due to dyspnea, the patient was hospitalized several times due to psychiatric disease, including severe depression and acute stress reaction. Still, none of these episodes was coupled to chest pain or severe dyspnea. Additionally, hospitalizations due to psychiatric illness and dyspnea were registered with a period of several months in between them. This suggests a physical TTS trigger in our patient, in this case acute COPD exacerbation, even if a combination of emotional and physical triggers could also be possible. Interestingly, all the TTS episodes started during the night hours, which also was the time of the day when the patient felt more intensified muscular pain and anxiety. In theory, both conditions, chronical pain and psychiatric illness, might predispose for increased levels of catecholamines and other stress hormones (possibly having an additive effect), which in turn might increase the risk for the development of TTS upon an external trigger. Suffering from both conditions for several years, our patient developed TTS first during her first event of severe dyspnea due to acute COPD exacerbation. This may have been the droplet that caused the beaker to overflow (Figure 2). Here, we suggest an explicatory model in which the patient's previous medical and psychiatric conditions predispose the development of TTS due to chronic increased stress levels with subsequent elevation of systemic catecholamines. Upon additional stressors or triggers, such as in this case severe dyspnea (with consequent hypoxemia, acidosis, and anxiety), the further catecholamine elevation might initiate a cascade of mechanisms resulting in manifest TTS.

3.5. Outcome. Although originally considered a less severe condition, TTS is nowadays considered a serious clinical condition with potentially poor prognosis as early and late mortality can be similar to those observed in ACS [37]. Typical type TTS and atypical type TTS appears to have comparable in-hospital mortality and a similar prognosis at long-term follow-up [38]. Additionally, a recent study revealed that patients with TTS secondary to neurological diseases had the worst prognosis [24]. Moreover, patients

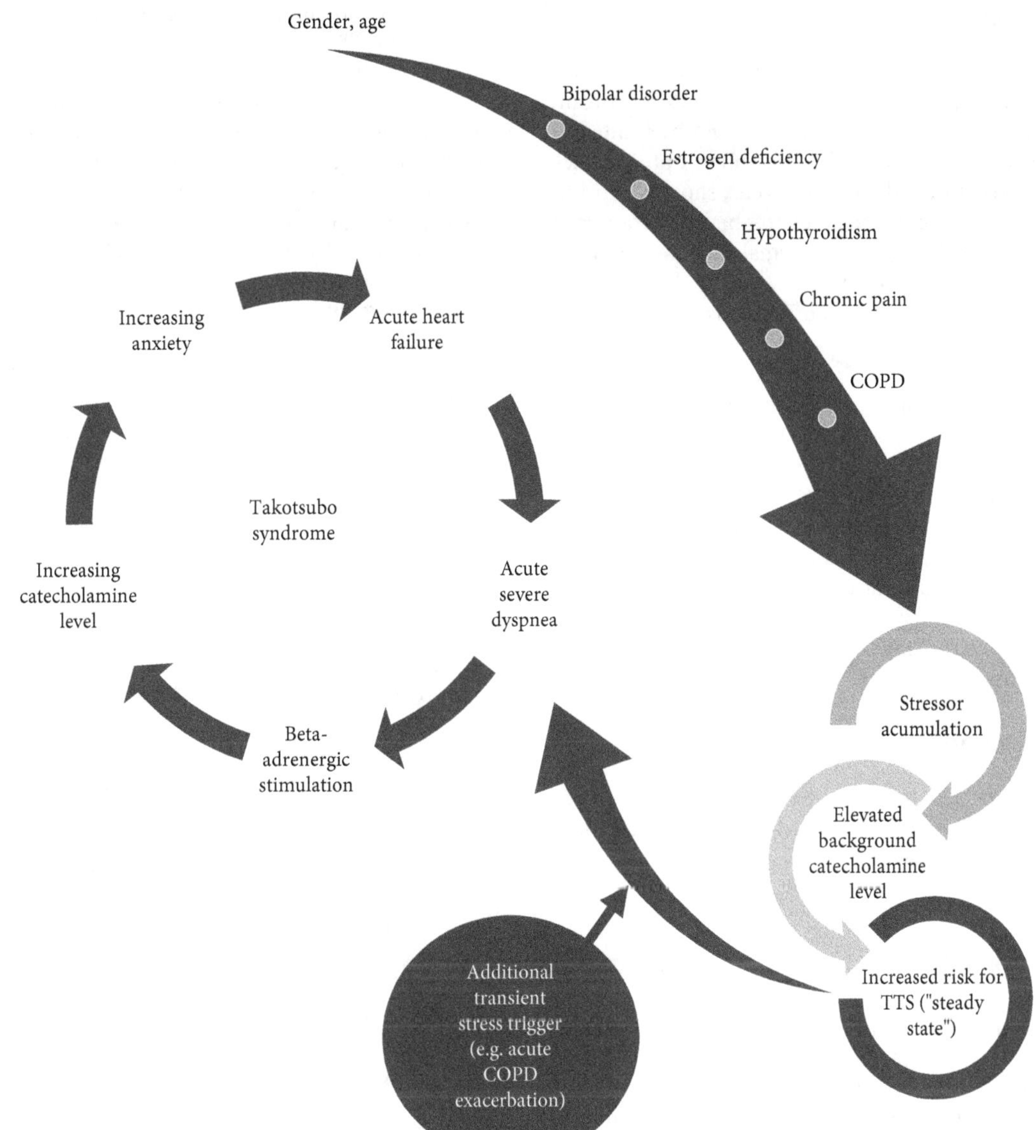

FIGURE 2: Recurrent Takotsubo syndrome in a 70-year-old female COPD patient. A 70-year-old female patient with several underlying medical and psychiatric conditions presented to the ER in 4 different occasions due to severe acute dyspnea related to acute COPD exacerbation. In all occasions, new ECG abnormalities, elevated cardiac troponin levels, and ECHO-verified acute heart failure were observed. Coronary angiography was performed without signs of coronary stenosis. COPD: chronic obstructive pulmonary disease; ECG: electrocardiogram; ER: emergency room.

with emotional stressors showed the most favorable outcome when compared to ACS patients and TTS patients secondary to physical stressors; a novel classification for TTS has also been proposed (InterTAK Classification) based on the type of triggering event [24].

Among others, physical triggers and admission LVEF < 45% are connected to adverse in-hospital outcome [3]. Moreover, a high heart rate is associated with increased mortality in TTS [39]. All these features were observed in our patient. However, common in-hospital complications, such as cardiac arrhythmias, ventricular thrombus, and cardiogenic shock were absent. On the contrary, our patient was fully recovered clinically before leaving the hospital (4 to 16 days, Table 2). Why our patient recovered rapidly is undetermined, but possibly it could be related to the main physical stressor, acute COPD exacerbation, for which there are effective therapeutic management strategies. Besides fatigue and shortness of breath, our patient does not show clinical signs related to cardiac dysfunction. These symptoms are nonspecific and could more likely be caused by her other medical conditions, specially COPD. Curiously, the HEROIC study revealed that post-TTS patients can develop a persistent, long-term heart failure phenotype in which fatigue and shortness of breath are common [40, 41]. The importance of this reported heart failure phenotype in recurrent TTS has to date not been investigated.

4. Conclusions

Acute COPD exacerbations might induce TTS in patients with concomitant psychiatric conditions and/or chronic pain. If so, the use of a beta-2 agonist should be limited or avoided in these patients and other treatment options, such as inhaled ipratropium and corticosteroids, should be prioritized. The patients might also have the benefit of an early ECHO if electrocardiographic abnormalities are observed, cardiac troponin levels are elevated, or if chest pain is described. However, "bronchogenic TTS" has been described as an atypical form of TTS, which might lack chest pain as a cardinal symptom [10].

This case report exemplifies the difficulties of the diagnosis of TTS on the onset of acute COPD exacerbation. In order to the prevent recurrence, improve acute treatment, and change the prognosis of "bronchial TTS," further research and elucidation of the involved mechanisms are demanded. Until then, the recently published InterTAK diagnostic algorithm in TTS is a promising diagnostic tool that, if it had been made available a few years earlier, could have led our patient's medical history towards an early TTS diagnosis with less morbidity and possibly less recurrence.

Acknowledgments

The authors would like to thank the patient for her written informed consent. Several (nonfundamental) facts have been changed in order to preserve the patient's anonymity.

References

[1] L. P. McGarvey, M. John, J. A. Anderson, M. Zvarich, and R. A. Wise, "Ascertainment of cause-specific mortality in COPD: operations of the TORCH Clinical Endpoint Committee," *Thorax*, vol. 62, no. 5, pp. 411–415, 2007.

[2] J. B. Soriano, A. A. Abajobir, K. H. Abate et al., "Global, regional, and national deaths, prevalence, disability-adjusted life years, and years lived with disability for chronic obstructive pulmonary disease and asthma, 1990–2015: a systematic analysis for the Global Burden of Disease Study 2015," *The Lancet Respiratory Medicine*, vol. 5, no. 9, pp. 691–706, 2017.

[3] C. Templin, J. R. Ghadri, J. Diekmann et al., "Clinical features and outcomes of Takotsubo (stress) cardiomyopathy," *The New England Journal of Medicine*, vol. 373, no. 10, pp. 929–938, 2015.

[4] J.-R. Ghadri, I. S. Wittstein, A. Prasad et al., "International expert consensus document on Takotsubo syndrome (part I): clinical characteristics, diagnostic criteria, and pathophysiology," *European Heart Journal*, vol. 39, no. 22, pp. 2032–2046, 2018.

[5] K. Kato, A. R. Lyon, J.-R. Ghadri, and C. Templin, "Takotsubo syndrome: aetiology, presentation and treatment," *Heart*, vol. 103, no. 18, pp. 1461–1469, 2017.

[6] K. Singh, K. Carson, Z. Usmani, G. Sawhney, R. Shah, and J. Horowitz, "Systematic review and meta-analysis of incidence and correlates of recurrence of takotsubo cardiomyopathy," *International Journal of Cardiology*, vol. 174, no. 3, pp. 696–701, 2014.

[7] O. S. Kotsiou, A. Douras, D. Makris, N. Mpaka, and K. I. Gourgoulianis, "Takotsubo cardiomyopathy: a known unknown foe of asthma," *The Journal of Asthma*, vol. 54, no. 8, pp. 880–886, 2017.

[8] J. R. Ghadri, R. D. Bataisou, J. Diekmann, T. F. Lüscher, and C. Templin, "First case of atypical takotsubo cardiomyopathy in a bilateral lung-transplanted patient due to acute respiratory failure," *European Heart Journal: Acute Cardiovascular Care*, vol. 4, no. 5, pp. 482–485, 2015.

[9] R. Manfredini, F. Fabbian, A. D. Giorgi et al., "Heart and lung, a dangerous liaison—tako-tsubo cardiomyopathy and respiratory diseases: a systematic review," *World Journal of Cardiology*, vol. 6, no. 5, pp. 338–344, 2014.

[10] A. Rajwani, Z. Adam, and J. A. Hall, "Bronchogenic stress cardiomyopathy: a case series," *Cardiology*, vol. 130, no. 2, pp. 106–111, 2015.

[11] J. E. Madias, ""Bronchogenic stress cardiomyopathy", a subset of Takotsubo syndrome," *Cardiology*, vol. 131, no. 3, pp. 160–160, 2015.

[12] A. Rajwani, Z. Adam, and J. A. Hall, "Authors' reply to the letter by Madias entitled "Bronchogenic stress cardiomyopathy", a subset of Takotsubo syndrome'," *Cardiology*, vol. 131, no. 3, pp. 161–161, 2015.

[13] I. Katsa, P. Christia, D. Massera, and R. Faillace, "Recurrent stress cardiomyopathy during COPD exacerbation: are beta-adrenergic agonists only to blame?," *Cureus*, vol. 9, no. 4, article e1166, 2017.

[14] I. Mendoza and G. M. Novaro, "Repeat recurrence of takotsubo cardiomyopathy related to inhaled beta-2-adrenoceptor agonists," *World Journal of Cardiology*, vol. 4, no. 6, pp. 211–213, 2012.

[15] J. R. Ghadri, M. Jaguszewski, R. Corti, T. F. Lüscher, and C. Templin, "Different wall motion patterns of three consecutive episodes of takotsubo cardiomyopathy in the same patient," *International Journal of Cardiology*, vol. 160, no. 2, pp. e25–e27, 2012.

[16] J.-R. Ghadri, I. S. Wittstein, A. Prasad et al., "International expert consensus document on Takotsubo syndrome (part II): diagnostic workup, outcome, and management," *European Heart Journal*, vol. 39, no. 22, pp. 2047–2062, 2018.

[17] I. S. Wittstein, D. R. Thiemann, J. A. C. Lima et al., "Neurohumoral features of myocardial stunning due to sudden emotional stress," *The New England Journal of Medicine*, vol. 352, no. 6, pp. 539–548, 2005.

[18] F. Pelliccia, J. C. Kaski, F. Crea, and P. G. Camici, "Pathophysiology of Takotsubo syndrome," *Circulation*, vol. 135, no. 24, pp. 2426–2441, 2017.

[19] S. Roshanzamir and R. Showkathali, "Takotsubo cardiomyopathy a short review," *Current Cardiology Reviews*, vol. 9, no. 3, pp. 191–196, 2013.

[20] T. Ueyama, K. Kasamatsu, T. Hano, Y. Tsuruo, and F. Ishikura, "Catecholamines and estrogen are involved in the pathogenesis of emotional stress-induced acute heart attack," *Annals of the New York Academy of Sciences*, vol. 1148, no. 1, pp. 479–485, 2008.

[21] P. A. Komesaroff, M. D. Esler, and K. Sudhir, "Estrogen supplementation attenuates glucocorticoid and catecholamine responses to mental stress in perimenopausal women," *The Journal of Clinical Endocrinology and Metabolism*, vol. 84, no. 2, pp. 606–610, 1999.

[22] S. Aggarwal, R. Papani, and V. Gupta, "Can thyroid break your heart? Role of thyroid in Takotsubo cardiomyopathy: a single

center retrospective study," *International Journal of Cardiology*, vol. 184, pp. 545-546, 2015.

[23] S. Aggarwal, R. Papani, and V. Gupta, "The role of thyroid in Takotsubo cardiomyopathy," *International Journal of Cardiology*, vol. 188, p. 34, 2015.

[24] J. R. Ghadri, K. Kato, V. L. Cammann et al., "Long-term prognosis of patients with Takotsubo syndrome," *Journal of the American College of Cardiology*, vol. 72, no. 8, pp. 874–882, 2018.

[25] A. R. Lyon, P. S. C. Rees, S. Prasad, P. A. Poole-Wilson, and S. E. Harding, "Stress (Takotsubo) cardiomyopathy—a novel pathophysiological hypothesis to explain catecholamine-induced acute myocardial stunning," *Nature Clinical Practice Cardiovascular Medicine*, vol. 5, pp. 22–29, 2008.

[26] F. Melão, J. P. L. Nunes, M. Vasconcelos et al., "Stress-induced cardiomyopathy associated with ipratropium bromide therapy in a patient with chronic obstructive pulmonary disease," *Revista Portuguesa de Cardiologia*, vol. 33, no. 3, pp. 175.e1–175.e4, 2014.

[27] K. A. Sluka and D. J. Clauw, "Neurobiology of fibromyalgia and chronic widespread pain," *Neuroscience*, vol. 338, pp. 114–129, 2016.

[28] R. C. Ziegelstein, "Depression and tako-tsubo cardiomyopathy," *The American Journal of Cardiology*, vol. 105, no. 2, pp. 281-282, 2010.

[29] H. Nabi, M. Hall, M. Koskenvuo et al., "Psychological and somatic symptoms of anxiety and risk of coronary heart disease: the health and social support prospective cohort study," *Biological Psychiatry*, vol. 67, no. 4, pp. 378–385, 2010.

[30] A. Dias, E. Franco, V. M. Figueredo, K. Hebert, and H. C. Quevedo, "Occurrence of Takotsubo cardiomyopathy and use of antidepressants," *International Journal of Cardiology*, vol. 174, no. 2, pp. 433–436, 2014.

[31] E. Grof, G. M. Brown, P. Grof, and G. R. Van Loon, "Effects of lithium administration on plasma catecholamines," *Psychiatry Research*, vol. 19, no. 1, pp. 87–92, 1986.

[32] M. Kitami, H. Oizumi, S. J. Kish, and Y. Furukawa, "Takotsubo cardiomyopathy associated with lithium intoxication in bipolar disorder: a case report," *Journal of Clinical Psychopharmacology*, vol. 34, no. 3, pp. 410-411, 2014.

[33] J. R. Ghadri, A. Sarcon, J. Diekmann et al., "Happy heart syndrome: role of positive emotional stress in takotsubo syndrome," *European Heart Journal*, vol. 37, no. 37, pp. 2823–2829, 2016.

[34] T. Hiestand, J. Hänggi, C. Klein et al., "Takotsubo syndrome associated with structural brain alterations of the limbic system," *Journal of the American College of Cardiology*, vol. 71, no. 7, pp. 809–811, 2018.

[35] L. Chen, Y. Wang, C. Niu et al., "Common and distinct abnormal frontal-limbic system structural and functional patterns in patients with major depression and bipolar disorder," *NeuroImage: Clinical*, vol. 20, pp. 42–50, 2018.

[36] D. E. Fleck, J. A. Welge, J. C. Eliassen, C. M. Adler, M. P. DelBello, and S. M. Strakowski, "Factor analysis of regional brain activation in bipolar and healthy individuals reveals a consistent modular structure," *Journal of Affective Disorders*, vol. 234, pp. 14–19, 2018.

[37] B. Redfors, R. Vedad, O. Angerås et al., "Mortality in takotsubo syndrome is similar to mortality in myocardial infarction - A report from the SWEDEHEART registry," *International Journal of Cardiology*, vol. 185, pp. 282–289, 2015.

[38] J. R. Ghadri, V. L. Cammann, L. C. Napp et al., "Differences in the clinical profile and outcomes of typical and atypical Takotsubo syndrome," *JAMA Cardiology*, vol. 1, no. 3, pp. 335–340, 2016.

[39] M. Böhm, V. L. Cammann, J. R. Ghadri et al., "Interaction of systolic blood pressure and resting heart rate with clinical outcomes in takotsubo syndrome: insights from the International Takotsubo Registry," *European Journal of Heart Failure*, vol. 20, no. 6, pp. 1021–1030, 2018.

[40] C. Scally, A. Rudd, A. Mezincescu et al., "Persistent long-term structural, functional, and metabolic changes after stress-induced (Takotsubo) cardiomyopathy," *Circulation*, vol. 137, no. 10, pp. 1039–1048, 2018.

[41] D. K. Dawson, "Takotsubo: the myth of rapid and complete recovery," *European Heart Journal*, vol. 39, no. 42, pp. 3762-3763, 2018.

22

The Role of Genetic Testing in the Evaluation of Dilated Cardiomyopathies

Kolade M. Agboola[1], **Trevon McGill**[2], **Barry A. Boilson**[1], **Naveen L. Pereira**[1] **and Jacob C. Jentzer**[1]

[1]*Department of Cardiovascular Medicine, Mayo Clinic College of Medicine, Rochester, MN 55905, USA*
[2]*Department of General Internal Medicine, Mayo Clinic College of Medicine, Rochester, MN 55905, USA*

Correspondence should be addressed to Jacob C. Jentzer; jentzer.jacob@mayo.edu

Academic Editor: Ertugrul Ercan

We present an adolescent African American male admitted to the cardiac intensive care unit with cardiogenic shock and acute respiratory failure. Through an overview of his presentation, diagnostic workup, and treatment, we demonstrate the clinical utility of genetic testing in the evaluation of unexplained dilated cardiomyopathies.

1. History of Presentation

Mr. A is a 19-year-old adopted African American male who presented to our cardiac intensive care unit with cardiogenic shock and acute respiratory failure requiring intubation.

The patient initially presented to an outside hospital with a several week history of chest pain and progressive shortness of breath and was hospitalized for 10 days prior to transfer. He was started on noninvasive positive-pressure ventilation for hypoxemic respiratory failure and severe acute respiratory syndrome. Coronavirus-2 (SARS-CoV-2) PCR testing was negative. He did not tolerate noninvasive ventilation, necessitating intubation and mechanical ventilation. Following intubation, he developed profound bradycardia and suffered a brief pulseless electrical activity cardiac arrest with return of spontaneous circulation after two minutes of cardiopulmonary resuscitation.

The patient was transferred to our cardiac intensive care unit while he was intubated, sedated, and supported on vasopressors. The history of present illness was provided by the patient's mother, who reported that the patient was previously relatively active and enjoyed playing sports. However, over the past few months, the patient had asked his mother for rides to the basketball court when he previously walked, and he had been bringing a chair to sit and rest on when he plays. He did not report any overt signs of shortness of breath, palpitations, or chest pain.

Initial physical examination revealed a well-developed, well-nourished young African American male without syndromic features. He was sedated with an endotracheal tube in place. Breath sounds were coarse bilaterally. Cardiovascular examination demonstrates a regular tachycardia, normal first and second heart sounds, and no appreciable murmurs or gallop. His extremities were cool to touch, and he had mild pretibial pitting edema bilaterally.

2. Past Medical History

Medical history was significant for developmental delay of unknown etiology, major depressive disorder, and anxiety. Cardiovascular risk factors include diabetes mellitus type 2 and morbid obesity. Family history was not available due to the patient's adopted status.

3. Differential Diagnosis

The range of possible etiologies for a young adult with cardiogenic shock and acute respiratory failure includes

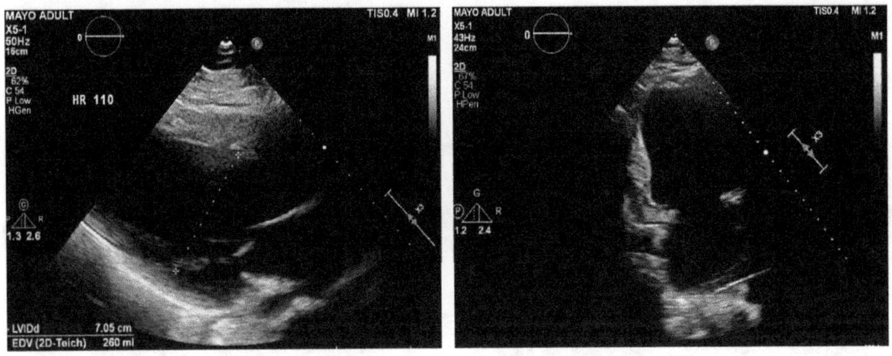

(a) (b)

Figure 1: Transthoracic echocardiogram images in the (a) parasternal long axis and (b) apical 2-chamber views demonstrating profound left ventricular dilatation, as well as left atrial enlargement.

pulmonary embolism, acute fulminant myocarditis, acute myocardial infarction triggered by drug use or spontaneous coronary dissection, and acute decompensated heart failure from cardiomyopathy.

4. Investigations

Transthoracic echocardiogram revealed a severely enlarged left ventricle with biplane ejection fraction of 20% and severe global hypokinesis (Figure 1). There was mild right ventricular chamber enlargement with mildly decreased systolic function. Cardiac troponin levels were mildly elevated, and urine drug screen was negative. The patient underwent right heart catheterization with endomyocardial biopsy. Pathology did not show evidence of myocarditis or active inflammation. Cardiac magnetic resonance imaging demonstrated a severely enlarged left ventricular chamber size with left ventricular ejection fraction 32% and global hypokinesis (Figure 2). No myocardial edema was appreciated and delayed postcontrast images revealed no late gadolinium enhancement. Viral screening for enterovirus, parvovirus B19, varicella-zoster, cytomegalovirus, herpes simplex virus-1, herpes simplex virus-2, and SARS-CoV-2 was performed, all of which were negative. Genetic testing was offered given the patient's extremely young age and the severe degree of systolic dysfunction. Sequencing using a cardiomyopathy-specific gene panel, which tests for variants within a total of 67 genes, demonstrated heterozygosity for a rare variant that was likely pathogenic involving the RBM20 gene, which encodes a splicing factor that targets multiple cardiac genes including titin. The specific variant is a single nucleotide polymorphism which replaces a cytosine nucleotide with a thymine nucleotide, resulting in a premature translational stop codon and absent or markedly disrupted protein production.

5. Management

The patient's cardiogenic shock and decompensated heart failure were managed with aggressive diuresis and intermittent inotropic support. The patient developed recurrent atrial arrhythmias and ultimately underwent atrial flutter ablation. He did not have a significant ventricular arrhythmia burden during his hospitalization. Once he was hemodynamically stable without inotropic support, guideline-directed medical therapy with a beta blocker, angiotensin receptor-neprilysin inhibitor, and aldosterone antagonist was initiated. Respiratory recovery was hindered by critical illness myopathy and prolonged intubation requiring tracheostomy placement to liberate from the ventilator.

6. Discussion

Dilated cardiomyopathy (DCM) is the second most common etiology of heart failure with reduced ejection fraction after ischemic cardiomyopathy, with an estimated prevalence of 30% to 40% of cardiomyopathies [1]. Approximately 30% to 50% of DCMs are due to familial cardiomyopathies with an identifiable genetic cause found in up to 40% of these, and genetically determined DCM is perhaps the single most common cause of DCM [1]. However, our understanding of the underlying genetic mechanisms of DCM remains poorly understood and underexplored. Although there is now great ability to test for genetic variants with whole exome or genome sequencing, the clinical significance of findings and associated phenotypes is often unknown.

RNA binding motif 20 (RBM20) is a splicing factor responsible for alternative splicing of several proteins expressed within cardiomyocytes, including the sarcomeric protein titin [2]. Truncating variations in the gene encoding titin are among the most common genetic causes of DCM and can be seen in 10 to 20 percent of patients with DCM [3]. Additionally, RBM20 controls splicing of many proteins involved in intracellular calcium handling, thereby leading to a propensity for ventricular arrhythmia in the setting of abnormal RBM20 function [4]. There are specific exons in which genetic variation has been demonstrated to be particularly deleterious. For example, transcription errors in exons 9 and 10 are associated with high penetrance of cardiomyopathy with a high arrhythmia burden, including atrial and ventricular tachyarrhythmias [4]. Animal models with RBM20 knockout mice have demonstrated increased intracellular calcium levels and increased sarcoplasmic reticulum calcium content compared to wild-type controls; these findings are also seen with heterozygous loss of RBM20 [5].

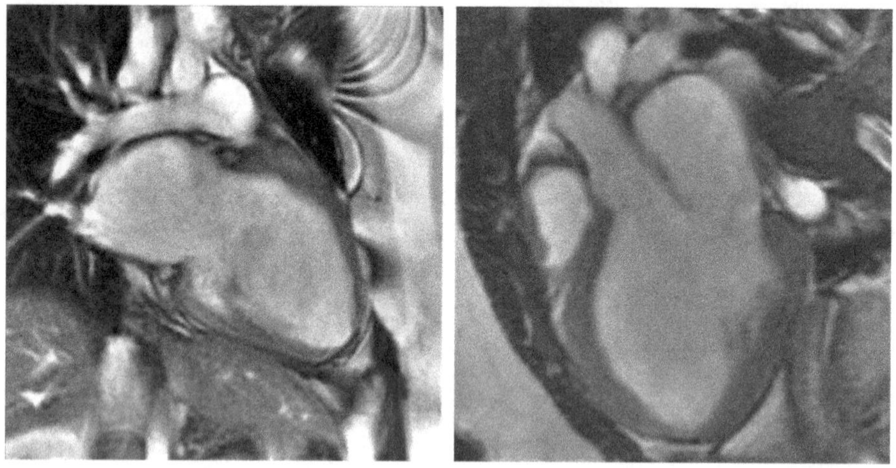

Figure 2: Cardiac magnetic resonance imaging video clips depicting severe left ventricular enlargement and markedly reduced left ventricular systolic function.

A similar phenotype is observed among humans with RBM20 genetic variation. A database study of DCM patients reveals a relatively younger age at diagnosis among individuals with a RBM20 variant. Additionally, patients with RBM20-associated cardiomyopathy are more likely to endorse a family history of DCM, suggesting a high degree of penetrance associated with this specific variant. Of note, a family history of sudden cardiac death was reported in 51% of RBM20 registry patients [4]. An increased burden of arrhythmia including atrial fibrillation, nonsustained ventricular tachycardia, and ventricular tachycardia necessitating implantable cardioverter-defibrillator (ICD) placement has been described among RBM20 DCM patients [4].

Interestingly, we present a patient ultimately found to have a genetic variant involving exon 2 of RBM20 who presents with an aggressive DCM accompanied by significant atrial arrhythmias, requiring catheter ablation. Pathogenic variations in exons 6-9 of RBM20 have previously been identified in individuals with DCM [6]. However, to the best of our knowledge, variants in the exon 2 gene have not previously been characterized as penetrant with regard to DCM and arrhythmia.

7. Conclusion

We present the case of an adolescent male presenting with new acute decompensated DCM resulting in cardiogenic shock. With rapid advances in genetic medicine and the availability of genetic diagnostics, providers can more readily integrate genetic testing into clinical practice. This case demonstrates the utility of genetic testing in the evaluation and treatment of DCM. With the use of such advances, we are now able to better characterize and understand the underlying genetic mechanisms of heart failure thus offering a molecular diagnosis to patients with DCM. Furthermore, understanding the role of genetics in DCM will ultimately allow for enhanced familial counseling, prognostication, and treatment for patients in addition to providing insights into normal cardiac function [7]. Identification of potentially arrhythmogenic genetic variants associated with DCM may facilitate decision-making regarding ICD implantation or the use of a wearable defibrillator in the early postdiagnosis period. As in our case due to the high arrhythmia risk conferred by his specific genetic variant, the patient was outfitted with a LifeVest wearable defibrillator prior to discharge. Although this practice is not recommended in the management guidelines for patients with RMB20 variants, we felt it was reasonable to recommend as the patient's true arrhythmia burden was unknown at the time of discharge. Future research will be needed to better characterize the divergent natural history of genetically determined DCM as a function of the affected gene and specific mutation, to help clinicians predict which patients may develop progressive or end-stage heart failure requiring early consideration for transplant.

8. Learning Objectives

(1) To understand the significance of genetics in idiopathic nonischemic cardiomyopathy

(2) To investigate the implication of RNA binding motif 20 variations in the pathogenesis of dilated cardiomyopathy

(3) To demonstrate the benefit and utility of genetic testing in the evaluation and treatment of individuals with idiopathic dilated cardiomyopathy

Additional Points

Tweet. Check out our case report demonstrating the utility of genetic testing in individuals with dilated cardiomyopathies and its implications on patient management.

Acknowledgments

A special thank you to all the contributing authors, as well as all the individuals that participated in the care of the patient discussed in our case. Additionally, we would not be able to provide this exceptional level of care without the support of our institution, Mayo Clinic Rochester. Lastly, we would like to thank the patient and his family for allowing us to share their story in the hope of advancing the field of medicine and science.

References

[1] E. M. McNally and L. Mestroni, "Dilated cardiomyopathy: genetic determinants and mechanisms," *Circulation Research*, vol. 121, no. 7, pp. 731–748, 2017.

[2] W. Guo, S. Schafer, M. L. Greaser et al., "RBM20, a gene for hereditary cardiomyopathy, regulates titin splicing," *Nature Medicine*, vol. 18, no. 5, pp. 766–773, 2012.

[3] U. Tayal, S. Newsome, R. Buchan et al., "Phenotype and clinical outcomes of titin cardiomyopathy," *Journal of the American College of Cardiology*, vol. 70, no. 18, pp. 2264–2274, 2017.

[4] V. N. Parikh, C. Caleshu, C. Reuter et al., "Regional variation in RBM20 causes a highly penetrant arrhythmogenic cardiomyopathy," *Circulation: Heart Failure*, vol. 12, no. 3, article e005371, 2019.

[5] M. M. G. van den Hoogenhof, A. Beqqali, A. S. Amin et al., "RBM20 mutations induce an arrhythmogenic dilated cardiomyopathy related to disturbed calcium handling," *Circulation*, vol. 138, no. 13, pp. 1330–1342, 2018.

[6] M. M. Refaat, S. A. Lubitz, S. Makino et al., "Genetic variation in the alternative splicing regulator RBM20 is associated with dilated cardiomyopathy," *Heart Rhythm*, vol. 9, no. 3, pp. 390–396, 2012.

[7] A. N. Rosenbaum, K. E. Agre, and N. L. Pereira, "Genetics of dilated cardiomyopathy: practical implications for heart failure management," *Nature Reviews Cardiology*, vol. 17, no. 5, pp. 286–297, 2020.

23

Profound Iron Deficiency Anemia and Irreversible Dilated Cardiomyopathy in a Child

Samuel G. Wittekind,[1,2] Hugo R. Martinez,[1] Chet Villa,[1,2] Matthew Bacon,[1,2] Adrienne M. Hammill,[2,3] and Angela Lorts[1,2]

[1]*Cincinnati Children's Hospital Medical Center, Heart Institute, Cincinnati, OH, USA*
[2]*Department of Pediatrics, University of Cincinnati College of Medicine, Cincinnati, OH, USA*
[3]*Cincinnati Children's Hospital Medical Center, Division of Hematology, Cincinnati, OH, USA*

Correspondence should be addressed to Samuel G. Wittekind; samuel.wittekind@cchmc.org
Academic Editor: Kathleen Ngu

Iron deficiency anemia has been associated with a secondary and potentially reversible cardiomyopathy. The pathophysiologic paradigm has been that the hematologic disease begets cardiac dysfunction. There may be, however, a point at which myocardial injury is irreversible in susceptible individuals. We present the case of a 4-year-old, developmentally normal, child who presented with iron deficiency anemia and a dilated cardiomyopathy with congestive heart failure. Despite appropriate correction of the anemia, the patient developed decompensated heart failure requiring milrinone therapy and eventual heart transplantation. This report will alert clinicians to the potential for irreversible adverse cardiac remodeling and the importance of close pediatric cardiology consultation and serial assessment in order to implement appropriate heart failure therapy.

1. Introduction

Anemia is highly prevalent in heart failure (HF) and is associated with increased morbidity in adults and children [1–3]. Iron deficiency anemia, in particular, has been implicated in the development of a secondary cardiomyopathy [4, 5] though a definitive pathogenesis has not been identified. Mechanisms linking anemia and HF might include (1) hemodilution in the setting of high-output HF, (2) elevated sympathetic tone, (3) impaired oxygen delivery and myocardial oxygen extraction, (4) renal dysfunction, and (5) poor dietary intake of micronutrients essential for myocardial function. Previous reports of high-output HF reversing with correction of the iron deficiency anemia [4, 5] are encouraging; however, such recovery should not be assumed. We present the case of a young child with severe anemia and cardiac dysfunction to highlight the diagnostic challenge of determining causation versus association. We also highlight the vital importance of differentiating high- and low-output HF states in this setting since they can change over time with major treatment implications.

2. Case Presentation

A previously healthy 4-year-old, 14 kg boy presented to the emergency department with several days of malaise, pallor, and tachypnea. He had a brief febrile illness one week prior to the onset of these symptoms. He was found to have severe microcytic anemia (hemoglobin 1.9 g/dL, MCV 46.4 fL) with iron deficiency (reticulocyte 4.4%, ferritin 1.1 ng/mL, iron 8 mg/dL, and RDW 35.3%) and normal micronutrient levels otherwise including selenium. Due to a poor appetite for solid food that began one year earlier, he was favoring liquids and was drinking roughly 60 fluid ounces per day of cow's milk. There was no evidence of gastrointestinal blood loss. On physical exam, he was developmentally appropriate, well perfused, and had signs of congestive HF including pitting edema of the lower extremities. The initial transthoracic echocardiogram

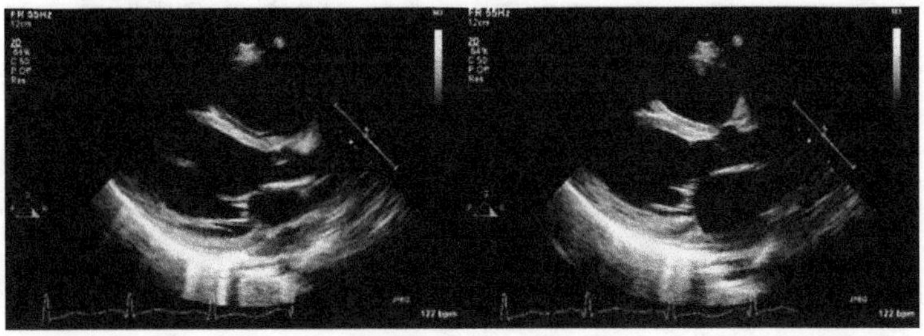

(a)

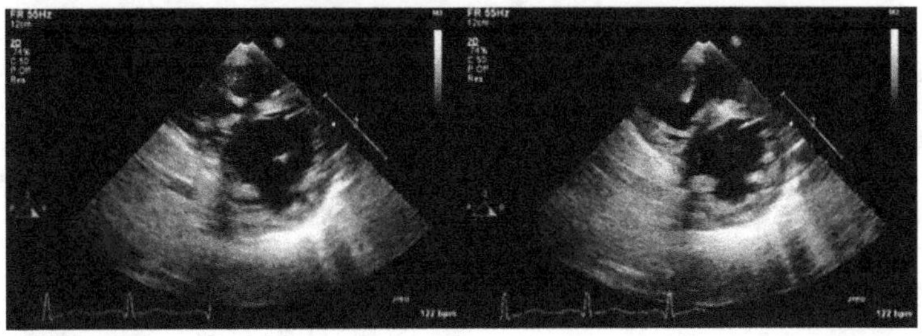

(b)

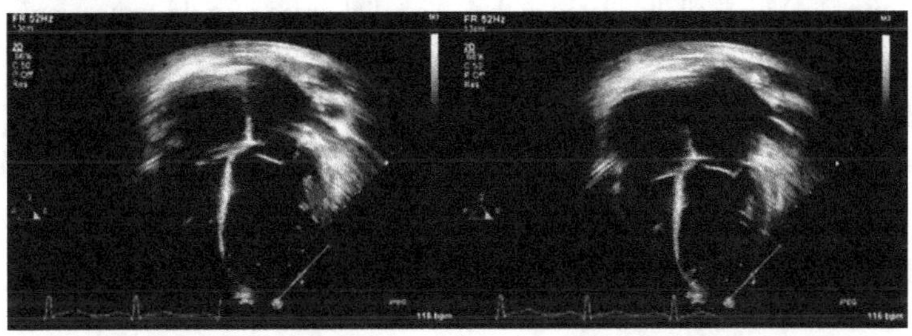

(c)

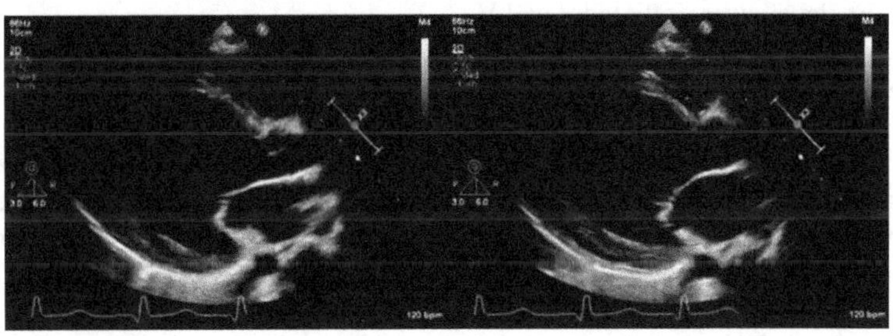

(d)

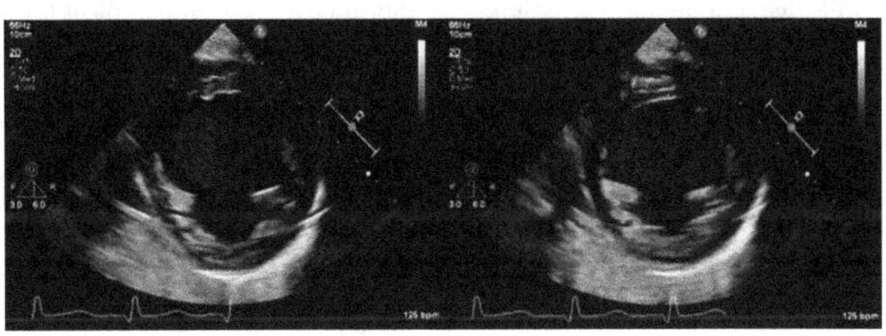

(e)

FIGURE 1: Continued.

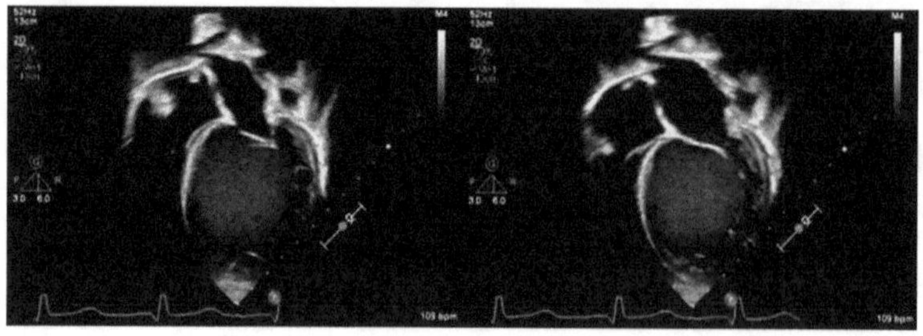

(f)

Figure 1: Transthoracic echocardiography (TTE) demonstrating LV size and systolic function at initial presentation (a–c) and 4 months later on milrinone therapy awaiting heart transplantation (d–f). The heart became progressively more dilated and dysfunctional over time. (a) Parasternal long axis view (PLAX) at end-diastole (left) and end-systole (right). (b) Parasternal short axis (PSAX) view at end-diastole (left) and end-systole (right). (c) Apical 4-chamber (A4C) view at end-diastole (left) and end-systole (right). (d) PLAX view at end-diastole (left) and end-systole (right). (e) PSAX view at end-diastole (left) and end-systole (right). (f) A4C view at end-diastole (left) and end-systole (right).

revealed a dilated left ventricle (LV) (LVEDD 4.61 cm, z-score + 5.85) with moderate LV systolic dysfunction (LVEF 33%). In addition, the left atrium (LA) was mildly dilated with an indexed volume of 39.5 mL/m^2 (normal < 30 mL/m^2), and there was mild mitral regurgitation (MR). A 12-lead ECG demonstrated sinus rhythm with left ventricular hypertrophy; there was no arrhythmia on telemetry. He was transfused with packed red blood cells over two days to a hemoglobin of 8.5 g/dL along with furosemide to prevent transfusion-related circulatory overload and given a replacement dose of intravenous iron dextran followed by supplemental oral ferrous sulfate. His appetite improved dramatically with correction of the anemia. Enalapril was initiated for LV reverse remodeling which he tolerated well. Screening for the common viral etiologies of myocarditis by serum PCR testing was negative. Given that he had not seen a primary care provider since he was 18 months of age, the patient was discharged home with wraparound services and close follow-up with hematology and cardiology. The discharge diagnosis was cow's milk-induced iron deficiency anemia with associated cardiac dysfunction.

The patient returned to the cardiology clinic 2 weeks later with signs of worsening congestive HF including fatigue, abdominal discomfort with decreased appetite, weight up 2 kg, liver edge 4 cm below the right costal margin, a serum B-type natriuretic peptide of 9,724 pg/mL, and a low mixed venous oxygen saturation. The echocardiogram demonstrated signs of worsening dilated cardiomyopathy (DCM) including an indexed LA volume 78.9 ml/m^2, LVEDD 4.96 cm (z-score + 6.66 H), LVEF 15%, and moderate MR. The hemoglobin had normalized to 12.3 g/dL by this time. He was admitted for intravenous diuretics and milrinone infusion for decompensated, low-output HF. Over a period of 2 months, he remained symptomatic, the LV further dilated without an improvement in systolic function, and he developed signs of congestive hepatopathy. Serial echocardiographic images demonstrating the progressive LV dilation are shown in Figure 1. Milrinone therapy was continued while he was listed status 1B for heart transplantation. He received an orthotopic heart transplant 2 months after listing (4.5 months after initial presentation) with an excellent outcome.

Histopathology on the explanted heart showed essentially normal appearing myocardial fibers with patchy, subendocardial areas of mild hypertrophy. There was no suggestion of myocardial fiber disarray, interstitial fibrosis, storage disorder, or inflammation. Electron microscopy demonstrated normal myocardial ultrastructure with no evidence of mitochondriopathy. Genetic testing for 47 genes implicated in DCM (Invitae, San Francisco, CA) was negative for known pathologic variants. Echocardiographic screenings of first-degree relatives have been negative to date.

3. Discussion

There are unique features of this case that challenge the pathophysiologic paradigm of iron deficiency itself leading to cardiac dysfunction. Firstly, his age at presentation makes him an outlier for the cow's milk-induced iron deficiency anemia commonly seen in toddlers between the ages of 1 and 3 years [6]. The chronic refusal of solid foods may have been a symptom of HF as it is well known that feeding difficulties and associated abdominal discomfort are often how HF presents in children [7]. Next, the LV was considerably dilated at presentation beyond what is typical for iron deficiency cardiomyopathy. Additionally, the LA was dilated at the time which is evidence of chronically elevated LV filling pressure [8]. Finally, there was rapid disease progression to the point of requiring advanced HF therapies after appropriate correction of the anemia. Notably, the lack of impressive histopathologic findings as well as the negative gene panel is common in pediatric DCM [9] and should not be taken as strong evidence against a primary cardiomyopathy. It seems most likely from the available evidence that iron deficiency anemia and DCM progressed in tandem and compounded each other in this case.

This case highlights the importance of regular pediatric primary care visits to review diet and screen for anemia in high-risk patients [6]. To our knowledge, this is the first report of a patient requiring advanced HF therapy despite appropriate correction of profound iron deficiency anemia. An expectation that the heart will recover may not be valid in all cases; there may be a "point of no return" in this type of cardiomyopathy. Furthermore, suspicion for a primary cardiomyopathy should be heightened when the heart is significantly dilated and dysfunctional at presentation since there are major prognostic and treatment implications. After correction of the anemia in this clinical scenario, close pediatric cardiology consultation and serial assessment of cardiac function can identify decompensation and promptly institute life-saving HF therapy when needed.

Abbreviations

DCM: Dilated cardiomyopathy
HF: Heart failure
kg: Kilogram
LA: Left atrium
LV: Left ventricle
LVEDD: Left ventricular end-diastolic diameter
LVEF: Left ventricular ejection fraction
MCV: Mean corpuscular volume
MR: Mitral regurgitation
RDW: Red cell distribution width.

Acknowledgments

We acknowledge Anita Gupta, MD, for her consultation regarding interpretation of the myocardial pathology specimens.

References

[1] J. F. Goldberg, M. D. Shah, P. F. Kantor et al., "Prevalence and severity of anemia in children hospitalized with acute heart failure," *Congenital Heart Disease*, vol. 11, no. 6, pp. 622–629, 2016.

[2] D. Higgins, J. Otero, C. Jefferis Kirk et al., "Iron laboratory studies in pediatric patients with heart failure from dilated cardiomyopathy," *The American Journal of Cardiology*, vol. 120, no. 11, pp. 2049–2055, 2017.

[3] G. C. Mueller, E. L. Schlueter, F. Arndt, A. Dodge-Khatami, J. Weil, and T. S. Mir, "Prevalence of anemia in children with congestive heart failure due to dilated cardiomyopathy," *International Journal Of Pediatrics*, vol. 2012, Article ID 452909, 4 pages, 2012.

[4] N. Hegde, M. W. Rich, and C. Gayomali, "The cardiomyopathy of iron deficiency," *Texas Heart Institute Journal*, vol. 33, no. 3, pp. 340–344, 2006.

[5] G. Doros, A. M. Ardelean, A. Popoiu, C. Olariu, R. Stroescu, and M. Gafencu, "*GP78 Dilated cardiomyopathy with ross iii heart failure induced by severe iron deficiency anaemia post long term cow milk excess*," BMJ Publishing Group Ltd, 2019.

[6] R. D. Baker and F. R. Greer, "Clinical report - diagnosis and prevention of iron deficiency and iron-deficiency anemia in infants and young children (0-3 years of age)," *Pediatrics*, vol. 2010-2576, 2010.

[7] R. Kirk, A. I. Dipchand, D. N. Rosenthal et al., "The International Society for Heart and Lung Transplantation Guidelines for the management of pediatric heart failure: executive summary," *The Journal of Heart and Lung Transplantation*, vol. 33, no. 9, pp. 888–909, 2014.

[8] A. Rossi, M. Cicoira, L. Zanolla et al., "Determinants and prognostic value of left atrial volume in patients with dilated cardiomyopathy," *Journal of the American College of Cardiology*, vol. 40, no. 8, pp. 1425–1430, 2002.

[9] J. A. Towbin, A. M. Lowe, S. D. Colan et al., "Incidence, causes, and outcomes of dilated cardiomyopathy in children," *JAMA*, vol. 296, no. 15, pp. 1867–1876, 2006.

24

105 Inappropriate ICD Shocks in a Patient with Dilated Cardiomyopathy and Broca's Aphasia

Christian Georgi, Michael Neuß, Viviane Möller, Martin Seifert, and Christian Butter

Heart Center Brandenburg-Department of Cardiology and Medical School Brandenburg Theodor Fontane, Bernau bei Berlin, Germany

Correspondence should be addressed to Christian Georgi; c.georgi@immanuel.de

Academic Editor: Hajime Kataoka

With a growing number of ICD recipients, device complications are seen more frequently in the clinical setting and outpatient departments. Among the most severe are ICD infections and inappropriate therapies caused by oversensing of atrial tachycardias or lead fracture. We report on a 76-year-old female patient with dilative cardiomyopathy and Broca's aphasia after stroke, who experienced 105 consecutive inappropriate ICD shocks due to cluster missensing of her fractured ICD lead. The diagnosis was complicated and delayed by patient's aphasia emphasizing the need for intensified remote monitoring along with regular in-person visits, especially in people with intellectual or communication disabilities.

1. Introduction

The implantable cardioverter-defibrillator (ICD) has been proven to be an effective therapy in the primary and secondary prevention of sudden cardiac death [1].

Yet inappropriate ICD therapies, mainly due to oversensing or SVTs, remain a great problem in device therapy. A lately published meta-analysis reports of inappropriate therapies in around 10% of patients with ICDs within the first year after implantation [2]. It is well known that ICD shocks, both appropriate and inappropriate, have a negative impact on morbidity and mortality [3, 4].

Beyond mortality rates, ICD shocks, especially inappropriate therapies, are found to cause a decline in the quality of life and reduced daily activity and increased general anxiety in postshock patients [5].

A reduction of inappropriate therapies therefore should be achieved by intensive treatment of the underlying disease, optimal ICD programming, and close monitoring of patients at high risk.

In this context, remote monitoring (RM) is a promising complement to conventional in-clinic follow-ups with the potential to dramatically reduce inappropriate therapies [6], although structural deficits concerning data overload, functional responsibility, and imprecise workflows need to be improved. In particular, for people in rural areas, in patients with impaired mobility or mental status, RM offers the chance for improved safety and quality of life. So far, remote control has not been fully implemented in the follow-up of ICD patients in Northern America and Europe, though [7].

We report on an aphasic patient with more than one hundred inappropriate shocks within a few hours that could have been prevented by more frequent expert consultations and connecting her to a remote monitoring program.

2. Case Report

A 76-year-old female patient was admitted to our emergency department early in the morning with suspected acute coronary syndrome. The patient had suffered from a major stroke causing Broca's aphasia three months prior to this admission and was referred to us from a nearby neurorehabilitation clinic. Initial ECG showed no signs of acute ischemia, but troponin I levels were about 1000-fold elevated. History taking was complicated by patient's aphasia, but she did not appear to be in acute pain at the time of admission.

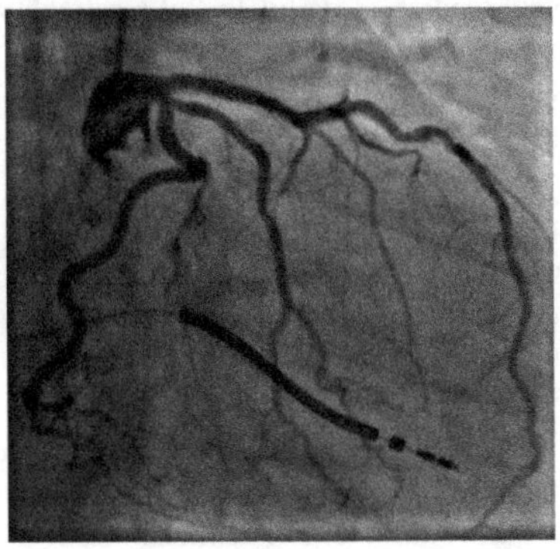

FIGURE 1: Angiogram of the patient coronaries showing no culprit lesion or significant stenosis.

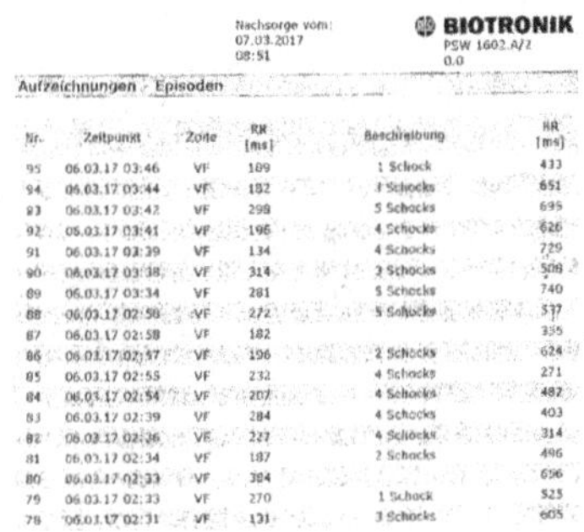

Nachsorge vom: 07.03.2017 08:51 — BIOTRONIK PSW 1602.A/2 0.0

Aufzeichnungen - Episoden

Nr.	Zeitpunkt	Zone	RR [ms]	Beschreibung	RR [ms]
95	06.03.17 03:46	VF	189	1 Schock	433
94	06.03.17 03:44	VF	182	[illegible] Schocks	651
93	06.03.17 03:42	VF	298	5 Schocks	695
92	06.03.17 03:41	VF	196	4 Schocks	626
91	06.03.17 03:39	VF	134	4 Schocks	729
90	06.03.17 03:38	VF	314	3 Schocks	508
89	06.03.17 03:34	VF	281	5 Schocks	740
88	06.03.17 02:58	VF	272	5 Schocks	537
87	06.03.17 02:58	VF	182		355
86	06.03.17 02:57	VF	196	2 Schocks	624
85	06.03.17 02:55	VF	232	4 Schocks	271
84	06.03.17 02:54	VF	207	4 Schocks	482
83	06.03.17 02:39	VF	284	4 Schocks	403
82	06.03.17 02:36	VF	227	4 Schocks	314
81	06.03.17 02:34	VF	187	2 Schocks	496
80	06.03.17 02:33	VF	384		696
79	06.03.17 02:33	VF	270	1 Schock	525
78	06.03.17 02:31	VF	131	3 Schocks	605

FIGURE 2: Last page of the ICD memory showing 54 shocks in 1:15 h.

With a history of heart failure and an implanted single-chamber ICD, the patient was brought to the catheter lab to undergo coronary angiogram, where no culprit lesion could be detected (Figure 1).

In a phone consultation with the rehab clinic's doctor in charge, he described how the patient had multiple episodes of acute chest and back pain with "electrical twitches" for the course of several hours during the past night. Pain medication was administered and the pain interpreted as musculoskeletal but no other diagnostic or therapeutic steps were taken. Eventually, in the morning, a troponin test was done and found positive, so the patient was referred.

Subsequently, we performed an ICD interrogation, which revealed an EOS (end of service) status and multiple inappropriate ICD therapies in the time between 00:07 AM and 03:46 AM until the battery of the Biotronik ICD was depleted and the device eventually stopped antitachycardia therapy. In summary, the patient suffered 105 consecutive inappropriate ICD shocks within 219 minutes (Figure 2), to our knowledge, the highest shock incidence in such a short period of time. The shocks were caused by cluster missensing on her right ventricular lead (Figure 3), presumably resulting from an insulation defect near the header. Further episodes of oversensing due to clusters could be seen over the preceding five months, occasionally followed by antitachycardia pacing but no shock therapy.

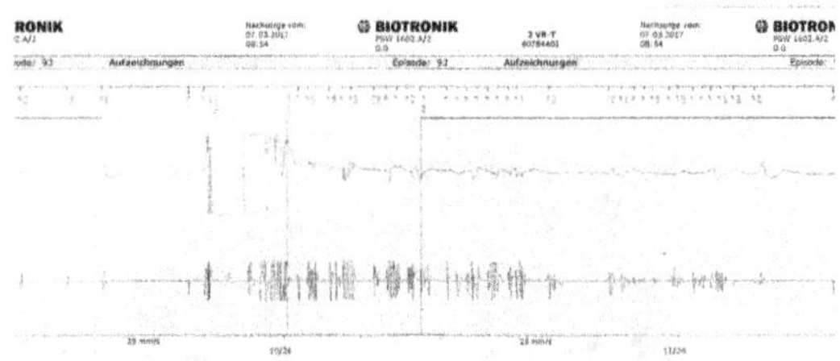

FIGURE 3: Inappropriate shock. Typical high-frequency signals (cluster) in the PS channel indicating a lead insulation problem.

The ICD was implanted in 2008 and exchanged for EOL (end of life) in 2015. The last ambulatory interrogation was in September 2016, just before the first episodes of cluster missensing occurred. The next appointment was scheduled for March 2017 but postponed due to the prolonged hospital stay after apoplexy. The technical analysis of the explanted ICD did not show any technical abnormalities; the chest X-ray revealed no sign of lead fracture.

After discussing the case with patient's family, the defective lead was disconnected, and at the request of the patient and her family, a new ICD and lead were implanted and the patient enrolled in our remote monitoring program.

3. Discussion

Since the first transvenous ICD was implanted in 1980 [8], there is a steadily growing number of ICD implantations and patients with long-lasting devices [9]. In the year 2023, there is an estimated 1.4 million pacemaker and ICD implantations worldwide [10]. Simultaneously, the lead- and generator-associated complications increased over the last years. Lead-associated complications include thrombosis and infection as well as fracture and insulation problems with the risk of inappropriate therapies. From large clinical trials, we know that about 5-20% of patients with ICDs receive inappropriate therapy, mainly due to the missensing of supraventricular arrhythmias, oversensing of external noise, or lead fracture/insulation defects [4]. The psychological impact of inappropriate ICD shocks was investigated in several studies. Among the most frequent side effects are anxiety disorders, posttraumatic stress disorders, panic attacks, depression, nightmare, and insomnia [11].

This case demonstrates possible pitfalls of ICD supply in elderly or handicapped people. The inability of the patient to communicate properly and missing awareness of the staff led to the dreadful course of events. The suspected short circuit between the lead and the scorched battery (Figure 4) might have reduced the current delivered to the whole body and weakened the pain; still the delay in therapy was unnecessary and avoidable. Immediate ECG monitoring would have helped to discover the cause for shock delivery and could have led to shock suppression by simply applying a magnet.

Retrospectively, the earlier access to remote monitoring could have prevented the massive amount of shocks, since the first asymptomatic cluster episodes could be detected

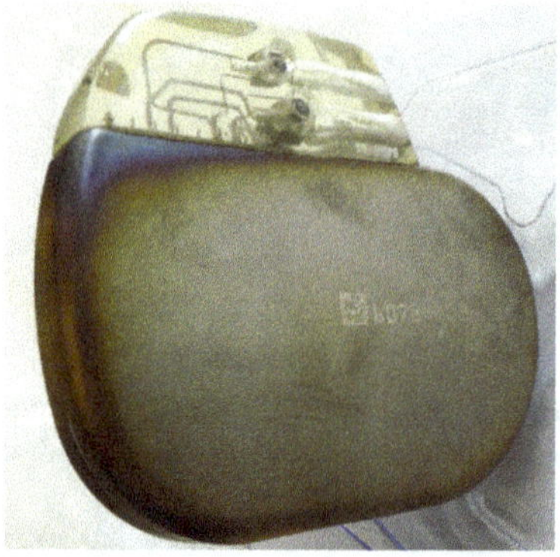

Figure 4: Scorched battery of the Biotronik ICD (Iforia 3 VR and Linox SD lead) due to an assumed lead insulation defect near the header.

already some months before the incident described. A significant reduction of the "first-incidence-to-action time" through remote monitoring has been described by many authors [12–14]. The TRUST study demonstrated a median delay of 1 day from occurrence of the event to physician evaluation, compared to 1 month with conventional follow-up [15]. They also confirmed a cost benefit from an economical perspective. Still the need for additional manpower to analyze the huge amount of data, legal issues, and lack of standardization remain open problems [16].

4. Conclusion

Regular in-person visits with cardiologists remain the foundation of appropriate ICD follow-up. Remote monitoring programs, though, are a very useful tool to supplement conventional follow-up and should be established whenever suitable. The transmission of technical data to experts is known to be very effective to detect early malfunctions of implantable devices as ICDs and pacemakers. This clearly helps to avoid inappropriate therapies, detects lead and battery problems, and discovers atrial fibrillation or other arrhythmias.

An increasing number of patients with ICDs, pacemakers, and CRTs require sufficient manpower and technical resources to guarantee high-quality monitoring. Moreover, further training programs for outpatient departments and GPs should be installed since there is a significant lack of knowledge concerning ICD function and troubleshooting.

References

[1] C. M. Tracy, A. E. Epstein, D. Darbar et al., "2012 ACCF/AHA/HRS focused update of the 2008 guidelines for device-based therapy of cardiac rhythm abnormalities: a report of the American College of Cardiology Foundation/American Heart Association Task Force on Practice Guidelines," *Heart rhythm*, vol. 9, no. 10, pp. 1737–1753, 2012.

[2] I. Basu-Ray, J. Liu, X. Jia et al., "Subcutaneous versus transvenous implantable defibrillator therapy: a meta-analysis of case-control studies," *JACC: Clinical Electrophysiology*, vol. 3, no. 13, pp. 1475–1483, 2017.

[3] J. E. Poole, G. W. Johnson, A. S. Hellkamp et al., "Prognostic importance of defibrillator shocks in patients with heart failure," *The New England Journal of Medicine*, vol. 359, no. 10, pp. 1009–1017, 2008.

[4] A. J. Moss, C. Schuger, C. A. Beck et al., "Reduction in inappropriate therapy and mortality through ICD programming," *The New England Journal of Medicine*, vol. 367, no. 24, pp. 2275–2283, 2012.

[5] S. F. Sears, L. Rosman, S. Sasaki et al., "Defibrillator shocks and their effect on objective and subjective patient outcomes: results of the PainFree SST clinical trial," *Heart rhythm*, vol. 15, no. 5, pp. 734–740, 2018.

[6] S. Ploux, C. D. Swerdlow, M. Strik et al., "Towards eradication of inappropriate therapies for ICD lead failure by combining comprehensive remote monitoring and lead noise alerts," *Journal of cardiovascular electrophysiology*, vol. 29, no. 8, pp. 1125–1134, 2018.

[7] R. Ganeshan, A. D. Enriquez, and J. V. Freeman, "Remote monitoring of implantable cardiac devices: current state and future directions," *Current opinion in cardiology*, vol. 33, no. 1, pp. 20–30, 2018.

[8] M. Mirowski, P. R. Reid, M. M. Mower et al., "Termination of malignant ventricular arrhythmias with an implanted automatic defibrillator in human beings," *The New England Journal of Medicine*, vol. 303, no. 6, pp. 322–324, 1980.

[9] M. J. Raatikainen, D. O. Arnar, K. Zeppenfeld et al., "Statistics on the use of cardiac electronic devices and electrophysiological procedures in the European Society of Cardiology countries: 2014 report from the European Heart Rhythm Association," *EP Europace*, vol. 17, Supplement 1, pp. i1–75, 2015.

[10] M. Jager, C. Jordan, A. Theilmeier et al., "Lumbar-load analysis of manual patient-handling activities for biomechanical overload prevention among healthcare workers," *The Annals of occupational hygiene*, vol. 57, no. 4, pp. 528–544, 2013.

[11] J. Jordan, G. Titscher, L. Peregrinova, and H. Kirsch, "Manual for the psychotherapeutic treatment of acute and post-traumatic stress disorders following multiple shocks from implantable cardioverter defibrillator (ICD)," *GMS Psycho-Social-Medicine*, vol. 10, article Doc09, 2013.

[12] A. Lazarus, "Remote, wireless, ambulatory monitoring of implantable pacemakers, cardioverter defibrillators, and cardiac resynchronization therapy systems: analysis of a worldwide database," *Pacing and clinical electrophysiology*, vol. 30, Supplement 1, pp. S2–S12, 2007.

[13] S. Spencker, N. Coban, L. Koch, A. Schirdewan, and D. Muller, "Potential role of home monitoring to reduce inappropriate shocks in implantable cardioverter-defibrillator patients due to lead failure," *EP Europace*, vol. 11, no. 4, pp. 483–488, 2009.

[14] L. Guedon-Moreau, D. Lacroix, N. Sadoul et al., "A randomized study of remote follow-up of implantable cardioverter defibrillators: safety and efficacy report of the ECOST trial," *European Heart Journal*, vol. 34, no. 8, pp. 605–614, 2013.

[15] N. Varma, A. E. Epstein, A. Irimpen, R. Schweikert, C. Love, and TRUST Investigators, "Efficacy and safety of automatic remote monitoring for implantable cardioverter-defibrillator follow-up: the Lumos-T Safely Reduces Routine Office Device Follow-up (TRUST) trial," *Circulation*, vol. 122, no. 4, pp. 325–332, 2010.

[16] M. Bertini, L. Marcantoni, T. Toselli, and R. Ferrari, "Remote monitoring of implantable devices: should we continue to ignore it?," *International Journal of Cardiology*, vol. 202, pp. 368–377, 2016.

25

Role of Cardiac Magnetic Resonance in Detecting Biventricular Apical Hypertrophic Cardiomyopathy

Nathan Zaher,[1] Hammam Shereef,[2] Rashid Al Hussain,[1] John Dawdy,[3] Diane Levine,[1] and M. Chadi Alraies[3]

[1]Department of Internal Medicine, Wayne State University/Detroit Medical Center, Michigan, USA
[2]Department of Internal Medicine, Beaumont Hospital-Dearborn, Michigan, USA
[3]Division of Cardiology, Wayne State University/Detroit Medical Center, Michigan, USA

Correspondence should be addressed to Hammam Shereef; hammam.shereef@beaumont.org

Academic Editor: Luigi Sciarra

Apical Hypertrophic Cardiomyopathy (ApHCM) is a rare variant of hypertrophic cardiomyopathy with a low prevalence in the general population. ApHCM with right ventricular involvement (BiApHCM) is largely unreported and may not be detected with conventional transthoracic echocardiogram (TTE) alone. Cardiac Magnetic Resonance (CMR) has been demonstrated to be a proficient imaging modality to diagnose BiApHCM. We present a case of BiApHCM that was diagnosed with TTE and further characterized by CMR. This imaging modality may be utilized more in the future to help diagnose and detect the prevalence of BiApHCM.

1. Introduction

Apical Hypertrophic Cardiomyopathy (ApHCM) is a rare variant of hypertrophic cardiomyopathy involving the left ventricle. ApHCM with right ventricular (RV) involvement (BiApHCM) is largely unreported and may not be detected with transthoracic echocardiogram (TTE). Cardiac Magnetic Resonance Imaging (C-MRI) has superior sensitivity and provides additional important details related to cardiac thickness and function. We herein present a case of BiApHCM that was diagnosed with TTE and further characterized by C-MRI. This imaging modality provides superior quality and may be considered for screening purposes in appropriately selected patients with clinically suggestive findings and negative echocardiograms. It has also been shown to be a better determinate of LV wall thickness which has a significant impact on management decisions and patient outcomes.

2. Case Description

A 55-year-old man presented to the Emergency Department (ED) with palpitations, shortness of breath, and nonexertional pleuritic chest pain and was found to be in atrial fibrillation. His vitals were stable, and there was a systolic grade 3/6 murmur loudest at the left sternal border on physical exam. A 12-lead EKG was obtained and revealed underlying atrial fibrillation rhythm with increased voltage criteria of left ventricular hypertrophy and right bundle branch block with RSR pattern in V2 and V4 (Figure 1). A TTE was ordered and demonstrated hyperdynamic systolic function and exuberant apical hypertrophy with right ventricular involvement (Figure 2). Offline longitudinal strain analysis was performed at appropriate frame rates and was consistent with BiApHCM (Figure 3). A C-MRI, without and with contrast, demonstrated nonobstructive cardiomyopathy with RV thickening (Figures 4–6). The thickening was pronounced

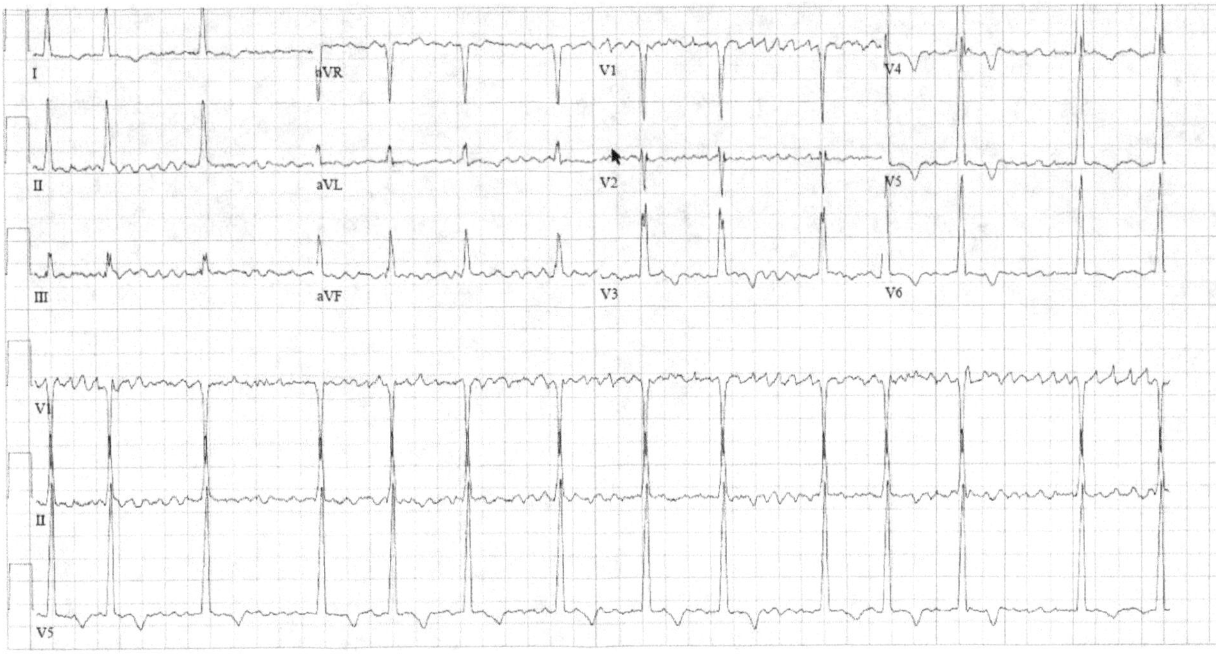

FIGURE 1: 12-lead EKG showed absence of *P* wave, baseline fibrillary waves, increased LVH by Sokolow-Lyon criteria, and RSR pattern in V2 and V3.

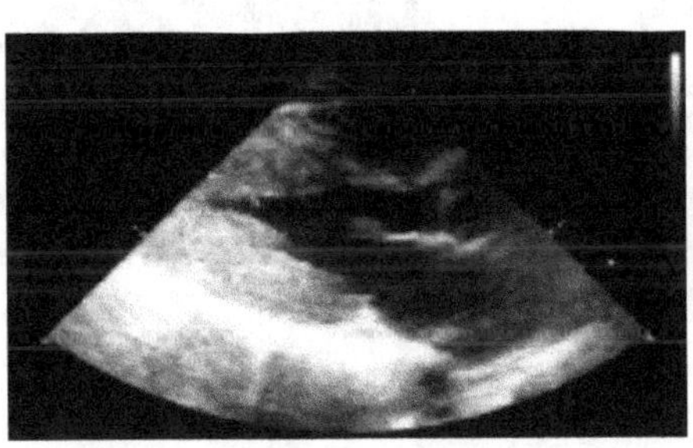

(a)

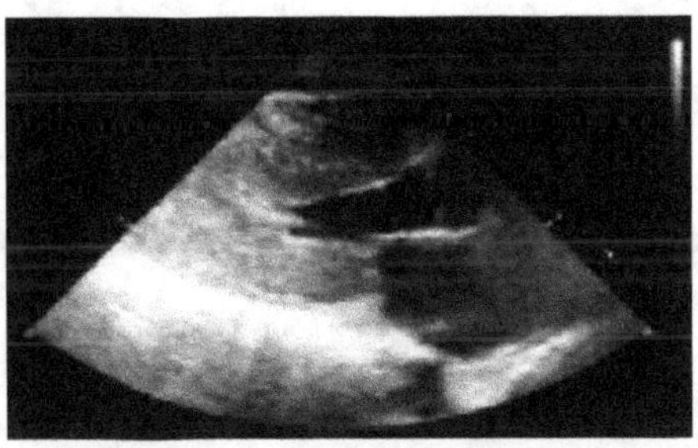

(b)

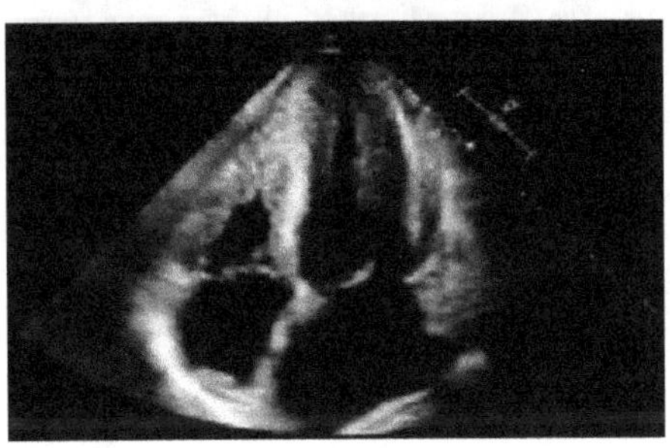

(c)

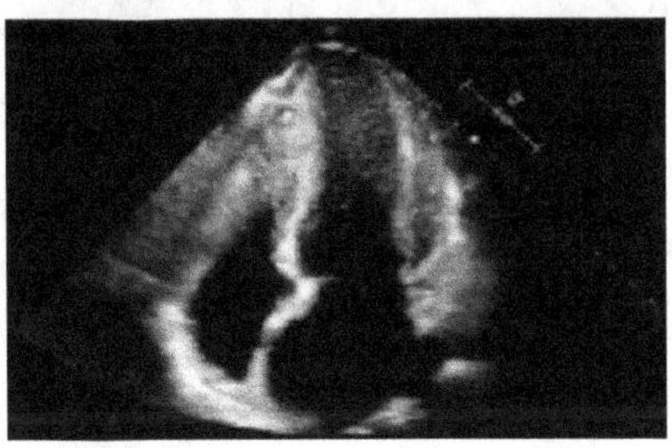

(d)

FIGURE 2: 2D echocardiography parasternal long-axis view in diastole (a) and systole (b) along with apical 4-chamber view in diastole (c) and systole (d) showing apical hypertrophy in both left and right ventricles (first attachment).

in the midapical area with a wall measurement of 6.5 + 1.3 mm at the midapical segment. The patient was managed with metoprolol both for rate control of atrial fibrillation and to maximize diastolic filling time and cardiac output. He was instructed to follow-up as an outpatient for genotyping/cascade screening.

3. Discussion

Apical Hypertrophic Cardiomyopathy (ApHCM), a rare form of HCM, manifests as hypertrophy of the left ventricular apex and has nonobstructive physiology. Research has found sarcomere mutations can cause apical hypertrophy,

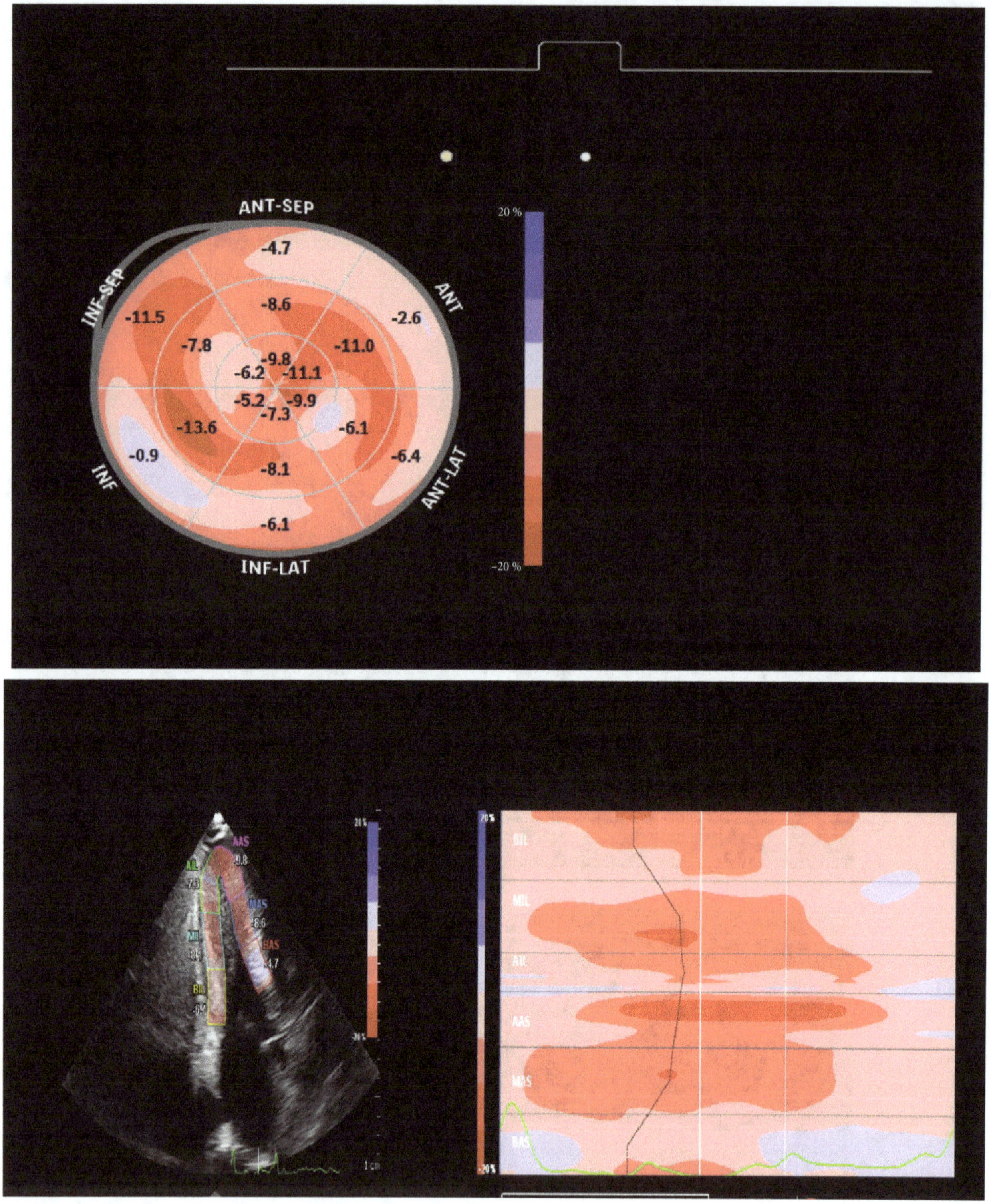

FIGURE 3: The longitudinal strain bull's eye plot showing concentric hypertrophy and normal EF is characterized by a mildly reduced average global and prominently reduced longitudinal strain of multiple nine segments.

such as the cardiac actin Glu101Lys [1]. The apical variant is most commonly seen in the Japanese population with a report of 15-25% prevalence in documented case series of HCM, in comparison to only 3% of patients with HCM in the general population [2]. Diagnostic studies include left ventriculography, contrast transthoracic echocardiogram (TTE), Computed-Tomography (CT), and Cardiovascular Magnetic Resonance (CMR) [3].

Obstruction in BiApHCM is due to midsystolic contact of the prominent RV muscle bundles in the RV outflow tract.

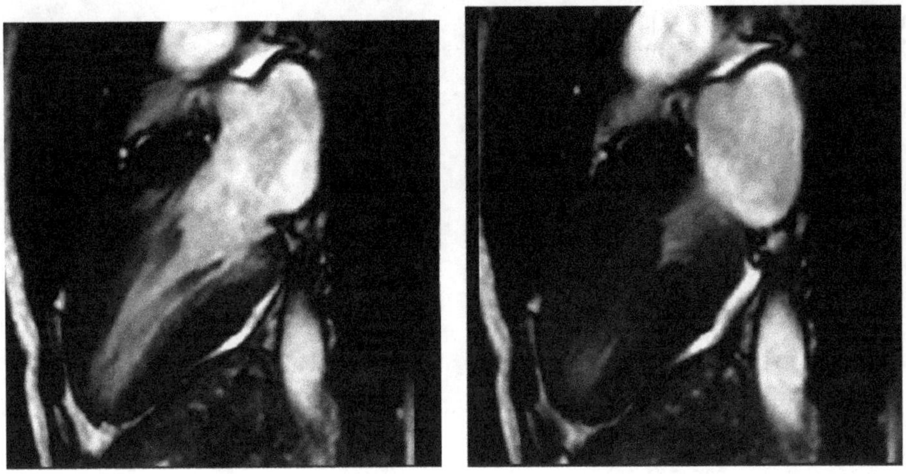

(a) (b)

FIGURE 4: (a) Severe concentric left ventricular hypertrophy with focal maximum thickness of myocardium 20 mm in the mid anterior wall. (b) Globally hyperdynamic left ventricular systolic function with calculated LV EF 80% and near obliteration of mid and distal segments in systole.

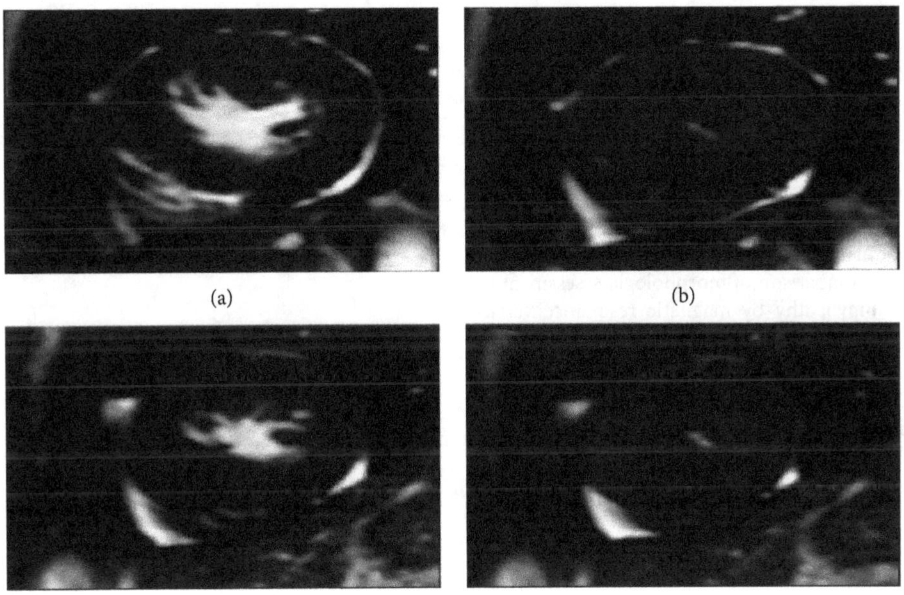

(a) (b) (c) (d)

FIGURE 5: MRI short-axis view showing mid-LV chamber at the end of diastole (a) with obliteration of cavity in end systole (b). MRI short-axis view showing apex in end diastole (c) with obliteration of cavity in systole (d). Hypertrophy can be appreciated in both the left and right ventricles.

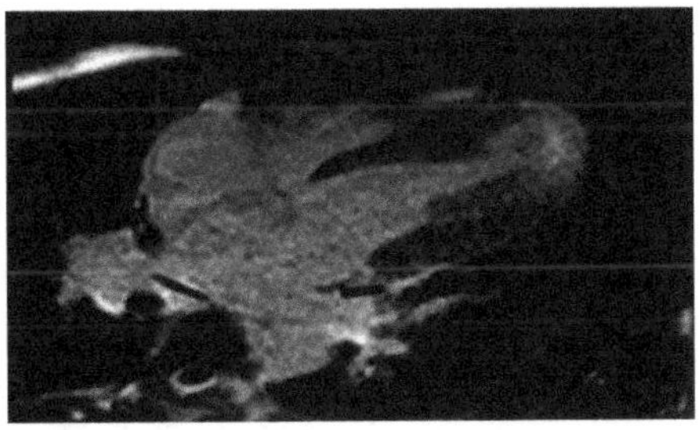

FIGURE 6: A 4-chamber long axis inversion recovery showing late gadolinium enhancement in the apex.

Patient presentation and approach to treatment in BiApHCM are similar to that of left-sided ApHCM. First-line therapy is an AV nodal blocking agent. Those who remain symptomatic can be offered resection of accessory RV muscles in the outflow tract [4, 5]. Despite being the most sensitive and accurate imaging modality for BiApHCM, C-MRI has not been widely obtained due to cost-related limitations [6]. One study involving 330 myocardial segments showed that thickness could be measured by echocardiography in 221 (67%) vs. 320 (97%) with C-MRI. Reliance on routine echocardiography as the sole imaging modality to rule out ApHCM has led to underreporting of this condition with potentially suboptimal outcomes [7]. This is also of important clinical significance as patients with massive LVH (>30 mm) are often considered high risk and should be considered for ICD therapy [8].

References

[1] M. Arad, M. Penas-Lado, L. Monserrat et al., "Gene mutations in apical hypertrophic cardiomyopathy," *Circulation*, vol. 112, no. 18, pp. 2805–2811, 2005.

[2] A. M. H. Ho, P. T. Chui, A. P. W. Lee, and S. Wan, "Hypertrophic cardiomyopathy apical variant," *Cleveland Clinic Journal of Medicine*, vol. 81, no. 9, pp. 517–519, 2014.

[3] T. Doctorian, W. J. Mosley, and B. Do, "Apical hypertrophic cardiomyopathy: case report and literature review," *American Journal of Case Reports*, vol. 18, pp. 525–528, 2017.

[4] H. Sanoussi, N. Kourireche, L. Oukerraj, and M. Cherti, "Right ventricle outflow obstruction in biventricular hypertrophic cardiomyopathy in amyloidosis," 2017, https://www.ejcrim.com/index.php/EJCRIM/article/view/733.

[5] X. Guo, C. Fan, L. Tian, and Y. Liu, "Abstract 12176: outcomes and genetic characteristics of hypertrophic cardiomyopathy with severe right ventricular hypertrophy," 2017, https://www.ahajournals.org/doi/abs/10.1161/circ.132.suppl_3.1217.

[6] S. Cardozo, ""International+Journal+of+Cardiology'[Jour] - PubMed - NCBI." National Center for Biotechnology Information, U.S. National Library of Medicine," 2016, http://www.ncbi.nlm.nih.gov/pubmed?term=International+journal+of+cardiology[Jour]&cmd=detailssearch.

[7] G. Pons-Lladó, F. Carreras, X. Borrás, J. Palmer, J. Llauger, and A. Bayés de Luna, "Comparison of morphologic assessment of hypertrophic cardiomyopathy by magnetic resonance versus echocardiographic imaging," *The American Journal of Cardiology*, vol. 79, no. 12, pp. 1651–1656, 1997.

[8] M. S. Maron, I. Olivotto, S. Betocchi et al., "Effect of left ventricular outflow tract obstruction on clinical outcome in hypertrophic Cardiomyopathy," *New England Journal of Medicine*, vol. 348, no. 4, pp. 295–303, 2003.

26

Takotsubo Cardiomyopathy in Dextrocardia with Situs Inversus

A. Ganes and L. Segan

Department of Cardiology, Barwon Health, Bellerine Street, Geelong, VIC 3220, Australia

Correspondence should be addressed to A. Ganes; anand.ganes@barwonhealth.org.au

Academic Editor: Kathleen Ngu

Takotsubo cardiomyopathy (TTC) is an acute reversible form of left ventricular (LV) systolic dysfunction extending beyond a coronary artery vascular territory usually due to physical or psychological stressors. Dextrocardia with situs inversus is a rare embryologic anomaly whereby the heart and aorta are mirrored on the contralateral side. We describe a case of a 93-year-old female with dextrocardia who presented with chest pain, atrial fibrillation with rapid ventricular response, and transient inferior ST elevation. Coronary angiography demonstrated an eccentric mid right coronary artery (RCA) lesion and apical ballooning consistent with concurrent takotsubo cardiomyopathy (TTC). To our knowledge, this is the first reported case of this dual pathology in a patient with dextrocardia, highlighting the procedural and diagnostic complexity in the setting of a rare anatomicvariant.

1. Introduction

Takotsubo cardiomyopathy (TTC) is an acute reversible form of symmetrical left ventricular systolic dysfunction extending beyond a coronary artery vascular territory, often occurring in postmenopausal women and frequently in the context of physical or psychological stressors [1, 2]. It is a recognised acute coronary syndrome (ACS)mimic, accounting for 2 % of ACS presentations [3]. While the aetiology of this condition is incompletely understood, it is believed to be precipitated by an increase in the level of circulating plasma catecholamines [1]. Historically, the diagnosis was made during coronary angiography in the absence of obstructive coronary artery disease (OCAD); however, the coexistence of TTC and OCAD is increasingly recognised [4–7].

We present a rare case of simultaneous TTC and OCAD in a patient with situs inversus dextrocardia, reinforcing that the presence of OCAD should not preclude a diagnosis of TTC. Moreover, the coexistence of TTC and OCAD in a patient with situs inversus dextrocardia raises unique diagnostic and procedural challenges not previously described.

2. Case Description

A 93-year-old female with known situs inversus dextrocardia presented with chest pain, increased work of breathing and a productive cough for the preceding 24 hrs. She was tachypnoeic (respiratory rate of 30 breaths per minute), hypoxic (oxygen saturation of 88% on room air), and in atrial fibrillation (AF) with rapid ventricular response. She was normotensive and afebrile. She had dual heart sounds with no murmurs and coarse crepitations in right upper and lower lung fields. Her admission ECG demonstrated inferior ST-segment elevation (Figure 1) in the setting of AF with rapid ventricular response. Her ECG had hallmark features of dextrocardia (loss of praecordial R wave progression and a dominant S wave). Chest X-ray demonstrated multifocal pneumonia and a rightward-facing cardiac apex, a right-sided aortic arch, and a right-sided gastric bubble consistent with situs inversus dextrocardia (Figure 2). Laboratory investigations revealed an acute inflammatory process with elevated neutrophil count ($16.3 \times 10^9 cells/L$), C-reactive protein (CRP 293 mg/L) and subsequent sputum culture detecting *Haemophilus Influenzae*. Initial Troponin I was elevated (0.74 μg/L), which incremented to 4.25 μg/L after

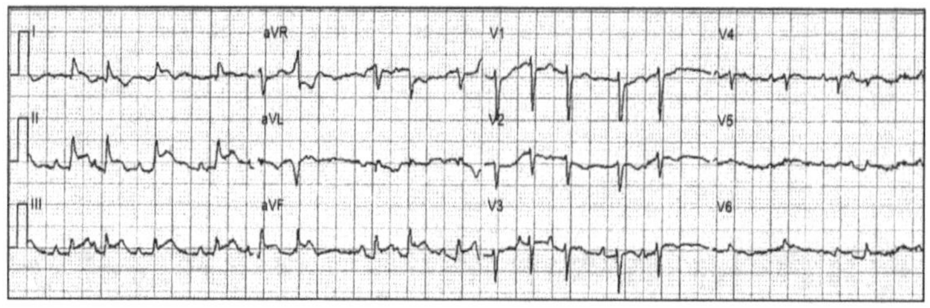

FIGURE 1: Admission standard 12-lead electrocardiogram (ECG) demonstrating inferior ST elevation, atrial fibrillation with rapid ventricular response, and features associated with dextrocardia (loss of praecordial R wave progression, dominant praecordial S wave).

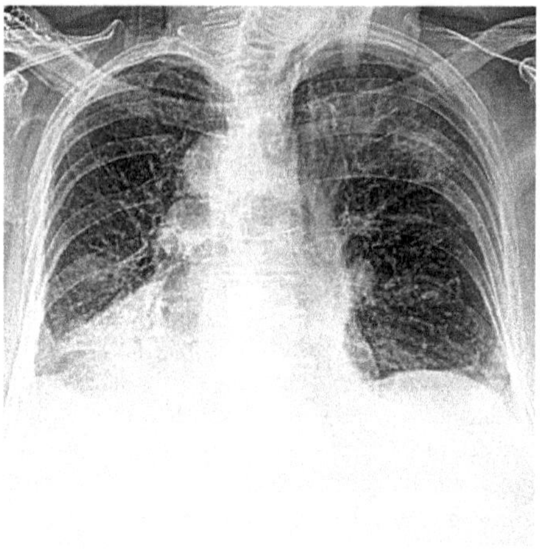

FIGURE 2: Chest X-ray demonstrating multifocal pneumonia, right-sided aortic arch, cardiac silhouette, and gastric bubble.

6 hours (normal range <0.05 μg/L). Coronary angiography demonstrated an eccentric mid-RCA stenosis (Figure 3(a)) with mild bystander disease. The RCA originated from the left coronary cusp and was engaged with a traditional Judkins Right 4.0 catheter with conventional angiographic image acquisition. The left coronary system (arising from the right coronary cusp) was engaged using a Judkins left 3.5 diagnostic catheter using traditional angiographic angulation. She spontaneously reverted to sinus rhythm at the time of angiography, with resolution of chest discomfort and ECG changes (Supplementary Figure 1). Left ventriculography demonstrated symmetrical apical ballooning with basal sparing consistent with an apical-variant TTC (Figure 3(b)). A decision was made against intervention as the RCA lesion was deemed high risk, the symptoms had resolved with recovery of sinus rhythm and the finding of TTC. Apical modified transthoracic echocardiography (TTE) confirmed severe hypokinesis of the apical segments consistent with left ventriculography. Guideline-directed pharmacotherapy was initiated including an Angiotensin-Converting Enzyme Inhibitor (ACEi) and beta-blocker. Intravenous antibiotics were administered for 48 hours and then de-escalated to oral therapy for multifocal pneumonia with interval improvement in chest X-ray and inflammatory markers (Supplementary Table 1). She was transferred to a subacute rehabilitation unit following a protracted medical admission.

3. Discussion

Situs inversus dextrocardia is a rare congenital condition whereby the internal viscera are mirrored to the contralateral side, with an estimated prevalence of <0.0001% in the general population [8, 9]. Undertaking cardiac investigations in the setting of anatomical variations is challenging, requiring careful consideration of impact on diagnostic accuracy and interpretation. Dextrocardia is identified on a standard 12-lead ECG by hallmark features including dominant S waves in praecordial leads with poor R wave progression, right axis deviation, T wave inversion in lead I and a VL and a positive QRS complex in aVR [10]. Right-sided ECG is recommended to aid in interpretation of the praecordial leads [11]. In our case, the right-sided ECG demonstrated appropriate R wave progression in the praecordial leads (Supplementary Figure 1).

ECG findings in TTC and OCAD are often indistinguishable [12] with invasive angiography being the gold standard diagnostic tool [13]. This is further complicated by marked anatomic variation, requiring careful consideration of procedural technique, equipment, and image acquisition to formulate a diagnosis. Literature regarding the approach to invasive coronary angiography insitus inversus dextrocardia is variable, describing a limited user experience with catheter selection, catheter engagement strategy, and modified image acquisition techniques, including mirror image fluoroscopic views and double inversion techniques [14–18]. Acquiring adequate TTE images is also extremely challenging and requires contralateral imaging with a mirror-image technique [19].

Historically, the Mayo Clinic Framework guidelines dictated that a diagnosis of TTC could not be made in the presence of OCAD [20]. Recent literature recognises an increasing incidence of dual pathology in a proportion of presentations, suggesting that these conditions are not mutually exclusive [20–23] and this enhanced understanding is now reflected in contemporary literature [23, 24].

In this case, TTC appeared to be triggered by a combination of pneumonia, tachyarrhythmia, and underlying coronary artery disease. The decision not to intervene on the RCA lesion was made on the basis of multiple physical stressors likely leading to demand ischaemia within a fixed stenosis, with complete symptom and electrographic resolution following the restoration of sinus rhythm. TTC was also likely a consequence of systemic illness and haemodynamic stress.

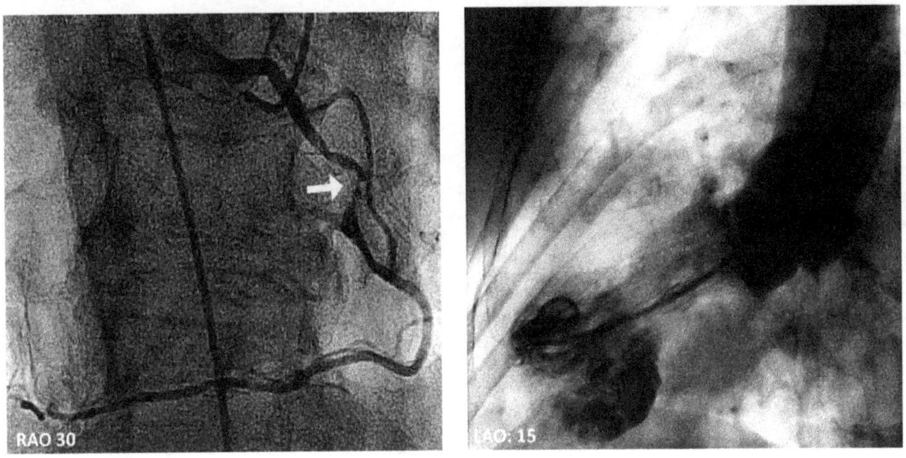

FIGURE 3: (a) Coronary angiography demonstrating RCA arising from left coronary cusp with an eccentric mid-RCA stenosis (depicted by white arrow). (b) Left ventriculography demonstrating apical ballooning in keeping with TTC.

In cases with coexistent TTC and OCAD, the diagnosis can be clarified with the use of cardiac MRI whereby TTC and myocardial ischaemia have distinctly different characteristics [25].

4. Conclusion

We describe a patient with situs inversus dextrocardia presenting with TTC and concurrent OCAD. This case highlights that the presence of coronary artery disease should not preclude a diagnosis of TTC in the appropriate context and the procedural and diagnostic complexities of recognising dual pathology in the setting of situs inversus dextrocardia.

Supplementary Materials

Supplementary Figure 1. (a) Right-sided ECG depicting inferior STE with reciprocal T wave inversion in I, a VL leads. (b) Standard ECG after resolution of atrial fibrillation and inferior ST segment elevation. Supplementary Table 1: trend of biochemistry from admission to discharge. Elevated biochemistry findings are underlined. *(Supplementary Materials)*

References

[1] I. S. Wittstein, D. R. Thiemann, J. A. C. Lima et al., "Neurohumoral features of myocardial stunning due to sudden emotional stress," *The New England Journal of Medicine*, vol. 352, no. 6, pp. 539–548, 2005.

[2] J. Abraham, J. O. Mudd, N. Kapur, K. Klein, H. C. Champion, and I. S. Wittstein, "Stress cardiomyopathy after intravenous administration of catecholamines and beta-receptor agonists," *Journal of the American College of Cardiology*, vol. 53, no. 15, pp. 1320–1325, 2009.

[3] K. Komamura, M. Fukui, T. Iwasaku, S. Hirotani, and T. Masuyama, "Takotsubo cardiomyopathy: pathophysiology, diagnosis and treatment," *World Journal of Cardiology*, vol. 6, no. 7, pp. 602–609, 2014.

[4] D. Haghi, T. Papavassiliu, K. Hamm, J. J. Kaden, M. Borggrefe, and T. Suselbeck, "Coronary artery disease in takotsubo cardiomyopathy," *Circulation Journal*, vol. 71, no. 7, pp. 1092–1094, 2007.

[5] C. Henriquez, R. Landau, N. Sabharwal et al., "Unusual Sequence of Events in a Case of Takotsubo Syndrome," *Case Reports in Cardiology*, vol. 2018, Article ID 5498052, 3 pages, 2018.

[6] N. Mencer, L. T. Justice, W. Black, and K. Litton, "A Rare Case of Takotsubo Syndrome and Acute Coronary Syndrome of the Right Coronary Artery," *Case Reports in Cardiology*, vol. 2019, Article ID 9128273, 4 pages, 2019.

[7] S. W. Sharkey, A. Kalra, T. D. Henry et al., "Coexistence of acute takotsubo syndrome and acute coronary syndrome," *Catheterization & Cardiovascular Interventions*, 2019.

[8] G. Supriya, S. Saritha, and S. Madan, "Situs inversus totalis–a case report," *IOSR Journal of Applied Physics*, vol. 3, no. 6, pp. 2278–4861, 2013.

[9] C. M. Bohun, J. E. Potts, B. M. Casey, and G. G. S. Sandor, "A population-based study of cardiac malformations and outcomes associated with dextrocardia," *American Journal of Cardiology*, vol. 100, no. 2, pp. 305–309, 2007.

[10] T. Tanawuttiwat, S. Vasaiwala, and M. Dia, "Mirror Mirror," *The American Journal of Medicine*, vol. 123, no. 1, pp. 34–36, 2010.

[11] P. Kligfield, L. S. Gettes, J. J. Bailey et al., "Recommendations for the standardization and interpretation of the electrocardiogram: part I: the electrocardiogram and its technology a scientific statement from the American Heart Association Electrocardiography and Arrhythmias Committee, Council on Clinical Cardiology; the American College of Cardiology Foundation; and the Heart Rhythm Society endorsed by the International Society for Computerized Electrocardiology," *Journal of the American College of Cardiology*, vol. 49, no. 10, pp. 1109–1127, 2007.

[12] J. Namgung, "Electrocardiographic findings in takotsubo cardiomyopathy: ECG evolution and its difference from the ECG of acute coronary syndrome," *Clinical Medicine Insights: Cardiology*, vol. 8, pp. 29–34, 2014.

[13] J.-R. Ghadri, I. S. Wittstein, A. Prasad et al., "International expert consensus document on Takotsubo syndrome (part II): diagnostic workup, outcome, and management," *European Heart Journal*, vol. 39, no. 22, pp. 2047–2062, 2018.

[14] H.-S. Lo, M.-L. Chen, P.-C. Chou, and H.-C. Chiou, "Successful percutaneous coronary intervention in a patient with dextrocardia and situs inversus," *Acta Cardiologica Sinica*, vol. 20, no. 3, pp. 191–196, 2004.

[15] N. Kakouros, S. J. Patel, S. Redwood, and B. S. Wasan, "Triple-vessel percutaneous coronary revascularization in situs inversus dextrocardia," *Cardiology Research and Practice*, vol. 2010, Article ID 606327, 4 pages, 2010.

[16] P. K. Goel and N. Moorthy, "Trans-radial primary percutaneous coronary intervention in dextrocardia using double inversion technique," *Journal of Cardiology Cases*, vol. 8, no. 1, pp. e31–e33, 2013.

[17] G. J. Sinner, B. George, and A. W. Messerli, "Transradial approach to coronary angiography and percutaneous intervention in patients with dextrocardia," *The Journal of Invasive Cardiology*, vol. 31, no. 5, pp. E83–E88, 2019.

[18] P. K. Goel, "Double-inversion technique for coronary angiography viewing in dextrocardia," *Catheterization and Cardiovascular Interventions*, vol. 66, no. 2, pp. 281–285, 2005.

[19] Y. Li, R. Liu, and X. Zhang, "Dextrocardia: why significant left-axis deviation?," *Circulation*, vol. 136, no. 17, pp. 1662–1664, 2017.

[20] K. A. Bybee, T. Kara, A. Prasad et al., "Systematic review: transient left ventricular apical ballooning: a syndrome that mimics ST-segment elevation myocardial infarction," *Annals of Internal Medicine*, vol. 141, no. 11, pp. 858–865, 2004.

[21] C. E. Alfonso, "Takotsubo cardiomyopathy and coronary artery disease: a meaningful coincidence?," *Journal of the American Heart Association*, vol. 5, no. 12, article e005131, 2016.

[22] J. E. Madias, "Why the current diagnostic criteria of Takotsubo syndrome are outmoded: A proposal for new criteria," *International Journal of Cardiology*, vol. 174, no. 3, pp. 468–470, 2014.

[23] A. Prasad, A. Lerman, and C. S. Rihal, "Apical ballooning syndrome (Tako-Tsubo or stress cardiomyopathy): a mimic of acute myocardial infarction," *American Heart Journal*, vol. 155, no. 3, pp. 408–417, 2008.

[24] J.-R. Ghadri, I. S. Wittstein, A. Prasad et al., "International Expert Consensus Document on Takotsubo Syndrome (Part I): Clinical Characteristics, Diagnostic Criteria, and Pathophysiology," *European Heart Journal*, vol. 39, no. 22, pp. 2032–2046, 2018.

[25] I. Eitel, F. von Knobelsdorff-Brenkenhoff, P. Bernhardt et al., "Clinical characteristics and cardiovascular magnetic resonance findings in stress (takotsubo) cardiomyopathy," *Journal of the American Medical Association*, vol. 306, no. 3, pp. 277–286, 2011.

27

Recurrence of LV Thrombus in a Patient with Severe Ischaemic Cardiomyopathy Anticoagulated with Apixaban

Azhar Farooqui,[1,2] **Tin Lwin**,[1,3] **Daniel Costa**,[1] **Simon Hetherington**,[1,4] **and Raj Mattu**[1,5]

[1]*Department of Cardiology, Kettering General Hospital NS Foundation Trust, Rothwell Road, Kettering, NN16 8UZ, UK*
[2]*University Hospitals of Leicester NHS Trust, Leicester, UK*
[3]*Department of Cardiology, Castle Hill Hospital, UK*
[4]*University of Leicester, Leicester, UK*
[5]*University College London, London, UK*

Correspondence should be addressed to Azhar Farooqui; amfarooqui91@gmail.com

Academic Editor: Yigit Canga

Background. Anticoagulation with warfarin remains the mainstay treatment for left ventricular thrombi. Although successful thrombus resolution has been reported with direct oral anticoagulants' (DOACs') recurrence/progression while resuming Apixaban therapy is yet to be reported. *Case Presentation.* This case report describes left ventricular thrombus progression/recurrence in a patient anticoagulated with Apixaban undergoing implantable cardioverter defibrillator to cardiac resynchronisation therapy with defibrillator upgrade procedure. He was thereafter changed to warfarin. Contrast echocardiogram at 6 months follow-up did not identify the previously demonstrated mural thrombus. *Conclusion.* Prospective randomised control trials should be conducted in patients with left ventricular thrombus to compare anticoagulants, assess the efficacy and safety of DOACs, and evaluate uninterrupted DOAC versus transient withdrawal for cardiac device procedures.

1. Background

Left ventricular thrombus (LVT) complicates between 2.5 and 15% acute myocardial infarctions (MIs) [1]. Left ventricular (LV) failure also associates with LVT, especially amongst patients with left ventricular ejection fractions (LVEFs) less than 40% [2]. LVT relates to increased morbidity and mortality [2–4].

Anticoagulation with warfarin or low-molecular weight heparin (LMWH) remains the mainstay of treatment whilst successful thrombus resolution is reported with direct oral anticoagulants (DOACs) [2, 5]. Recurrence or progression of LVT after successful resolution while continuing Apixaban is yet to be reported. This case report describes LVT progression/recurrence in a patient anticoagulated with Apixaban undergoing ICD to CRT-D upgrade procedure.

2. Case Presentation

A 75 year-old gentleman was admitted for elective upgrade of his ICD to a CRT-D. He had a background of ischaemic cardiomyopathy, severe left ventricular systolic dysfunction (LVSD), ICD implant (2017), chronic obstructive pulmonary disease, hypothyroidism, glaucoma, and gout.

In 2017, he presented to the cardiology service with unexplained shortness of breath. Echocardiogram showed severe LVSD (LVEF < 30%) with extensive regional wall motion abnormalities (RWMAs) and akinesia of the apex. ECG showed sinus rhythm with narrow-complex QRS. His angiogram revealed significant coronary artery disease involving proximal chronic subtotal occlusion of the left anterior descending artery and focal tight stenosis of the midright coronary artery.

Cardiac magnetic resonance (CMR) demonstrated marked ischemic cardiomyopathy, severe LV dilation (EDD 62 mm, ESD 54 mm) and LVSD (EF 24%), transmural MI of midanteroseptum and true apex, partial MI of apical, inferior, anterior walls, and midinferoseptal and apical septal walls. The multidisciplinary team meeting (MDT) decided that surgical and percutaneous revascularisation were unsuitable. A small apical laminar thrombus was noted (Figure 1), whereupon the patient's dual antiplatelet therapy was changed to Apixaban 5 mg bd. A primary prevention ICD was implanted in 2017 for underlying ischaemic cardiomyopathy with severe LVSD. Optimisation of heart failure medications improved the symptoms from New York Heart Association class IV to II.

Repeat echocardiogram in 2019 showed unchanged severe LVSD; the previous apical laminar thrombus noted on CMR that was not identified on the echocardiogram. Given the akinetic apex, severe LVSD, and high risk for development of further intraventricular thrombus, Apixaban was continued.

During review in November 2019, it was noted that his narrow-complex tachycardia had changed to right bundle branch block with QRS duration of >150 ms. He met the criteria for upgrade to a CRT-D and was admitted for device upgrade. Post procedure ECHO demonstrated a mural thrombus at the left ventricular apex (1.8 × 1.1 cm) (Figures 2 and 3). The patient throughout remained compliant with medications and in sinus rhythm; the only times Apixaban was withheld was 48 hours prior to ICD implantation (2017) and 48 hours prior to ICD upgrade to CRT-D during current admission. He was thereafter changed to warfarin. Contrast ECHO at 6 months follow-up did not identify the previously demonstrated mural thrombus.

3. Discussion and Conclusion

Anticoagulation with DOACs is increasingly utilised as off-label alternatives to warfarin in managing patients with LVT, with several case reports and observational studies demonstrating successful resolution on follow-up imaging [6].

In a retrospective observational study involving echocardiographic surveillance of 108 patients receiving long-term anticoagulation after diagnosis of LVT [2], complete thrombus resolution was found on follow-up ECHO at 1-year in all patients that received a DOAC, in 75% of patients on warfarin and 40% of those on LWMH. Interpretation must remain cautious as significantly fewer patients received DOAC therapy compared to warfarin and LMWH treatment groups (3.7% vs. 87% vs. 9.3%, respectively).

In a further study where 35 of 52 patients (67%) treated with DOAC for LVT proceeded to imaging follow-up, 83% had complete resolution of LVT with mean duration to complete resolution being 264 days [5]. The authors of this study recommended limited interpretation in duration to LVT resolution given nonstandardised timing of their follow-up echocardiograms.

A systematic review of thirty articles involving patients diagnosed with LVT and treated with DOACs found that

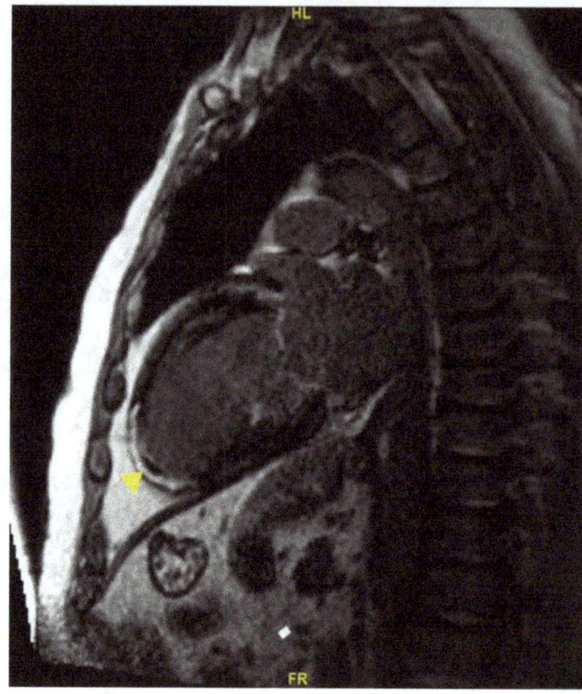

Figure 1: Delayed enhanced cardiac magnetic resonance image. Delayed enhanced cardiac MR (CMR) demonstrating an apical laminar thrombus (blocked arrow).

thrombus resolution rates were 81%, 100%, and 88.9% for rivaroxaban, apixaban and dabigatran, respectively, with a median time to resolution of 40, 36, and 24 days, respectively [6].

Little is published on formation of new LVT whilst taking DOAC therapy, with one article describing this at the time of our report. Degheim et al. described a patient who developed LVT whilst on rivaroxaban for atrial fibrillation with subsequent subacute parietal lobe infarction [7].

CMR is superior to ECHO (with or without contrast) at detecting LVT [8]. It is possible the LV laminar thrombus found in our patient at CMR may not have completely resolved and went undetected on follow-up echocardiograms.

It raises the prospect that whether transiently withholding Apixaban for 48 hours prior to device upgrade may be a factor in formation or extension into the mural LV thrombus subsequently identified, given our patient's significantly impaired LV and akinetic apex.

Predisposition to significant thrombophilia appears unlikely in our patient by observations of no personal or family history of clinical thromboembolism and background coagulation profiles (× 3) within normal limits.

Our observations raise the question as to whether patients diagnosed with LVT having underlying severe LVSD, significant RWMAs, or akinetic/aneurysmal apex should continue anticoagulation rather than withholding it prior to device upgrade procedures. In the event uninterrupted anticoagulation emerges as beneficial in LVT, it also remains to be determined as to what form this should take.

The BRUCE CONTROL 2 study [9] found no statistically significant difference in formation of clinically

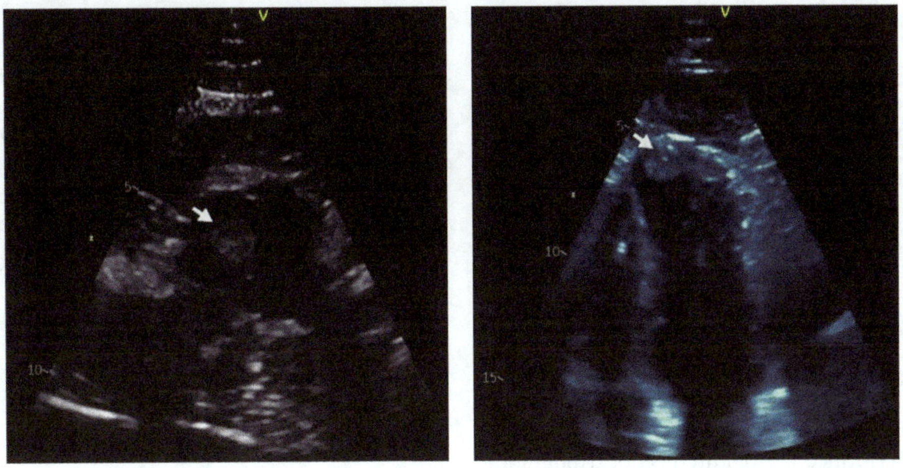

(a) (b)

FIGURE 2: Post device upgrade ECHO. (a) Parasternal short axis view and (b) apical 4-chamber view of transthoracic echocardiogram demonstrating the left ventricular apical thrombus (arrow).

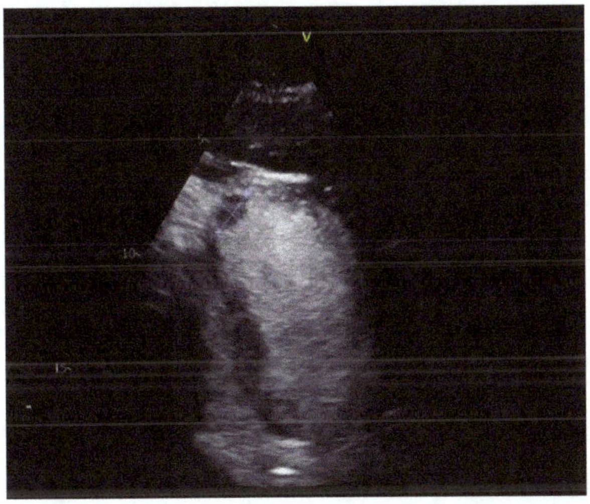

FIGURE 3: Contrast-enhanced transthoracic echocardiogram. Contrast ECHO demonstrating the left ventricular thrombus.

important hematoma postpacemaker or ICD-related procedures with continued compared to interrupted use of DOAC therapy.

The importance of the minimising risk of LVT formation is evidenced from patients with LVT having significantly increased risk of major adverse cardiovascular events (MACEs) and death, as highlighted in a present report from a single-centre French study examining 159 patients with LVT for effects of anticoagulation therapy on patient outcomes [4]. They received vitamin K antagonists (48.8%) followed by parenteral heparins (27.7%) and DOACs (22.6%). Antiplatelet therapy was also continued in 67.9% of patients. Total regression of LVT was observed in 62.3% and independently correlated with a smaller baseline thrombus area and a nonischemic cardiomyopathy.

With median follow-up of 632 days, 35.4% of patients with total LVT regression and 40.0% of patients with persistent LVT experienced MACE. Compared with other patients, those with LVT regression had lower risk of mortality, while anticoagulation therapy for more than 3 months and LVEF ≥35% were independently associated with lower rates of MACE.

At a median follow-up with ECHO of approximately 1 year, 76% of thrombi had regression from baseline. Independent predictors of complete resolution were nonischemic cardiomyopathy and smaller thrombus size at baseline.

While patients with LVT are at increased risk of adverse outcomes, there is also a lower mortality risk in patients showing LVT regression.

Nonpharmacologic mechanisms have also been suggested to aid the formation or progression of left ventricular thrombi in patient with aneurysmal apex. Fakhry and Siddique [10] suggested biventricular pacing-promoted ballooning of the left ventricular apex in their patient, leading to nonlaminar flow, stasis, and eventually leading to the formation of LVT.

In conclusion, prospective randomised control trials should be conducted in patients with LV thrombus to compare anticoagulants, assess the efficacy and safety of DOACs, and evaluate uninterrupted DOAC versus transient withdrawal for cardiac device procedures. This data may yield factors that enable individualised anticoagulation regime's periprocedure in LV thrombus.

3.1. Learning Objective. In this case report, the authors highlight to be mindful that LVT may propagate/recur in patients on DOAC therapy and transient withholding of DOAC therapy for cardiac device procedures may increase possible risk.

Abbreviations

LVT: Left ventricular thrombus
LMWH: Low molecular weight heparin
DOAC: Direct oral anticoagulants.
ICD: Implantable cardioverter defibrillator
CRT-D: Cardiac resynchronisation therapy with defibrillator

LVSD: Left ventricular systolic dysfunction
RWMA: Regional wall motion abnormalities
ECHO: Echocardiogram
CMR: Cardiac magnetic resonance
MACEs: Major adverse cardiovascular events.

Consent

A written consent has been obtained from the patient to publish this content.

Authors' Contributions

AF, TL, and RM were involved in writing of the manuscript. DC arranged and performed the required echocardiographic imaging. SH was the patient's primary cardiologist and helped with reviewing and revising the manuscript. RM was also the supervising author for the paper. All authors were involved in the critical review and the final assessment of the paper prior to submission. Detailed affiliation of the authors can be found on the title page of the manuscript.

References

[1] A. M. Garber, R. J. Mentz, H. Al-khalidi, L. K. Shaw, M. Fiuzat, and C. O'connor, "Clinical predictors and outcomes of patients with left ventricular thrombus following ST-segment elevation myocardial infarction," *Journal of Thrombosis and Thrombolysis*, vol. 41, no. 3, pp. 365–373, 2016.

[2] C. P. McCarthy, S. Murphy, R. V. Venkateswaran et al., "Left ventricular thrombus: contemporary etiologies, treatment strategies, and outcomes," *Treatment Strategies, and Outcomes, JACC*, vol. 73, no. 15, pp. 2007–2009, 2019.

[3] T. C. Crawford, W. T. Smith IV, E. J. Velazquez, S. M. Taylor, J. G. Jollis, and J. Kisslo, "Prognostic usefulness of left ventricular thrombus by echocardiography in dilated cardiomyopathy in predicting stroke, transient ischemic attack, and death," *American Chemical Journal*, vol. 93, no. 4, pp. 500–503, 2004.

[4] B. Lattuca, N. Bouziri, M. Kerneis et al., "Antithrombotic therapy for patients with left ventricular mural thrombus," *Journal of the American College of Cardiology*, vol. 75, no. 14, pp. 1676–1685, 2020.

[5] A. M. Fleddermann, C. H. Hayes, A. Magalski, and M. L. Main, "Efficacy of Direct Acting Oral Anticoagulants in Treatment of Left Ventricular Thrombus," *American Chemical Journal*, vol. 124, no. 3, pp. 367–372, 2019.

[6] M. Kajy, M. Shokr, and P. Ramappa, "Use of direct oral anticoagulants in the treatment of left ventricular thrombus," *American Journal of Therapeutics*, vol. 27, no. 6, pp. e584–e590, 2019.

[7] G. Degheim, A. Berry, and M. Zughaib, "Off label use of direct oral anticoagulants for left ventricular thrombus. Is it appropriate?," *American Journal of Cardiovascular Disease*, vol. 7, no. 5, pp. 98–101, 2017.

[8] J. W. Weinsaft, H. W. Kim, A. L. Crowley et al., "LV thrombus detection by routine echocardiography: insights into performance characteristics using delayed enhancement CMR," *JACC: Cardiovascular Imaging*, vol. 4, no. 7, pp. 702–712, 2011.

[9] D. H. Birnie, J. S. Healey, G. A. Wells et al., "Continued vs. interrupted direct Oral anticoagulants at the time of device surgery, in patients with moderate to high risk of arterial thrombo-embolic events (BRUISE CONTROL-2)," *European Heart Journal*, vol. 39, no. 44, pp. 3973–3979, 2018.

[10] M. A. Fakhry and S. Siddique, "A shocking discovery: apical thrombus formation post-cardiac resynchronization therapy placement," *CASE: Cardiovascular Imaging Case Reports*, vol. 4, no. 6, pp. 500–503, 2020.

A Rare Culprit of Simultaneous Arteriovenous Thromboembolism: Acute Viral Perimyocarditis

Christoph Sossou ,[1] Tobi Ogundare,[1] Ogechukwu Chika-Nwosuh ,[1] Amee Sodha,[2] Christopher Nnaoma ,[1] Cynthia McKinney,[3] and Jose Bustillo[4]

[1]*Internal Medicine Resident, Newark Beth Israel Medical Center, Newark, NJ, USA*
[2]*Teaching Attending Physician, Newark Beth Israel Medical Center, Newark, NJ, USA*
[3]*Medical Student, St. George's University School of Medicine, Grenada*
[4]*Associate Program Director, Internal Medicine, Newark Beth Israel Medical Center, Newark, NJ, USA*

Correspondence should be addressed to Christoph Sossou; chrisw05@gmail.com

Academic Editor: Expedito E. Ribeiro

Simultaneous arteriovenous embolism is extremely rare. Herein, we present a rare case of systemic arteriovenous emboli in a healthy 33-year-old male after an episode of acute viral perimyocarditis. The culprits are postulated to be viral-induced myocardial necrosis and resulting proinflammatory state in the setting of negative malignant, autoimmune, genetics, and chronic infectious conditions. The patient was successfully managed with guideline-directed medical therapy and safely discharged to a subacute rehabilitation facility.

1. Case Introduction

Simultaneous arteriovenous thromboembolism is an extremely rare phenomenon. This is a case of a 33-year-old male with dual cardiac chambers thrombi, complicated by arteriovenous thromboembolism, four months after an acute episode of viral perimyocarditis.

2. Case Description

A 33-year-old African-American man (BMI 22) presents to the emergency department of our facility with progressive dyspnea with mild exertion and bilateral lower extremity (LE) edema associated with paresthesia and pain. Four months prior, he was treated for viral perimyocarditis complicated by new onset heart failure with reduced left ventricular ejection fraction (LVEF ~ 30–35%).

He was noted to be afebrile, tachycardiac to (110 s) BPM, tachypneic (20 s) Br/min, pulse oximetry of 93% on room air, normotensive (110/70 mmHg) and oxygen saturation is 93% breathing ambient air. Cardiopulmonary exam revealed jugular venous distention, diffuse bilaterally crackles, bilateral pitting LE edema up to the knee, reduced femoral, and dorsalis pedis pulses. The rest of the exam was otherwise unremarkable. Initial laboratory findings were significant for neutrophil-predominant leukocytosis (WBC 19×10^3 mcL), elevated brain natriuretic peptide (BNP 2506 pg/mL), troponin-I 0.48 ng/mL (normal < 0.03), D-dimer 6.6 μg/mL (normal high < 0.46), erythrocyte sedimentation rate 110 mm/Hr (normal high 15), and C-reactive protein 12.7 mg/dL (normal high 0.99). Transthoracic echocardiogram showed severe global hypokinesis, moderate-to-severe systolic dysfunction, paradoxical septal motion, and multiple biventricular pedunculated mobile echodensities (about 2-3 centimeters in size) consistent with thrombi with trace pericardial effusion (Figure 1). Contrast-enhanced pulmonary embolism (CTPE) study revealed right lobar pulmonary embolus and bilateral small pleural effusions (Figure 2). Lower extremity computed tomography angiogram (CTA) revealed bilateral occlusion of the superficial femoral,

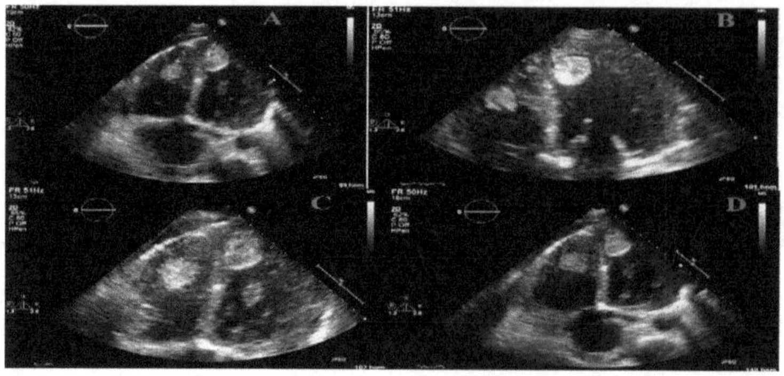

FIGURE 1: Transthoracic echocardiography, apical 4-chamber views, and multiple pedunculated 2-3 cm echodensities in the right and left ventricles consistent with intracardiac thrombi (a–d): moderate left ventricular hypertrophy (a), borderline LV dilatation (b), right ventricle appears moderately dilated (c), and intra-atrial septal deviated to the left (d). There is a small pericardial effusion.

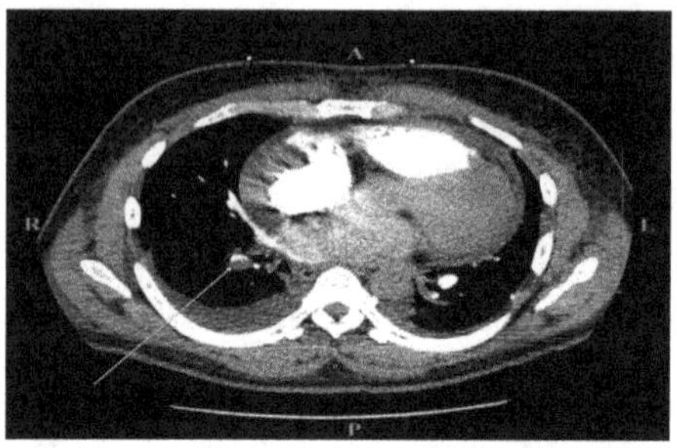

FIGURE 2: A contrast-enhanced chest computed tomography with pulmonary embolism protocol: large filling defect within the distal right lobar pulmonary artery, with thrombus extending into the right lower lobe branches (white arrow). The heart is markedly enlarged with a moderate pericardial effusion. Bibasilar consolidations and areas of linear atelectasis versus scarring/fibrosis at both lower lobes. Bilateral pleural effusions, larger on the right than the left. There is no pneumothorax or pneumomediastinum.

popliteal, posterior tibial, peroneal, and anterior tibial arteries (Figure 3). Patient underwent urgent embolectomy and thrombectomies, with successful restoration of adequate inflow. Contrast-enhanced cardiac MRI revealed diffuse patchy late enhancement of the epicardial layer of the myocardium and small pericardial effusion consistent with perimyocarditis (Figure 4). He was managed with intravenous furosemide, heparin drip, successfully transitioned to rivaroxaban, and safely discharged to a subacute rehabilitation facility, with significant improvement noted on subsequent follow-ups.

3. Case Discussion

Intracardial thrombi are common in patients with severe left ventricular systolic dysfunction, but multiple intracardial thrombi leading to simultaneous arteriovenous thromboembolic are extremely rare moderately reduced left ventricular ejection [1, 2]. The underlying mechanisms for intracardiac thrombogenesis have been postulated as a complication of blood stasis, hematological hypercoagulability, inflammatory conditions (i.e., viral myocarditis, vasculitis), cardiac dysrhythmias, myocardial infarction, cardiomyopathic states, or genetic conditions and deficiencies [1–6]. This is a unique case because unlike previously reported cases of multicardiac chamber thrombi, our patient only had a moderately reduced LVEF (30–35%) but with a higher clot burden. Concerning the possibility of hypercoagulability, a thrombophilia screen was performed before the initiation of heparin, revealing normal antithrombin III level, protein S, and protein C along with negative anticardiolipin, lupus anticoagulant, and beta 2 glycoprotein antibody. Genetic tests for factor V Leiden and prothrombin gene mutation were also unremarkable. Possible explanation in our case includes viral-induced myocardial necrosis (elevated troponin I) prompting chronic inflammatory state (elevated ESR and CRP). Acute viral perimyocarditis causes myocardial necrosis, which leads to chronic inflammatory state and stimulates systemic cytokines circulation, causing further endothelial injury, platelet activation, thrombi generation, and propagation. Acute viral myocarditis is also associated with increased tissue factor (TF); a low molecular weight glycoprotein initiates the clotting cascade and is considered to be a major regulator of coagulation, hemostasis, and thrombosis [1, 7].

The optimal management of intracardial thrombi remains uncleared [8]. Warfarin, the antithrombotic therapy of choice for intracardial thrombi management, has unpredictable pharmacodynamics and pharmacokinetics, making it an unattractive option. Thus, there is limited data on direct oral anticoagulant (DOAC) usage in intracardial thrombi; DOAC has a better safety profile compared to warfarin [4, 8, 9]. Direct oral anticoagulation (i.e., rivaroxaban) has been extensively studied in deep vein thrombosis, nonvalvular atrial fibrillation, and pulmonary embolism and has been used for many years for the prevention of stroke in patients with these conditions [8, 9]. Hence, it is reasonable to assume that if patients are compliants, DOAC could be a safer and effective alternative to warfarin in intracardial thrombi management. Our patient was optimized with guideline-directed heart failure therapy and safely discharged to subacute rehabilitation center on rivaroxaban 15 mg twice daily for 21 days and 10 mg once daily thereafter. The patient

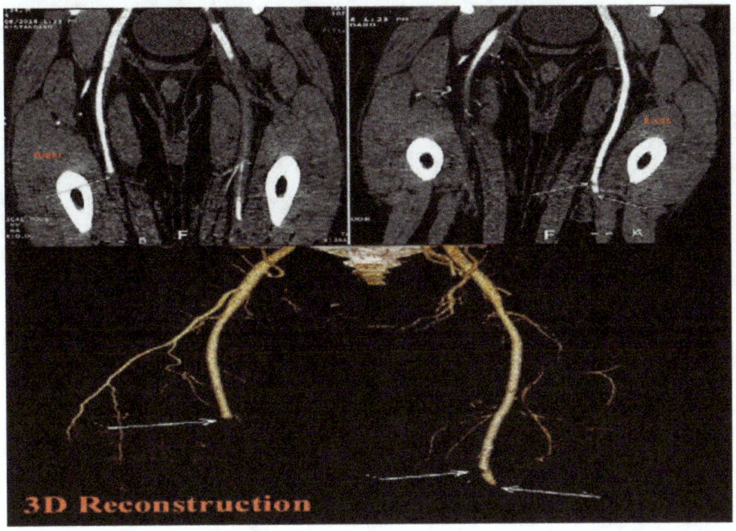

FIGURE 3: A computed tomography angiogram of bilateral lower extremity: severe occlusive bilateral superficial femoral arteries at the level of the mid thighs and occlusion of the right internal iliac artery. Mild reconstitution is seen on the right side anterior tibial artery with no flow in it seen distal to the ankle. No reconstitution is seen on the left side. No radiographic evidence of collateralization.

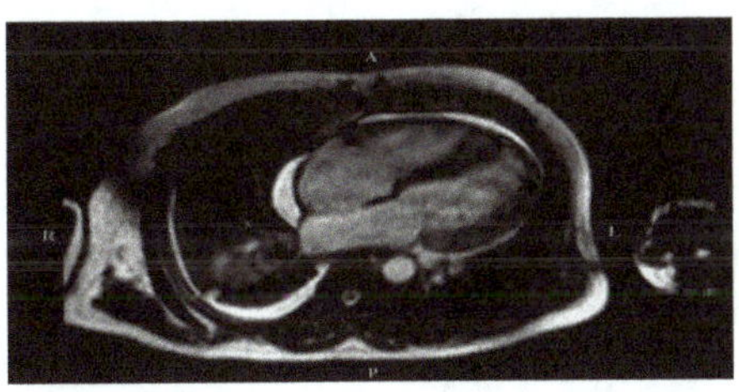

FIGURE 4: Contrast-enhanced cardiac MRI: contrast late enhancement study shows diffuse patchy contrast late enhancement mostly involving mid- and epicardial layer of myocardium, more at the midlateral wall and inferior wall which can be consistent with myocarditis. Small pericardial effusion.

has clinically improved and is free of any complication as noted in subsequent follow-up visits. This case illustrates a rare complication of acute viral perimyocarditis and highlights the need for a randomized controlled clinical trial involving the use of DOAC in patients with intracardiac thrombi.

4. Conclusion

This case illustrates a rare complication of acute viral perimyocarditis: intracardial thrombi complicated by simultaneous arteriovenous thromboembolic events. Besides warfarin, there are few data to guide clinicians' decision regarding choice of antithrombotic therapy in intracardial thrombi management. Our case demonstrates that DOAC is a safe and effective antithrombotic option. Nonetheless, randomized clinical trials are needed before DOAC can be universally recommended as the mainstay of antithrombotic therapy in intracardial thrombi management.

Authors' Contributions

All authors contributed significantly to this manuscript.

References

[1] D. L. Kasper, A. S. Fauci, S. L. Hauser, D. L. Longo, J. Jameson, and J. Loscalzo, *Harrison's Principle of Internal Medicine*, McGraw-Hill, New York, NY, USA, 19e edition, 2015.

[2] M. Koç, D. Y. Sahin, K. Tekin, and M. Caylı, "Development of biventricular large apical thrombi and cerebral embolism in a young woman with peripartum cardiomyopathy," *Türk Kardiyoloji Derneği Arşivi*, vol. 39, no. 7, pp. 591–594, 2011.

[3] F. Thuny, J. F,. Avierinos, B. Jop et al., "Massive biventricular thrombosis as a consequence of myocarditis: findings from 2-dimensional and real-time 3-dimensional echocardiography," *Circulation*, vol. 113, no. 25, pp. e932–e933, 2006.

[4] M. J. Kim, S. H. Hur, Y. S. Lee et al., "Intracardiac multichamber thrombi in a patient with combined protein C and protein S deficiencies," *International Journal of Cardiology*, vol. 100, no. 3, pp. 505-506, 2005.

[5] A. Porter, H. Kandalker, Z. Iakobishvili et al., "Left ventricular mural thrombus after anterior ST-segment-elevation acute myocardial infarction in the era of aggressive reperfusion therapy-still a frequent complication," *Coronary Artery Disease*, vol. 16, no. 5, pp. 275–279, 2005.

[6] R. H. Falk, E. Foster, and M. H. Coats, "Ventricular thrombi and thromboembolism in dilated cardiomyopathy: a prospective follow-up study," *American Heart Journal*, vol. 123, no. 1, pp. 136–142, 1992.

[7] S. Antoniak, U. Boltzen, A. Riad et al., "Viral myocarditis and coagulopathy: increased tissue factor expression and plasma thrombogenicity," *Journal of Molecular and Cellular Cardiology*, vol. 45, no. 1, pp. 118–126, 2008.

[8] E. Yildirim, K. Kalkan, E. Ipek, S. Demirelli, and E. Ermiş, "Successful resolution of left ventricular thrombus with apixaban treatment," *International Journal of the Cardiovascular Acad-*

emy, vol. 2, no. 2, pp. 57-58, 2016.

[9] H. Heidbuchel, P. Verhamme, M. Alings et al., "European Heart Rhythm Association practical guide on the use of new oral anticoagulants in patients with non-valvular atrial fibrillation," *Europace*, vol. 15, no. 5, pp. 625–651, 2013.

29

COVID-19 Induced Cardiomyopathy Successfully Treated with Tocilizumab

Ariyon Schreiber,[1] **Kalaimani Elango**,[1] **Christoph Sossou**,[1] **Sadaf Fakhra**,[2] **Shabada Asad**,[3] **and Chowdhury Ahsan**[1]

[1]*Department of Cardiology-University of Nevada, Las Vegas-Kirk Kirkorian School of Medicine, USA*
[2]*Department of Internal Medicine-University of Nevada, Las Vegas-Kirk Kirkorian School of Medicine, USA*
[3]*Department of Infectious Disease-University of Nevada, Las Vegas-Kirk Kirkorian School of Medicine, USA*

Correspondence should be addressed to Ariyon Schreiber; ariyon.schreiber@unlv.edu
and Kalaimani Elango; kalaimani.elango@unlv.edu

Academic Editor: Manabu Shirotani

Background. Currently, the literature regarding the management of COVID-19 induced cardiomyopathy with reduced ejection fraction is limited. In this case report, we present the first documented case of COVID-19 induced myocardial stunning leading to severely reduced LV systolic function that was reversed by the administration of corticosteroids and tocilizumab. *Case Summary.* A 39-year-old female with well controlled systemic hypertension, tested positive for SARS-CoV-2 RNA and underwent self-isolation for 14 days. Patient presented to our facility a month later with one-week history of progressively worsening generalized body aches, chills, fever, watery diarrhea, nausea with associated mild dry nonproductive cough, shortness of breath and nonspecific chest pain. Initial labs demonstrated that she was COVID-19 positive, elevated troponin (4.295 ng/ml), and elevated BNP (2,291 pg/ml). Her initial Transthoracic echocardiography demonstrated an Left ventricular ejection fraction (LVEF) of 20-25% with apical akinesis. After administration of tocilizumab and corticosteroids, patient demonstrated interval improvement with LVEF improving to 50-55% within days. Her labs confirmed these findings with improved troponin (0.858 ng/ml) and BNP (209 pg/ml). *Discussion.* This case demonstrates that it can be safe and efficacious to use tocilizumab and corticosteroids in patients with COVID-19 induced cardiomyopathy. These finding suggest that cytokine storm is the predominant mechanism by which COVID-19 induced cardiomyopathy occurs. Additional studies are required to determine the role of corticosteroids and tocilizumab in management of this condition.

1. Introduction

It has been demonstrated that SARS-CoV-2 (COVID-19) can induce myocardial injury consequent to left ventricular (LV) systolic dysfunction; however, the exact pathophysiology is not fully understood [1]. A number of mechanisms have been proposed. The most commonly proposed mechanism is myocardial injury as a result of cytokine storm [2]. This is manifested by a parallel rise in inflammatory biomarkers and cardiac troponins alongside consequent left ventricular systolic dysfunction. Acute inflammation can trigger plaque destabilization, resulting in acute coronary syndrome as well as oxygen supply and demand mismatch-induced myocardial injury similar to type 1 and type 2 myocardial infarctions [1]. Another mechanism which has been hypothesized is direct invasion of the myocardium by the virus itself resulting in acute cardiomyopathy. However, data supporting this hypothesis are limited to case reports or case series, none of which have documented definitive diagnosis with endomyocardial biopsy as there is a paucity of inflammatory and cellular infiltrate as seen in myocarditis [2, 3]. Furthermore, autopsy series have failed to demonstrate myocardial necrosis as a result of COVID-19 [2]. Despite the fact that myocardial damage in the setting of COVID-19 infection is likely related to an exaggerated inflammatory response, direct myocardial invasion cannot be excluded.

Currently, the literature regarding management of COVID-19 induced cardiomyopathies is limited [4]. To that end, we present a case of COVID-19 induced cardiomyopathy that was reversed by the administration of corticosteroids, tocilizumab, and a number of other supportive medications.

2. Case Presentation

A 39-year-old female with well-controlled systemic hypertension tested positive for SARS-CoV-2 via PCR and underwent self-isolation for 10 days. She was admitted to our facility a month later with a three-day history of progressively worsening generalized body aches, chills, fever, watery diarrhea, nausea, mild dry nonproductive cough, mild shortness of breath, and nonspecific chest pain. She had minimal oxygen requirements saturating well above 90% on 2 L nasal cannula.

Her vital signs were significant for hypotension (blood pressure 82/44 mmHg), sinus tachycardia (heart rate of 132 beats/min), and axillary body temperature of 101.5°F (38.6°C). Cardiovascular exam demonstrated S3, 2+ pulses, warm extremities with bilateral pitting edema. Pulmonary exam was unremarkable, and no significant clinical symptoms of congestive heart failure or fluid overload were identified.

Electrocardiogram (ECG) showed sinus tachycardia (Figure 1). Laboratory studies demonstrated positive SARS-CoV-2 RNA PCR, troponin-I 4.295 ng/mL, and BNP 2291 pg/mL. Inflammatory markers for lactate dehydrogenase (LDH), ferritin, C-reactive protein, procalcitonin, and IL-6 were also elevated (Table 1). Chest X-ray and computed tomography angiography of the chest were unremarkable. Blood cultures were negative and no antibiotics were given throughout her admission.

Cardiology was consulted regarding the patient's chest pain and elevated troponin. Transthoracic echocardiogram revealed left ventricular ejection fraction (LVEF) of 20-25% with LVIDd of 6.1 cm; apical akinesis but no pericardial effusion or significant valvular abnormalities (Figures 2 and 3).

After extensive discussion with our interdisciplinary team and the patient, she was started on tocilizumab 8 mg/kg once, dexamethasone 6 mg daily for 10 days, and furosemide 20 mg daily. She improved remarkably over a 72-hour period. She was subsequently started on guideline-directed medical therapy (GDMT) for systolic heart failure (i.e. losartan, carvedilol, and spironolactone).

On hospital day seven, repeat transthoracic echocardiogram demonstrated interval improvement with LVEF to 50-55%, (Figures 4) and improvement in lab values (Table 1). The patient was successfully discharged home on hospital day 9. She was seen in cardiology outpatient clinic a week later and in medicine clinic 2 weeks afterward exhibiting excellent health.

3. Discussion

We present a case of COVID-19 associated cardiomyopathy most likely related to cytokine storm, Takotsubo stress induced cardiomyopathy (TC), or an acute coronary syndrome whereafter the patient showed complete recovery through treatment with tocilizumab and supportive vasoactive medications.

The differential for patients with COVID-19 and concomitant signs of acute coronary syndrome (ACS) includes a very broad spectrum of disease classified as COVID-19 associated acute cardiovascular syndrome [1]. Although our patient presented with mild chest pain and elevated troponin, coronary angiography was not pursued due to the low suspicion for occult plaque rupture or coronary arterial disease given her age, mild symptoms, and lack of signs of ischemia on ECG. Furthermore, a number of anecdotal reports have described cases of acute myocardial injury characterized by marked cardiac troponin elevation accompanied by ST-segment elevation or depression on ECG and angiography, often without coronary artery disease or culprit lesions identified on heart catheterization [5].

TC is another possible etiology. The most widely accepted hypothesis is thought to be related to complex systemic responses to acute severe stress and the response of the cardiovascular system to sudden surges in endogenous or exogenously-administered catecholamines [6]. In primary TC, acute cardiac symptoms resulting from emotional or physical stress are the main reason for seeking medical attention [6]. In contrast, secondary TC develops in patients who are hospitalized for other reasons [6]. The intense sympathetic stimulation in these patients caused by the primary condition or its treatment results in the development of TC [7, 8]. Some of the commonly identified triggers for the development of secondary TC are respiratory conditions, intubation, medication use, epinephrine use, anxiety and beta-blocker withdrawal [6, 9–11]. Many of these triggers are typically present in patients with COVID-19 pneumonia; however none of them were present in our patient [6]. Although her overall course appears consistent with a TC with temporary apical akinesia, no angiography was performed and without angiographic evidence of absence of obstruction we were unable to diagnose her with Takotsubo stress induced cardiomyopathy.

Due to the similarity of myocardial injury patterns in other cardiovascular pathologies, exact etiology is often difficult to determine and our case is no exception [1].Although CT coronary angiography, cardiac MRI, and endomyocardial biopsy were not performed due to material limitations, we suspect that her overall condition was related to sequalae from cytokine storm as no other causes of cardiomyopathy were identified.

As discussed, cytokine activation appears to be a prominent feature of severe COVID-19 illness with marked elevations of IL-6 along with other inflammatory markers [1]. Tocilizumab is an IL-6 inhibitor that has been FDA approved for chimeric antigen receptor (CAR) T cell-induced cytokine release syndrome (CRS) and has shown promise in the treatment of COVID-19 associated acute

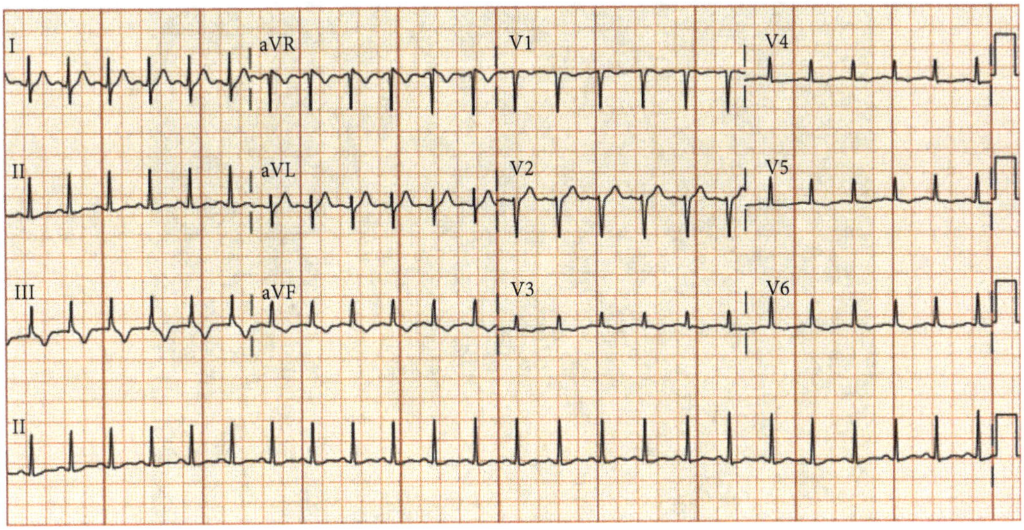

Figure 1: ECG from day of admission demonstrating sinus tachycardia without ST-T changes.

Table 1: Demonstrating all lab values during her Hospital course.

	Reference range	Hospital day 1	Hospital day 2	Hospital day 3	Hospital day 5	Hospital day 7	Hospital day 9
Troponin I (NG/ML)	0.020-0.040	4.295	4.294	0.858			
Brain Natiuretic peptide (pg/ml)	<99		2,291(H)			209(H)	
Lactate dehydrogenase (U/L)	125-243		229	294 (H)	229	330 (H)	208
C-reactive protein(mg/L)	<3.0		>200(H)	>200(H)	71.3(H)	37.7(H)	23.2(H)
D-dimer (MG/L)	<0.49		1.80 (H)	1.56(H)	0.96(H)	0.95(H)	1.25(H)
Ferritin (NG/ML)	7.0-271.0		408.6(H)	588.9(H)	304.8(H)	255.4	223.1
Intcrlcukin-6 (pg/ml)	0.00-12.2		46.5 (H)				

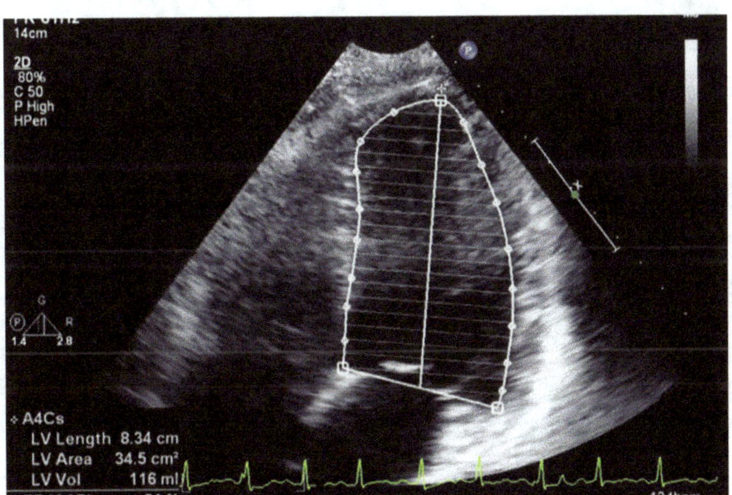

Figure 2: Simpson's method of disc's for measuring ejection fraction at the end of systole on admission.

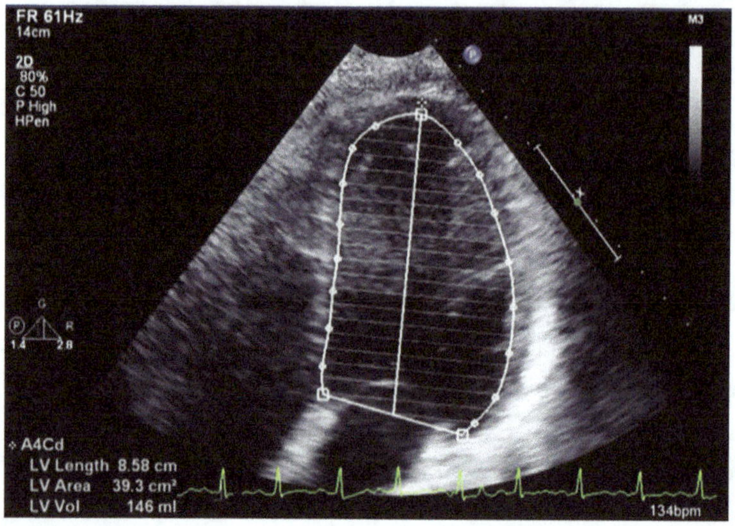

Figure 3: Simpson's method of disc's for measuring ejection fraction at the end of diastole on admission.

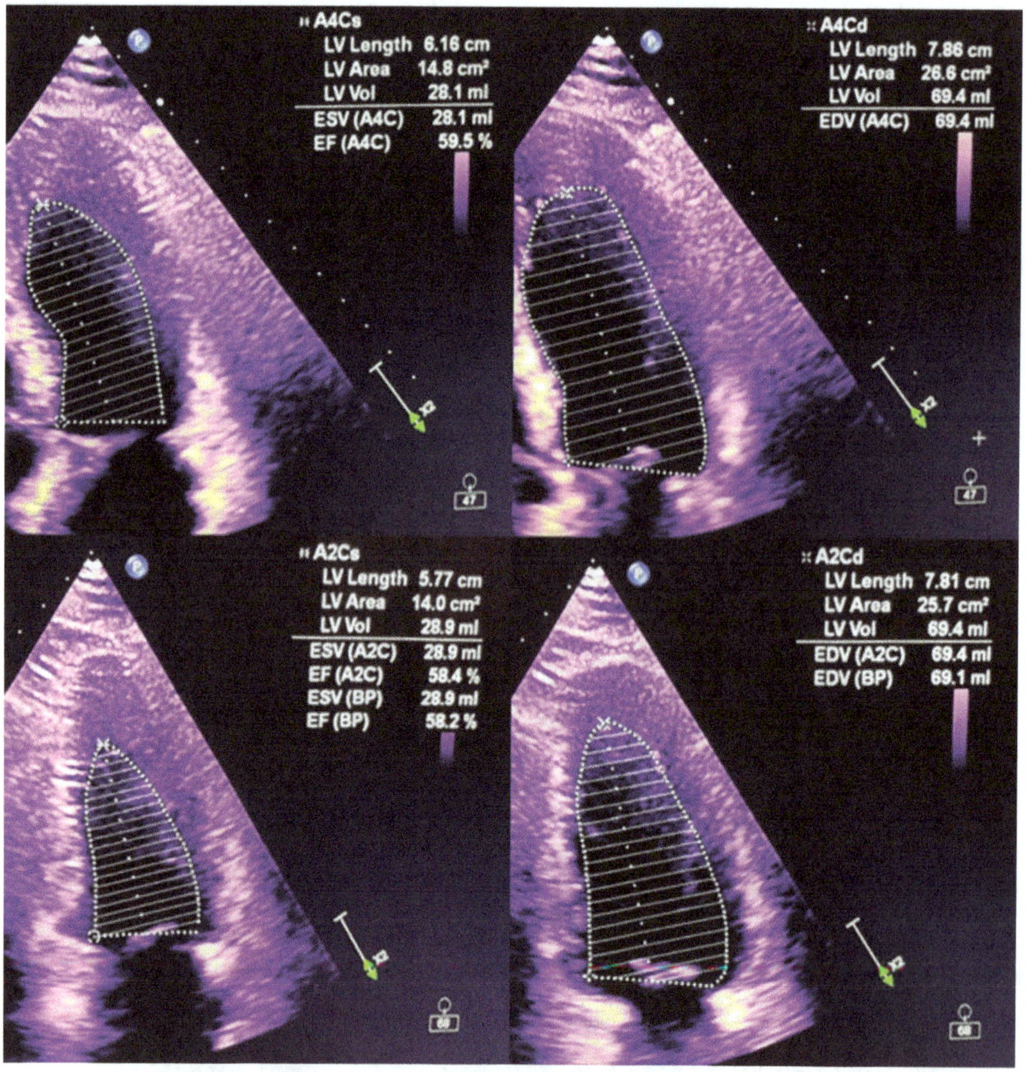

Figure 4: Simpson's method of disc's for measuring ejection fraction at end of systole and end of diastole on discharge demonstrating normal LVEF.

coronary syndrome [12, 13]. Several early small observational studies failed to show mortality benefit of tocilizumab in COVID-19 and expressed concern for secondary infections, increased transaminases, infusion reaction, and neutropenia [14–23]. However, more recent advancements from a well-designed multicenter study out of Oxford University using tocilizumab demonstrated shorter hospital stays and decreased need for mechanical ventilation [24].

To our knowledge, no current studies have been conducted to assess the efficacy of corticosteroid therapy on COVID-19 induced cardiomyopathy, specifically. Due to the lack of evidence regarding management for COVID-19 induced cardiomyopathy, we relied on evidence-based strategies employed to overcome cytokine storm caused by CAR therapy by increasing doses of corticosteroids [25].

We did not administer remdesivir or convalescent plasma due to the occurrence of symptoms more than a month beyond COVID-19 infection and quarantine; presentation of symptoms occurred after the viral phase which would thus make the use of antiviral therapy and convalescent plasma superfiluous [26]. Furthermore, despite the early promise for both of these treatments, the most recently published large trials have revealed no efficacy of either treatment against COVID-19 infection [27, 28].

This patient's prompt response to tocilizumab and corticosteroids appears to support the underlying hypothesis that cytokine storm is the primary mechanism by which COVID-19 induces cardiomyopathy and myocardial stunning. Presently, the exact pathologic mechanism of COVID-19 induced cardiomyopathy is unclear and evidence that COVID-19 invades the myocardium directly is limited to only a handful of case reports [2, 29–31].

4. Conclusion

SARS-CoV-2 continues to complicate the health of millions of people worldwide but guidelines for the management of COVID-19 associated cardiomyopathy have not yet been established. Nevertheless, we successfully employed treatment strategies for COVID-19 associated cardiomyopathy based on our understanding of the pathogenesis and from previous experience in treating COVID-19. Greater consistency and efficacy in its treatment will be undoubtedly uncovered from further successful investigation of the exact mechanism and appropriate management of COVID-19 associated cardiomyopathy. More data is required to determine the risks and benefits involved in using tocilizumab in the management of COVID-19 associated cardiomyopathy but the successful outcome of this case lends hope for a consensus and development of common guidelines for treatments of COVID-19 associated cardiomyopathy.

Consent

The authors confirm that written consent for submission and publication of this case report including images and associated text has been obtained from the patient in line with COPE guidance.

Authors' Contributions

Ariyon Schreiber and Kalaimani Elango equal authorship first author.

References

[1] V. Verma, S. Sondhi, R. Sharma, and K. Mahajan, "COVID-19 associated viral myocarditis: does it exist?," *Monaldi Archives for Chest Disease*, vol. 90, no. 4, p. 90(4), 2020.

[2] R. B. Azevedo, B. G. Botelho, J. V. G. Hollanda et al., "Covid-19 and the cardiovascular system: a comprehensive review," *Journal of Human Hypertension*, vol. 27, pp. 1–8, 2020.

[3] R. Kalyan, S. T. Chitturi, M. A. Al-Saadi, and M. Kassi, "Successful treatment of acute heart failure in COVID-19-induced cytokine storm with tocilizumab: a case report," *European Heart Journal-Case Reports*, vol. 4, no. FI1, pp. 1–6, 2020.

[4] R. M. Inciardi, L. Lupi, G. Zaccone et al., "Cardiac involvement in a patient with coronavirus disease 2019 (COVID-19)," *JAMA Cardiology*, vol. 5, no. 7, pp. 819–824, 2020.

[5] S. Hegde, R. Khan, M. Zordok, and M. Maysky, "Characteristics and outcome of patients with COVID-19 complicated by Takotsubo cardiomyopathy: case series with literature review," *Open Heart.*, vol. 7, no. 2, article e001360, 2020.

[6] H. Medina de Chazal, M. G. Del Buono, L. Keyser-Marcus et al., "Stress Cardiomyopathy Diagnosis and Treatment," *Journal of the American College of Cardiology*, vol. 72, no. 16, pp. 1955–1971, 2018.

[7] A. R. Lyon, E. Bossone, B. Schneider et al., "Current state of knowledge on Takotsubo syndrome: a position statement from the taskforce on Takotsubo syndrome of the heart failure Association of the European Society of cardiology," *European Journal of Heart Failure*, vol. 18, no. 1, pp. 8–27, 2016.

[8] E. A. Hessel, "Takotsubo cardiomyopathy and its relevance to anesthesiology: a narrative review," *Canadian Journal of Anaesthesia*, vol. 63, no. 9, pp. 1059–1074, 2016.

[9] C. Templin, J. R. Ghadri, J. Diekmann et al., "Clinical features and outcomes of Takotsubo (stress) cardiomyopathy," *The New England Journal of Medicine*, vol. 373, no. 10, pp. 929–938, 2015.

[10] K. Singh, K. Carson, R. Shah et al., "Meta-analysis of clinical correlates of acute mortality in Takotsubo cardiomyopathy," *The American Journal of Cardiology*, vol. 113, no. 8, pp. 1420–1428, 2014.

[11] R. Khera, K. Light-McGroary, F. Zahr, P. A. Horwitz, and S. Girotra, "Trends in hospitalization for Takotsubo cardiomyopathy in the United States," *American Heart Journal*, vol. 172, pp. 53–63, 2016.

[12] H. S. Chen, W. Wang, S. N. Wu, and J. P. Liu, "Corticosteroids for viral myocarditis," *Cochrane Database of Systematic Reviews*, vol. 2021, no. 4, article CD004471, 2021.

[13] J. C. Fitzgerald, S. L. Weiss, S. L. Maude et al., "Cytokine Release Syndrome After Chimeric Antigen Receptor T Cell Therapy for Acute Lymphoblastic Leukemia," *Critical Care Medicine*, vol. 45, no. 2, pp. e124–e131, 2017.

[14] Tocilizumab/IL-6 Inhibitors IDSA Home, 2021, https://www.idsociety.org/covid-19-real-time-learning-network/

therapeutics-and-interventions/Tocilizumab-IL-6-Inhibitors/.

[15] L. M. Kimmig, D. Wu, M. Gold et al., "IL6 inhibition in critically ill COVID-19 patients is associated with increased secondary infections," *Preprint. MedRxiv*, vol. 7, 2020.

[16] A. C. Gordon, P. R. Mouncey, F. Al-Beidh et al., "Interleukin-6 Receptor Antagonists in Critically Ill Patients with Covid-19 – Preliminary," *Report.Medrxiv*, vol. 2021, article 21249390, 2021.

[17] S. Gupta, W. Wang, S. S. Hayek et al., "Association between early treatment with tocilizumab and mortality among critically ill patients with COVID-19," *JAMA Internal Medicine*, vol. 181, no. 1, pp. 41–51, 2021.

[18] J. Malgie, J. W. Schoones, and B. G. Pijls, "Decreased Mortality in Coronavirus Disease 2019 Patients Treated With Tocilizumab: A Rapid Systematic Review and Meta-analysis of Observational Studies," *Clinical Infectious Diseases*, vol. 72, 2020.

[19] N. Biran, A. Ip, J. Ahn et al., "Tocilizumab among patients with COVID-19 in the intensive care unit: a multicentre observational study," *Lancet Rheumatol*, vol. 2, no. 10, pp. e603–e612, 2020.

[20] G. Guaraldi, M. Meschiari, A. Cozzi-Lepri et al., "Tocilizumab in patients with severe COVID-19: a retrospective cohort study," *Lancet Rheumatol*, vol. 2, no. 8, pp. e474–e484, 2020.

[21] E. C. Somers, G. A. Eschenauer, J. P. Troost et al., "Tocilizumab for Treatment of Mechanically Ventilated Patients With COVID-19," *Clinical Infectious Diseases*, vol. 73, no. 2, pp. e445–e454, 2020.

[22] J. H. Stone, M. J. Frigault, N. J. Serling-Boyd et al., "Efficacy of tocilizumab in patients hospitalized with Covid-19," *New England Journal of Medicine.*, vol. 383, no. 24, pp. 2333–2344, 2020.

[23] O. Hermine, X. Mariette, P. Tharaux et al., "Effect of tocilizumab vs usual Care in Adults Hospitalized with COVID-19 and moderate or severe pneumonia: a randomized clinical trial," *JAMA Internal Medicine*, vol. 181, no. 1, pp. 32–40, 2021.

[24] C. Salama, J. Han, L. Yau et al., "Tocilizumab in patients hospitalized with Covid-19 pneumonia," *New England Journal of Medicine.*, vol. 384, no. 1, pp. 20–30, 2021.

[25] R. Q. Le, L. Li, W. Yuan et al., "FDA approval summary: tocilizumab for treatment of chimeric antigen receptor T cell-induced severe or life-threatening cytokine release syndrome," *The Oncologist*, vol. 23, no. 8, pp. 943–947, 2018.

[26] D. C. Fajgenbaum and C. H. June, "Cytokine Storm," *The New England Journal of Medicine*, vol. 383, no. 23, pp. 2255–2273, 2020.

[27] O. Dyer, "Covid-19: Remdesivir has little or no impact on survival, WHO trial shows," *BMJ*, vol. 19, p. m4057, 2020.

[28] V. A. Simonovich, L. D. Burgos Pratx, P. Scibona et al., "A randomized trial of convalescent plasma in Covid-19 severe pneumonia," *The New England Journal of Medicine*, vol. 384, no. 7, pp. 619–629, 2021.

[29] COVID-19 Treatment Guidelines Panel, "Coronavirus Disease 2019 (COVID-19)," Treatment Guidelines. National Institutes of Health, 2020, https://www.covid19treatmentguidelines.nih.gov/.

[30] M. Dolhnikoff, J. F. Ferranti, R. A. de Almeida Monteiro et al., *SARS-CoV-2 in Cardiac Tissue of a Child with COVID-19-Related Multisystem Inflammatory Syndrome*, vol. 4, no. 10, 2020, The Lancet, Aug, 2020.

[31] G. Tavazzi, C. Pellegrini, M. Maurelli et al., "Myocardial Localization of Coronavirus in COVID-19 Cardiogenic Shock," *European Journal Heart Failure*, vol. 22, no. 5, pp. 911–915, 2020.

30

Sclerotherapy Induced Takotsubo Syndrome

Sunny Patel,[1] **Sepideh Nabatian**,[2] **and Michael Goyfman**[2]

[1]*Department of Medicine, Long Island Jewish Forest Hills, Northwell Health, New York, USA*
[2]*Department of Cardiology, Long Island Jewish Forest Hills, Northwell Health, New York, USA*

Correspondence should be addressed to Sunny Patel; spatel71@northwell.edu

Academic Editor: Aiden Abidov

A 66-year-old female was brought to the emergency department for acute-onset left-sided chest pain. Prior to arrival, she was at an outpatient appointment with a vascular surgeon for elective sclerotherapy treatment of her lower extremity varicose veins. After receiving an IV injection of polidocanol, she developed severe chest pain with left arm and jaw numbness for the first time in her life. Upon arrival to the ED, the patient reported that her symptoms had resolved. Electrocardiogram (ECG) on presentation was significant for T-wave inversions in leads V1-V3. An initial set of cardiac enzymes showed a troponin I level of 0.62 ng/mL, which subsequently increased to 2.26 ng/mL. Her echocardiogram was significant for mild left ventricular systolic dysfunction with apical hypokinesis (ejection fraction 50%). A repeat ECG showed new T-wave inversions compared to that from the time of admission. The patient eventually agreed to cardiac catheterization, which revealed patent vessels without coronary artery disease, supporting our diagnosis of Takotsubo syndrome and what is the first reported case of likely polidocanol-induced Takotsubo syndrome in the United States.

1. Introduction

Takotsubo syndrome is typically caused by significant emotional or physical stress and is considered nonischemic in nature. However, the condition can be diagnosed in patients with less typical presentations and histories as well. We present a case of a 66-year-old female who presented to the ED with severe chest pain and was later diagnosed with Takotsubo syndrome after being administered polidocanol, a commonly used sclerotherapy agent.

2. Case Report

A 66-year-old female with no significant past medical history was brought to the emergency department by emergency medical services (EMS) with a complaint of left-sided chest pain. She was in her usual state of health when she went to a scheduled appointment with a vascular surgeon for outpatient elective sclerotherapy for the cosmetic treatment of varicose veins. Shortly after being administered an injection of polidocanol, she began experiencing severe left-sided chest pain radiating to her left back with left arm numbness. She also complained of nausea, one episode of vomiting, pressure in her jaw, and lightheadedness. Prior to being transported to the emergency department by ambulance, she was given two doses of aspirin 81 mg.

On arrival to the emergency department, she reported that her symptoms had subsided. Her initial electrocardiogram (ECG) was remarkable for T-wave inversions in leads V1-V3 and sinus bradycardia at 54 beats per minute (Figure 1), with no prior ECG available for comparison. No ST-segment abnormalities were present. Initial laboratory studies were also notable for an elevated troponin I level of 0.62 ng/mL.

The patient was admitted to the inpatient telemetry unit for suspected acute coronary syndrome. Repeat assessment of her cardiac enzymes six hours after her initial bloodwork revealed that her troponin I level had risen to 2.26 ng/mL, at which point the patient had been started on continuous unfractionated intravenous heparin. She remained asymptomatic. The patient was offered cardiac catheterization but initially declined. In a third set of cardiac enzymes, her troponin I level had trended down to 1.15 ng/mL.

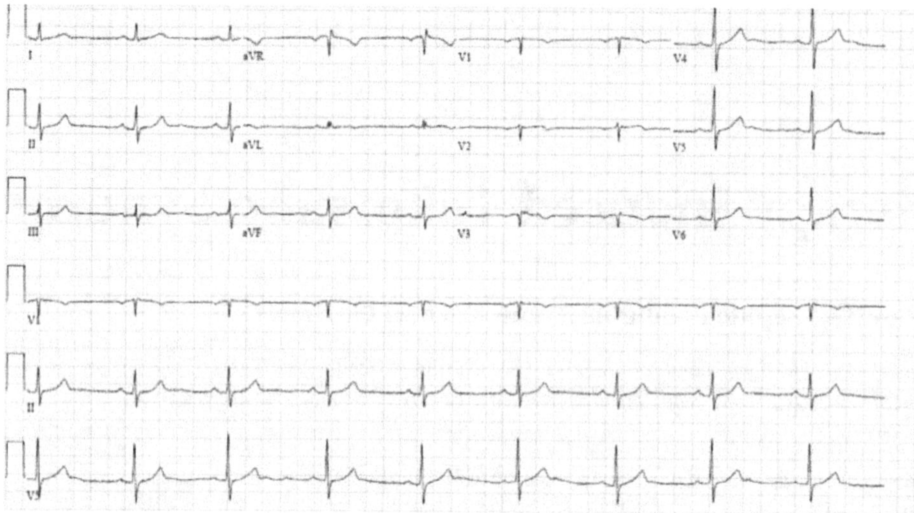

Figure 1: Initial ECG showing T-wave inversions in leads V1-V3.

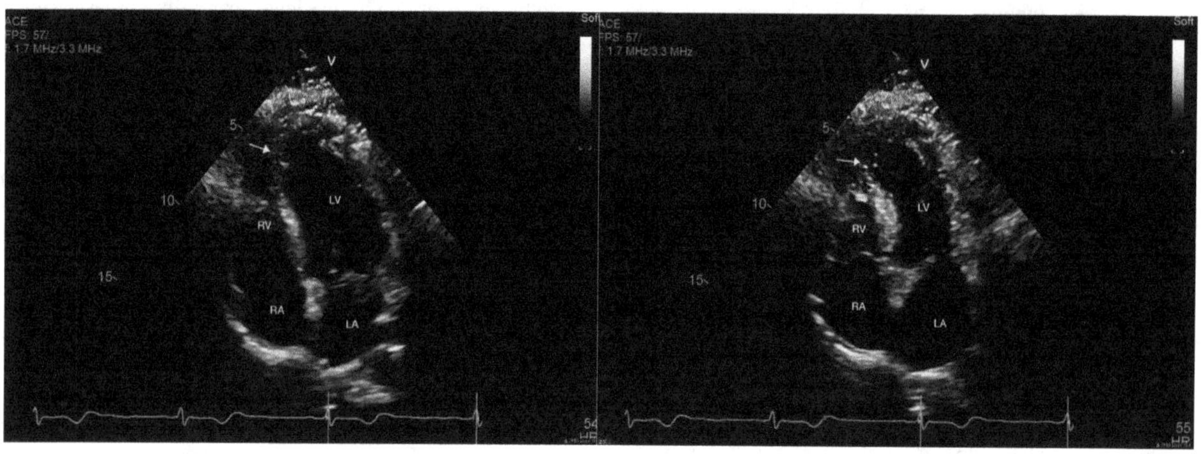

Figure 2: Transthoracic echocardiogram (TTE), revealing a hypokinetic cardiac apex. Yellow arrow on image of diastole (left) and systole (right) shows minimal apical wall motion during the cardiac cycle.

Further studies, including echocardiogram and nuclear stress testing, were pursued to better define her cardiovascular function. A transthoracic echocardiogram revealed an ejection fraction of 50%, suggestive of mild systolic dysfunction, in addition to the presence of apical hypokinesis (Figure 2). Grade II diastolic dysfunction was also noted. Her stress test confirmed an akinetic cardiac apex, as well as a small, severe-intensity, fixed defect, possibly suggestive of myocardial infarction. No areas of reversible ischemia were identified.

After completing her stress test, the patient stated that her left-sided chest pain had returned and was accompanied by shortness of breath. A repeat ECG again showed deeper T-wave inversions in leads V1-V3, in addition to new T-wave inversions in leads I, II, aVL, and V4-V6 (Figure 3). A CT angiogram of her chest with IV contrast was able to rule out an underlying pulmonary embolism and aortic dissection as potential sources of her chest pain.

After further discussion with the patient and her family, she eventually agreed to undergo cardiac catheterization. The procedure established that all vessels were patent, effectively ruling out an acute ischemic event and atherosclerotic disease as the source of her symptoms. In the setting of left ventricular systolic dysfunction, the absence of coronary artery disease, and elevated cardiac enzymes with T-wave inversions on ECG, the patient was diagnosed with Takotsubo syndrome. Her postprocedure course was uncomplicated, and the patient was ultimately discharged home on aspirin 81 mg and simvastatin 20 mg for preventative purposes, with instructions to follow up for a repeat echocardiogram as an outpatient.

3. Discussion

Takotsubo syndrome is a condition often associated with immense emotional or physical stress. The mechanism through which this develops is still ill-defined but has been theorized to be associated with a surge of neuroendocrine hormones in response to the stress [1]. At least 1-2% of cases of acute coronary syndrome with elevated cardiac enzyme levels are linked to the condition [2], and patients are

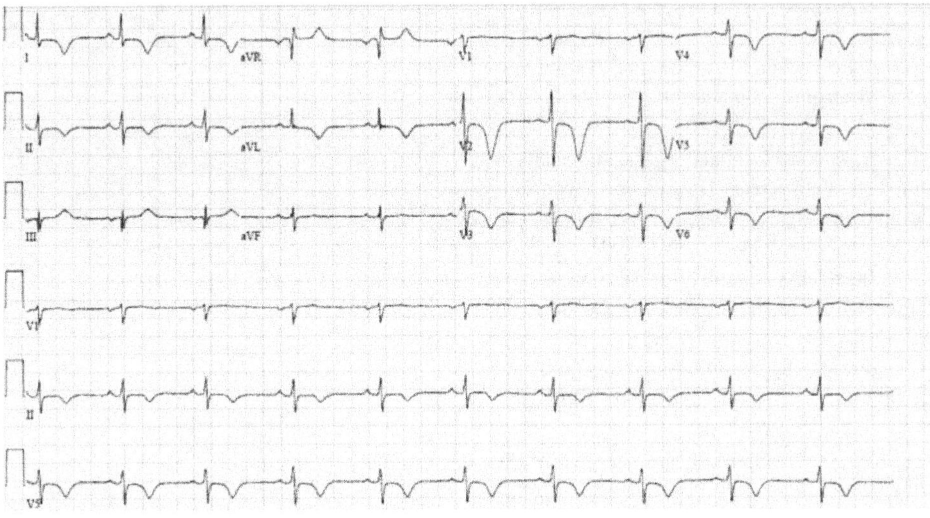

FIGURE 3: Repeat ECG again showing deeper T-wave inversions in leads V1-V3, with new T-wave inversions in leads I, II, aVL, and V3-V6.

typically expected to provide a history of recent onset stressors, which may include events such as loss of family members or financial hardship, among others.

The classic clinical presentation of a patient with Takotsubo syndrome is often identical to true acute coronary syndrome, involving symptoms of acute-onset substernal chest pain, with associated symptoms of dyspnea and occasionally syncope. Diagnostic tools including ECG, cardiac biomarkers, echocardiogram, cardiac catheterization, and more recently the InterTAK Diagnostic Score also play a role in delineating potential sources of a patient's symptoms. Takotsubo syndrome may be associated with ECG findings of ST-segment elevations or depressions, QT-segment prolongations, and T-wave inversions. Cardiac biomarkers, such as serum troponin levels, are commonly elevated. Furthermore, echocardiogram will usually reveal left ventricular systolic dysfunction, most commonly with apical wall motion abnormalities in the form of akinesis, hypokinesis, or dyskinesis. This is typically paired with a hyperdynamic cardiac base. However, variant forms have also been identified, including midventricular and reverse subtypes. In the former, akinesis is noted in the midventricle and is seen with a hyperdynamic base and apex. In the reverse subtype, the cardiac base is akinetic, while the apex is hyperdynamic [3]. Cardiac catheterization can be useful in identifying the presence of obstructive coronary artery disease, but it is important to note that the presence of some atherosclerotic disease does not exclude the diagnosis. In the case of our patient, cardiac catheterization confirmed patent vasculature without atherosclerotic disease, suggesting the previously noted fixed defect on her stress test was attributable to attenuation artifact.

The management of Takotsubo syndrome is not yet well established and primarily focuses on supportive care [4]. The use of angiotensin-converting enzyme (ACE) inhibitors, angiotensin receptor blockers (ARBs), and beta-blockers has been suggested in cases involving heart failure; however, there are currently no guidelines or randomized studies supporting the use of these medications [4]. Regardless, all patients diagnosed with Takotsubo syndrome should have repeat echocardiograms to monitor their cardiac function and overall recovery [5]. This is particularly important, as the mortality rate during long-term follow-up has been reported to be 5.6% [6].

While our patient's presenting complaint of chest pain is expected in a patient with Takotsubo syndrome, the history she provided is not. She had undergone no significant emotional stressors in the recent past. Rather, she informed us that her symptoms began shortly after being injected with a sclerotherapy agent for the cosmetic treatment of varicose veins. The agent in question was polidocanol, marketed in the United States under the trade names Asclera® and Varithena®. The intravenous injection is formulated to irreversibly damage the endothelial lining of blood vessels, which in turn causes vessel occlusion through the formation of a network of platelets, fibrin, and cellular debris [7]. The occluded vessel is then ultimately replaced with connective tissue over time, leading to the desired effect of diminishing the prominence of vein varicosities. Although polidocanol typically works locally, systemic effects can be observed. To date, there has only been one documented case of Takotsubo syndrome developing after an injection of polidocanol [8], as well as one other involving a similar agent called sodium tetradecyl sulfate [9]. Our case report highlights the first documented case of likely polidocanol-induced Takotsubo syndrome occurring in the United States.

The overall purpose of this case report is to highlight a rare but clinically significant iatrogenic outcome of a chemical injection routinely used in the outpatient setting. While the complication of Takotsubo syndrome secondary to polidocanol use is uncommon, it is essential that those administering and receiving the intravenous injection be made aware that this diagnosis remains a clinically relevant adverse outcome that can mimic major ischemic cardiac events.

References

[1] F. Pelliccia, J. C. Kaski, F. Crea, and P. G. Camici, "Pathophysiology of Takotsubo syndrome," *Circulation*, vol. 135, no. 24, pp. 2426–2441, 2017.

[2] V. Kurowski, A. Kaiser, K. von Hof et al., "Apical and Midventricular Transient Left Ventricular Dysfunction Syndrome (Tako-Tsubo Cardiomyopathy) Frequency, Mechanisms, and Prognosis," *Chest*, vol. 132, no. 3, pp. 809–816, 2007.

[3] P. Velankar and J. Buergler, "A mid-ventricular variant of Takotsubo cardiomyopathy," *Methodist DeBakey Cardiovascular Journal*, vol. 8, no. 3, pp. 37–39, 2012.

[4] S. Y-Hassan and P. Tornvall, "Epidemiology, pathogenesis, and management of Takotsubo syndrome," *Clinical Autonomic Research*, vol. 28, no. 1, pp. 53–65, 2018.

[5] J.-W. Lee and J.-Y. Kim, "Stress-induced cardiomyopathy: the role of echocardiography," *Journal of Cardiovascular Ultrasound*, vol. 19, no. 1, pp. 7–12, 2011.

[6] C. Templin, J. R. Ghadri, J. Diekmann et al., "Clinical features and outcomes of Takotsubo (stress) cardiomyopathy," *New England Journal of Medicine*, vol. 373, no. 10, pp. 929–938, 2015.

[7] A. Kitagawa, T. Yamamoto, N. Matsunaga et al., "Polidocanol sclerotherapy combined with transarterial embolization using n-butyl cyanoacrylate for extracranial arteriovenous malformations," *CardioVascular and Interventional Radiology*, vol. 41, no. 6, pp. 856–866, 2018.

[8] L. Auboire, J. Alexandre, V. Boccadamo, and C. Labbé, "Takotsubo syndrome induced by a polidecanol injection: a case report," *International Journal of Cardiology*, vol. 223, pp. 418-419, 2016.

[9] B. J. Potter, F. Gobeil, A. Oiknine, and P. Laramée, "Le premier cas de cardiomyopathie takotsubo associee a une sclerotherapie au tetradecylsulfate de sodium," *Canadian Journal of Cardiology*, vol. 26, no. 4, pp. e146–e148, 2010.

Monomorphic Ventricular Tachycardia as a Presentation of Giant Cell Myocarditis

Michael H. Chiu, Cvetan Trpkov, Saman Rezazedeh, and Derek S. Chew

Libin Cardiovascular Institute of Alberta, Cummings School of Medicine, University of Calgary, Alberta, Canada

Correspondence should be addressed to Michael H. Chiu; michael.chiu@ahs.ca

Academic Editor: Man-Hong Jim

Background. Idiopathic giant cell myocarditis (GCM) has a fulminant course and typically presents in middle-aged adults with acute heart failure or ventricular arrhythmia. It is a rare disorder which involves T lymphocyte-mediated myocardial inflammation. Diagnosis is challenging and requires a high index of suspicion since therapy may improve an otherwise uniformly fatal prognosis. *Case Summary.* A previously healthy 54-year-old female presented with hemodynamically significant ventricular arrhythmia (VA) and was found to have severe left ventricular dysfunction. Cardiac MRI demonstrated acute myocarditis, and endomyocardial biopsy showed giant cell myocarditis. She was treated with combined immunosuppressive therapy as well as guideline-directed medical therapy. A secondary prevention implantable cardioverter defibrillator (ICD) was implanted. *Discussion.* GCM is a rare, lethal myocarditis subtype but is potentially treatable. Combined immunosuppression may achieve partial clinical remission in two-thirds of patients. VA is common, and patients should undergo ICD implantation. More research is needed to better understand this complex disease. *Learning Objectives.* Giant cell myocarditis is an incompletely understood, rare cause of myocarditis. Patients present predominately with heart failure and dysrhythmia. Diagnosis is confirmed by histopathology, and immunosuppression may improve outcomes. ICD implantation should be considered. In the absence of treatment, prognosis is poor with a median survival of three months.

1. Introduction

Idiopathic giant cell myocarditis is a rare clinical entity first recognized in the early 1950s [1]. GCM has a fulminant course with an autoimmune pathophysiology in virus-negative GCM [2, 3]. Often fatal due to arrhythmia or heart failure, two-thirds of patients exhibit response to immunosuppressive therapy, and some undergo cardiac transplantation [2]. We report a case of a previously healthy female diagnosed with idiopathic giant cell myocarditis.

2. Case Report

A previously healthy 54-year-old female presented to emergency services with acute onset of malaise, nausea, palpitations, and presyncope. Her ECG showed monomorphic ventricular tachycardia at 230 bpm, and she underwent successful cardioversion. Hemodynamic stability was restored, and she was admitted to the cardiac intensive care unit.

Initial cardiovascular examination was pertinent for a positive abdominojugular reflux sign and a third heart sound. There was no clinical evidence of pulmonary or systemic congestion or low cardiac output state, and no other manifestations of systemic disorders were present.

ECG in sinus rhythm revealed a nonspecific intraventricular conduction delay with a QRS duration of 130 ms, a P wave of 1 mm in the lead II, a PR interval of 166 ms, and a QTc of 507 ms at a heart rate of 96 bpm. Transthoracic echocardiography showed left ventricular systolic dysfunction with an estimated ejection fraction of 35%, preserved right ventricular function, and no valvular abnormalities (aortic root dimension of 2.9 cm, left atrium of 3.2 cm, LV diastole of 4.9 cm, LV systole of 4.0 cm, fractional shortening of 18.6%, interventricular septum of 0.85 cm, posterior wall of 0.78 cm, left atrium volume index of 36.3 ml/m^2, left

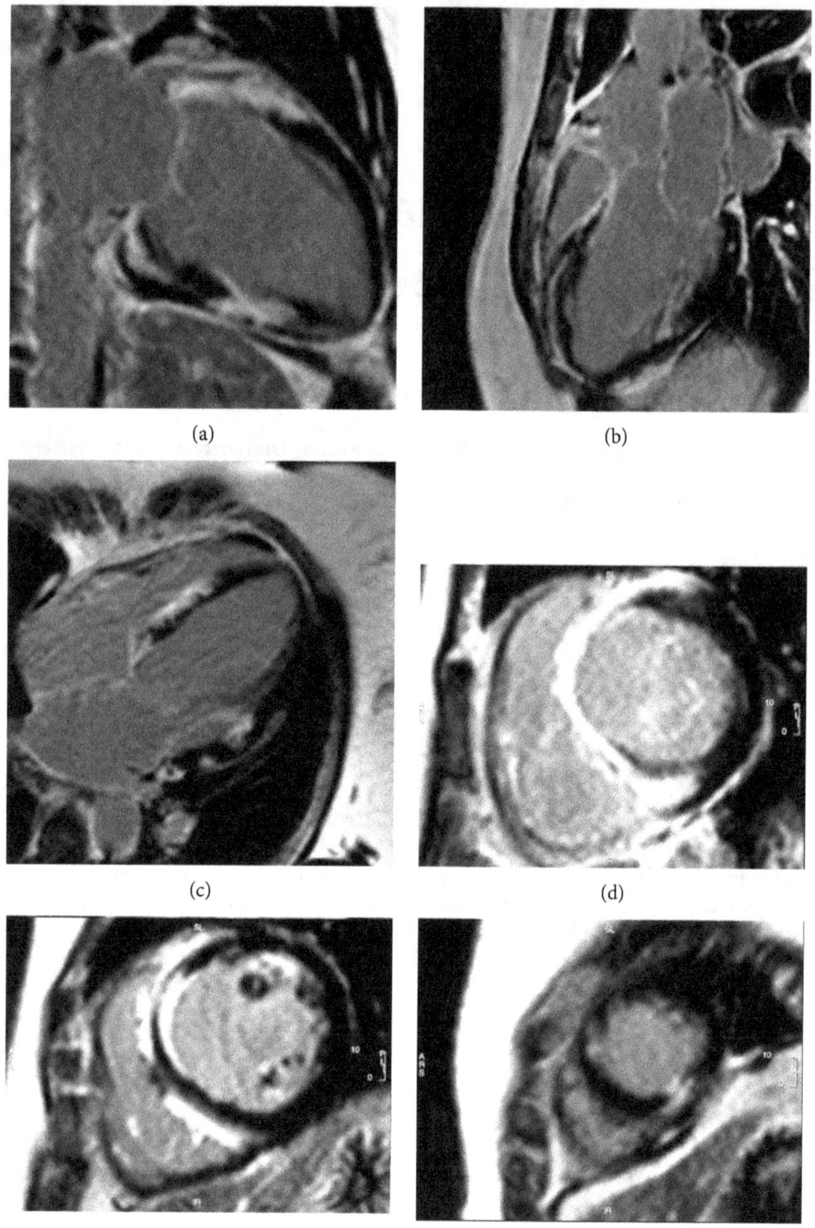

Figure 1: Cardiac myocardial resonance imaging demonstrating late gadolinium enhancement of the basal to midanterior, anteroseptal, inferoseptal, and inferior segments and apical inferior segments of the left ventricle. Patchy enhancement within the septum on the side of the ventricle: (a) 2-chamber view (b) 3-chamber view (c) 4-chamber view, (d) short-axis view at the base, (e) short-axis view at the level of the papillary muscles, and (f) short-axis view at the level of the apex.

ventricular mass of 79.3 grams/m^2, left ventricular outflow tract diameter of 2.2 cm, stroke volume of 39.9 ml, end diastolic volume (MOD-bp) of 128.5 ml, ejection fraction (MOD-bp) of 31.1%, cardiac output (LVOT) of 4.9 l/min, stroke volume (LVOT) of 57.3 cc, TAPSE of 2.2 cm, and RV S' velocity of 11.5 cm/sec). Coronary arteries were angiographically normal. On cardiac magnetic resonance imaging, there was extensive, midwall patchy late gadolinium enhancement consistent with acute myocarditis (Figure 1).

A serum blood work revealed a hemoglobin count of 141 g/l with an MCV of 92 fl, a platelet count of 182 × 10^9/l, a WBC of 12.3 × 10^9/l with a differential (neutrophil 8.2 × 10^9/l, lymphocytes 2.8 × 10^9/l, monocytes 0.9 × 10^9/l, eosinophils 0.3 × 10^9/l, and basophils 0.1 × 10^9/l), a high-sensitivity troponin T of 46 ng/l, an NT-proBNP of 261 ng/l, an ESR of 11 mm/h, and a CRP of 3.2 mg/l. An infectious panel was negative for cytomegalovirus, Epstein–Barr virus, hepatitis B, hepatitis C, herpes simplex virus, HIV, mumps, toxoplasmosis, and varicella.

Right ventricular endomyocardial biopsy was performed. This demonstrated features typical of GCM, including extensive myocyte damage, multinucleated giant cells, and mixed inflammatory cell infiltrate. There was no granuloma formation (Figure 2). Autoimmune and connective tissue disease

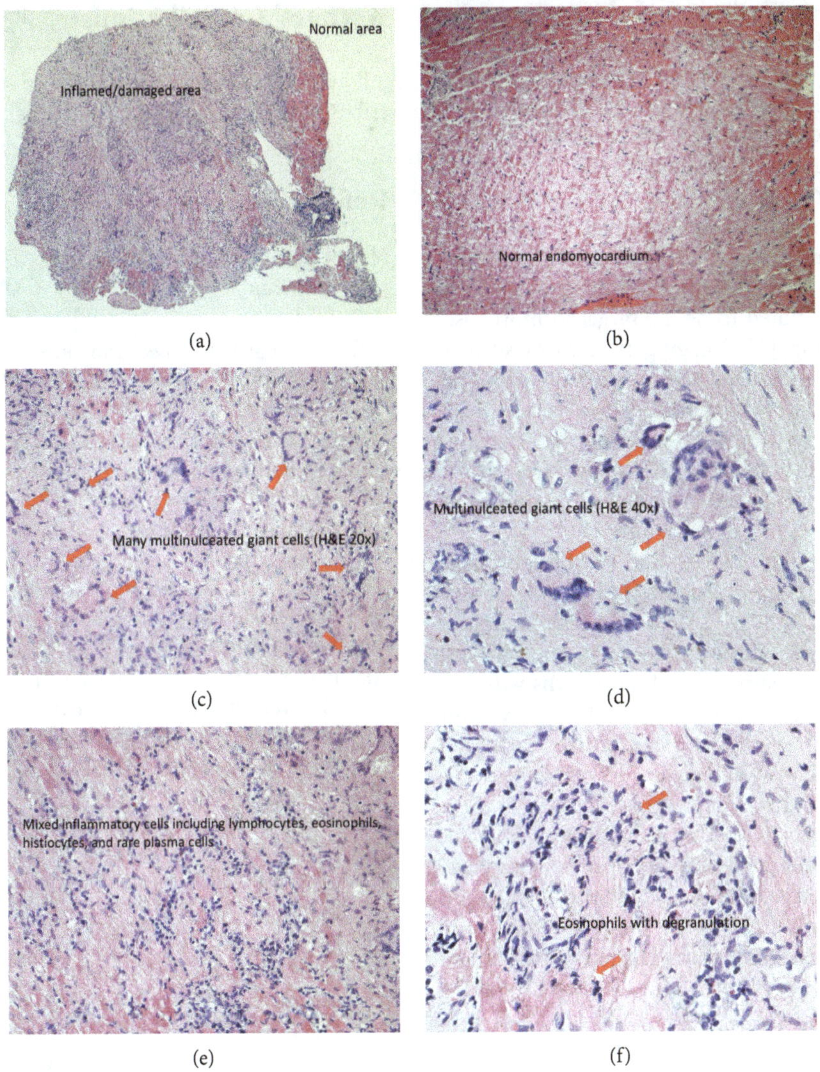

Figure 2: Pathological slides from the endomyocardial biopsy: (a) damaged and normal myocardium, (b) normal myocardium, (c) multinucleated giant cells (H&E staining 20x), (d) multinucleated giant cells (H&E staining 40x), (e) mixed inflammatory cells, and (f) eosinophils.

serology was unremarkable (negative anti-nuclear antibody, glomerular basement membrane antibody, anti-neutrophil cytoplasmic antibody, myeloperoxidase antibody, proteinase 3 antibody, and lymphotoxic antibody screening). Anti-heart autoantibodies were not tested on the patient and may be a limitation in the diagnosis of GCM.

The patient was treated with standard heart failure therapy including a beta-blocker, angiotensin receptor inhibitor, and mineral corticoid receptor antagonist. Once the diagnosis of GCM was confirmed, a combined immunosuppressive therapy with high-dose prednisone (60 mg daily), tacrolimus (alternating doses of 1 mg and 2 mg daily), and mycophenolate mofetil (1000 mg BID) was added. She also underwent implantation of a secondary prevention dual chamber ICD. In total, the diagnosis of GCM was established within 8 days of presentation, immunosuppressive therapy prescribed on day 9, and ICD implanted on day 14. Total hospital stay was 16 days, and there was no recurrence of VA or heart failure progression. She was discharged in stable condition and remained NYHA II at her follow-up appointments. Her echocardiogram at 6 and 12 months is unchanged with severe LV systolic dysfunction with minor regional variability and mild RV dysfunction. Repeat biopsy performed at 6 months demonstrated interstitial fibrosis and myocyte hypertrophy. Currently, our patient remains on her current immunosuppressive therapies aside from a tapering of her steroid dose to 5 mg daily.

3. Discussion

Idiopathic giant cell myocarditis (GCM) is presumed to be a T lymphocyte-mediated inflammatory disorder. An association with other autoimmune disorders such as thyroiditis and myasthenia gravis has been reported; however, it was found only among 20% of patients in a larger contemporary case series [2]. GCM affects men and women equally, with a mean age of onset of 42.6 years reported in the multicenter GCM study registry [2]. Common presentation includes heart failure and VA; however, it can also present as an acute myocardial infarction mimic or atrioventricular block [4].

Many cases are clinically diagnosed as idiopathic cardiomyopathy until autopsy or cardiac transplantation confirms GCM by histopathology [4]. Differential diagnosis includes sarcoidosis, but granulomata formation, which is absent in GCM, differentiates the two diseases. Repeated endomyocardial biopsy may be necessary to diagnose GCM, with higher sensitivity early in the disease process and in more fulminant cases with more extensive myocardial involvement [4, 5]. EMB has a reported sensitivity of 80% with a positive predictive value of 71% that increases with repeat biopsy [5]. Right ventricular septum was noted to be the target in most cases for myocardial sampling [4]. Imaging modalities such as echocardiography reveal reduced LV function and dilation. Contrast-enhanced cardiac MRI typically reveals areas of late gadolinium enhancement (scar) and increased T2-weighted signal (myocardial edema). ^{18}FDG-PET shows the areas of perfusion defects and inflammation and may be utilized to target biopsies to the sites of active inflammation [4].

Prognosis is poor with a median survival of 3 months in the absence of treatment. Sole corticosteroid use was associated with an improved survival of 3.8 months. Combined immunosuppression may be more effective than corticosteroids alone with a median survival of 11.5 months with steroids plus azathioprine and 12.6 months with cyclosporine [2, 4]. GCM is known to recur in transplanted hearts with infiltrates identified on biopsy at a mean of 3 years posttransplant [2, 6]. There are limited data to guide long-term treatment strategies; however, it may be necessary to continue immunosuppression indefinitely due a relapse risk described even eight years after initial diagnosis [7]. Idiopathic GCM is an organ-specific autoimmune disease thought to be due to autoimmunity to myosin, thus necessitating an individualized immunosuppressive regimen with most cases requiring lifelong therapy.

Although seemingly effective, combined immunosuppression achieves partial clinical remission in only two-thirds of patients and EMB frequently shows ongoing inflammation. The lack of complete remission suggests the pathophysiology, and optimal treatment is not fully understood [3, 4, 8]. GCM recurrences have even been reported among patients who underwent heart transplantation [4, 9]. Despite medical therapy, sustained VA is present in up to 50% of patients and ICD implantation is recommended [2, 4].

Experimental models have suggested that there may be two forms of giant cell myocarditis with macrophage-derived giant cells and with myocyte-derived giant cells with the appearance of multinucleated giant cells corresponding to the fulminant phase of inflammation and myocardial damage [10]. Diagnosis is typically made via endomyocardial biopsy. Combined immunosuppressive therapy, implantable cardioverter defibrillators, and guideline-based heart failure therapies improve the overall prognosis; however, more research is needed to better understand this complex disease.

Consent

The patient has agreed and provided consent for this case report.

Authors' Contributions

All authors participated in the care of this patient and contributed in the preparation of the figures and manuscript.

References

[1] B. Kean and M. T. Hoekenga, "Giant cell myocarditis," *The American Journal of Pathology*, vol. 28, no. 6, pp. 1095–1105, 1952.

[2] L. T. Cooper, G. J. Berry, and R. Shabetai, "Idiopathic giant-cell myocarditis — natural history and treatment," *New England Journal of Medicine*, vol. 336, no. 26, pp. 1860–1866, 1997.

[3] L. T. Cooper Jr., J. M. Hare, H. D. Tazelaar et al., "Usefulness of immunosuppression for giant cell myocarditis," *The American Journal of Cardiology*, vol. 102, no. 11, pp. 1535–1539, 2008.

[4] R. Kandolin, J. Lehtonen, K. Salmenkivi, A. Räisänen-Sokolowski, J. Lommi, and M. Kupari, "Diagnosis, Treatment, and Outcome of Giant-Cell Myocarditis in the Era of Combined Immunosuppression," *Circulation: Heart Failure*, vol. 6, no. 1, pp. 15–22, 2013.

[5] R. C. Shields, H. D. Tazelaar, G. J. Berry, and L. T. Cooper Jr., "The role of right ventricular endomyocardial biopsy for idiopathic giant cell myocarditis," *Journal of Cardiac Failure*, vol. 8, no. 2, pp. 74–78, 2002.

[6] V. V. Menghini, V. Savcenko, L. J. Olson et al., "Combined immunosuppression for the treatment of idiopathic giant cell myocarditis," *Mayo Clinic Proceedings*, vol. 74, no. 12, pp. 1221–1226, 1999.

[7] J. J. Maleszewski, V. M. Orellana, D. O. Hodge, U. Kuhl, H.-P. Schultheiss, and L. T. Cooper, "Long-term risk of recurrence, morbidity and mortality in giant cell myocarditis," *The American Journal of Cardiology*, vol. 115, no. 12, pp. 1733–1738, 2015.

[8] L. T. Cooper and C. ElAmm, "Giant cell myocarditis," *Herz*, vol. 37, no. 6, pp. 632–636, 2012.

[9] W. Gries, D. Farkas, G. Winters, and M. Costanzo-Nordin, "Giant cell myocarditis: first report of disease recurrence in the transplanted heart," *The Journal of Heart and Lung Transplantation*, vol. 11, no. 2, pp. 370–374, 1992.

[10] M. Kodama, Y. Matsumoto, M. Fujiwara et al., "Characteristics of giant cells and factors related to the formation of giant cells in myocarditis," *Circulation Research*, vol. 69, no. 4, pp. 1042–1050, 1991.

COVID-19 mRNA Vaccine-Associated Myocarditis Presenting as STEMI in a 48-Year-Old Male

Mohammad Dlewati[1] **Kyeeun Park,**[1] **Saumya Rawat,**[1] **Jorge Conte,**[1,2] **and Kashmira Bhadha**[1,2]

[1]*Division of Internal Medicine, Memorial Healthcare System, Hollywood, Florida, USA*
[2]*Division of Cardiology, Memorial Healthcare System, Hollywood, Florida, USA*

Correspondence should be addressed to Mohammad Dlewati; mdlewati@mhs.net

Academic Editor: Manabu Shirotani

Myocarditis has been recognized as a rare complication of coronavirus disease 2019 (COVID-19) mRNA vaccinations. Young adult and adolescent males < 30 years of age are the most commonly affected group, with decreased incidence with older age. This is a case of a 48-year-old male who presented with chest pain and EKG findings of STEMI shortly after receiving the second dose of the Moderna COVID-19 mRNA vaccine. Emergent left heart catheterization revealed normal coronaries. Subsequently, the patient had rapid resolution of his symptoms and improvement in serum markers. The exact etiology factors to this new and rare phenomenon are yet to be fully understood. This patient did have a history of previous viral myocarditis 7 years ago; however, it remains unclear if this could be a predisposing factor to the development of mRNA vaccine-associated myocarditis.

1. Introduction

The coronavirus disease 2019 (COVID-19) messenger RNA-(mRNA-) based vaccines (BNT162b2 mRNA-Pfizer-BioNTech and the mRNA-1273-Moderna) have a relatively benign side effect profile; usually associated with local reactions, fatigue, and headache. A more severe adverse effect, myocarditis, has recently been recognized as a rare complication with higher incidence than expected, usually after the second dose of the 2-dose series. Young adult and adolescent males < 30 years of age are the most commonly affected group, with decreased incidence with older age [1].

2. Case

A 48-year-old male presented to the emergency department with acute-onset typical chest pain. He reported having fevers, fatigue, and chills for the past 3 days which began shortly after receiving the second dose of the Moderna COVID-19 mRNA vaccine. Vital signs were within normal limits, his weight was 83 kg with a BMI of 30.5, and the rest of his general and cardiorespiratory physical exam were largely unremarkable. His medical history was one of health; however, 7 years prior, the patient was diagnosed with viral myocarditis after a flulike illness which resolved with supportive management and the patient had no sequelae. That episode was characterized by acute-onset chest pain consistent after having severe flulike symptoms for 1 to 2 weeks, elevated troponins, and no ischemic changes on EKG. A left heart catheterization with coronary angiography was done revealing normal and patent coronary arteries, and the specific offending virus was not identified. He was of Hispanic ethnicity and a lifelong nonsmoker and reported only rare alcohol consumption on social occasions. He worked in construction management, exercised one to two times per week, and had a family history positive for coronary artery disease.

Upon his current presentation, the patient was found to have ST elevations in the lateral leads (Figure 1) and was taken for emergent cardiac catheterization. Coronary

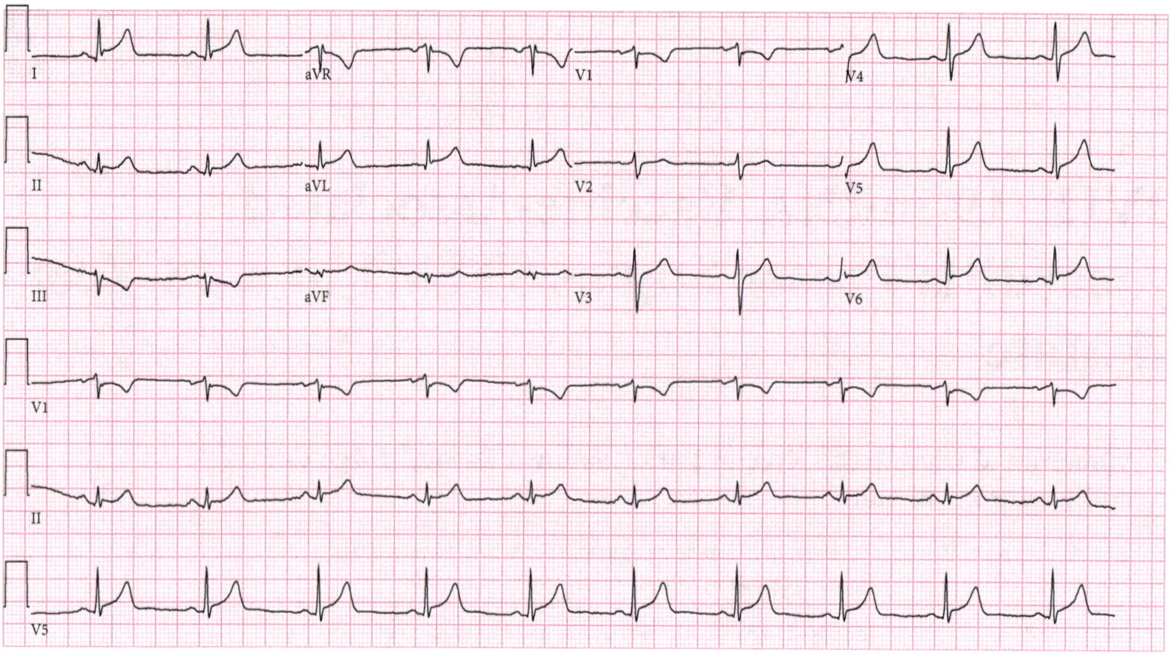

FIGURE 1: ST elevations in leads I, V4, V5, V6, aVL, and ST depression in lead III.

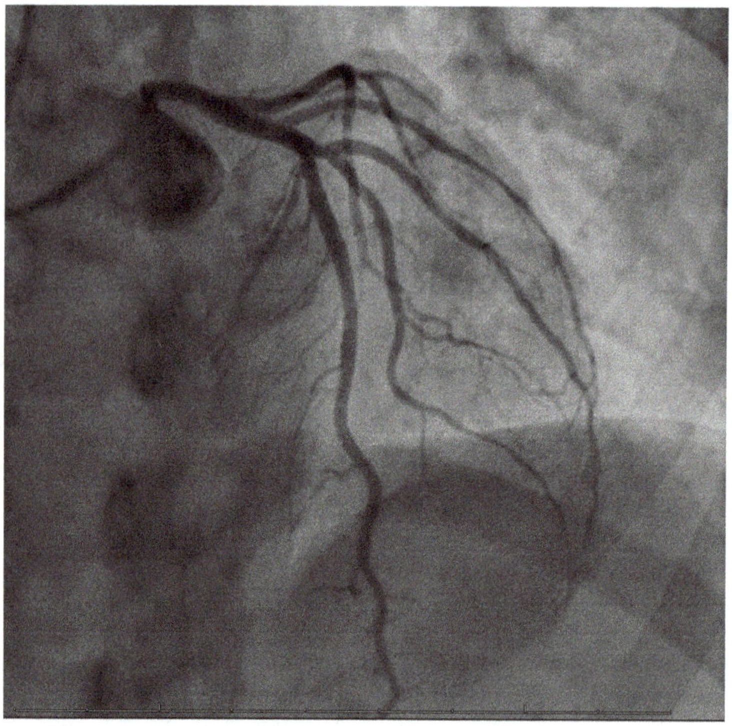

FIGURE 2: Image of patent left coronary system.

angiography revealed normal coronary arteries (Figure 2) with slow flow through the left anterior descending artery and anterolateral and apical hypokinesis, with an estimated ejection fraction of 40% on ventriculography. Pertinent laboratory testing is summarized in Table 1, including nasopharyngeal swab PCR testing for SARS-CoV-2 which resulted negative.

The next day, he had resolution of the chest pain along with resolution of his flulike symptoms. Troponins and CRP were trending down. He denied any dyspnea on exertion and subjectively felt that he was back in his usual state of health. Left ventricular biplane function ejection fraction on echocardiogram was similar to that estimated by ventriculography, and no pericardial effusion or thickening was

Table 1: Pertinent laboratory testing.

Diagnostic test	Result	Reference range and units
Troponin (presentation) (ng/mL)	4.40	≤0.045 ng/mL
Troponin (peak)	13.60	≤0.045 ng/mL
CRP	5.10	<1.00 mg/dL
ESR	21	0-20 mm/h
SARS-CoV-2 RT-PCR	Negative	Negative
Respiratory viral panel*	Negative	Negative
WBC	8.4	3.5-10.0 1000/μL
Absolute eosinophil count	0.15	0.03-0.44 10 * 3/μL
TSH	1.740	0.350-4.000 μ[IU]/mL

*Influenza A, flu A human H1, flu A human H3, INFLU A 2009 HINI Influenza B, RSV A, RSV B, parainfluenza-1, parainfluenza-2, parainfluenza-3, parainfluenza-4, metapneumovirus, rhinovirus, adenovirus B/E, adenovirus C, coronavirus 229E, coronavirus NL63, coronavirus HKU1, and coronavirus OC43.

noted. He was started on guideline-directed medical therapy with metoprolol succinate 25 mg, ramipril 2.5 mg, and atorvastatin 40 mg daily and was discharged after extensive counselling. At 3-month follow-up, the patient was feeling well with no symptoms of chest pain or shortness of breath including with exertion.

3. Discussion

In the current literature, patients with mRNA vaccine-associated myocarditis invariably presented with chest pain, usually 2 to 3 days after second-dose mRNA vaccine and had elevated cardiac troponin levels. Data from the largest study to date from Israel found that the estimated incidence of myocarditis was 2.13 cases per 100,000 persons, with the highest incidence among male patients between the ages of 16 and 29 years. Most cases of myocarditis were mild or moderate in severity. STEMI was the most common electrocardiographic presentation [1, 2]. This disease entity has been reported with both mRNA vaccines in use today, BNT162b2 mRNA-Pfizer-BioNTech and the mRNA-1273-Moderna. With or without treatment with corticosteroids, NSAIDs, and/or colchicine, almost all cases had resolution of symptoms and improvement in diagnostic markers [1].

In this case, the presentation and clinical course are compatible with those of majority of COVID-19 mRNA vaccine-associated myocarditis. Endomyocardial biopsy was not indicated due to the absence of acute-onset heart failure, hemodynamic compromise, ventricular arrhythmias, high-degree AV block, or failure to respond to medical therapy [3]. Cardiac MRI was appropriate in supporting the diagnosis of clinically suspected myocarditis. Unfortunately, this modality was unavailable at this facility. Longer follow-up is warranted to determine long-term effects and recurrence.

Only a few reports of acute thrombotic events post-mRNA COVID-19 vaccines exist and Kounis syndrome has been suggested as the pathophysiology. This along with temporally coincidental acute plaque rupture is an important differential diagnosis with life-threatening consequences if not promptly diagnosed and treated [4–6]. More reports of acute thrombotic events postvaccination for COVID-19 exist with the AZD1222 (Oxford University and AstraZeneca) adenoviral vector vaccine but this vaccine induces immunity by a different mechanism [7, 8].

As mRNA vaccine-associated myocarditis is a new phenomenon in clinical practice, there are many gaps in our understanding of the disease. Future research studies are needed to investigate the mechanism of development of mRNA vaccine-associated myocarditis, to explore predisposing factors for the development of myocarditis related to COVID-19 vaccines, and to provide guidance to those who have suffered this myocarditis on the safest future vaccination/booster strategy. This case also highlights the need to investigate if prior viral myocarditis is a predisposing factor to development of mRNA vaccine-related myocarditis.

Consent

Verbal consent was obtained from the patient. No written consent has been obtained as there is no patient identifiable data included in this case report.

References

[1] B. Bozkurt, I. Kamat, and P. J. Hotez, "Myocarditis with COVID-19 mRNA vaccines," *Circulation*, vol. 144, no. 6, pp. 471–484, 2021.

[2] G. Witberg, N. Barda, S. Hoss et al., "Myocarditis after COVID-19 vaccination in a large health care organization," *The New England Journal of Medicine*, vol. NEJMoa2110737, 2021.

[3] C. Tschöpe, L. T. Cooper, G. Torre-Amione, and S. Van Linthout, "Management of myocarditis-related cardiomyopathy in adults," *Circulation Research*, vol. 124, no. 11, pp. 1568–1583, 2019.

[4] J. Hinton, E. Briosa, A. Gala, and S. Corbett, "mRNA COVID-19 vaccine-related anaphylactoid reaction and coronary thrombosis," *Mayo Clinic Proceedings*, vol. 96, no. 12, pp. 3182-3183, 2021.

[5] J. G. Sung, P. S. Sobieszczyk, and D. L. Bhatt, "Acute myocardial infarction within 24 hours after COVID-19 vaccination," *The American Journal of Cardiology*, vol. 156, pp. 129–131, 2021.

[6] N. G. Kounis, I. Koniari, V. Mplani, S. N. Kouni, P. Plotas, and G. Tsigkas, "Acute myocardial infarction within 24 hours after

COVID-19 vaccination: is Kounis syndrome the culprit?," *The American Journal of Cardiology*, vol. 162, p. 207, 2022.

[7] O. Maadarani, Z. Bitar, M. Elzoueiry et al., "Myocardial infarction post COVID-19 vaccine - coincidence, Kounis syndrome or other explanation - time will tell," *JRSM Open*, vol. 12, no. 8, p. 205427042110252, 2021.

[8] L. Flower, Z. Bares, G. Santiapillai, and S. Harris, "Acute ST-segment elevation myocardial infarction secondary to vaccine-induced immune thrombosis with thrombocytopaenia (VITT)," *BML Case Reports*, vol. 14, no. 9, article e245218, 2021.

33

Serotonin Syndrome Induced Takotsubo Syndrome

Ian Lancaster, Jeffrey Steinhoff, Jose Mosco-Guzman, and Deep Patel

HCA Healthcare/USF Morsani College of Medicine GME/Largo Medical Center, USA

Correspondence should be addressed to Ian Lancaster; ian.lancaster.2@und.edu

Academic Editor: Muhammad Zia-Ul-Haq

Tako-tsubo syndrome is characterized by temporary systolic dysfunction of the left ventricle in the absence of coronary artery disease. Serotonin syndrome is a life-threatening condition associated with increased serotonergic activity in the central nervous system (CNS). We report a case of Tako-tsubo syndrome following seizures secondary to serotonin syndrome.

1. Introduction

Tako-tsubo syndrome is a temporary and reversible systolic dysfunction of the left ventricle's apical area, typically in the setting of an emotional or physical trigger [1]. The exact pathophysiologic mechanism of Tako-tsubo syndrome is unknown with multiple theories postulated including catecholamine-induced cardiotoxicity and microvascular dysfunction [1]. This condition can resemble an acute coronary syndrome (ACS) as both conditions may present with acute onset chest pain, dyspnea, and electrocardiogram changes, most notably acute ST segment elevations [2]. The diagnosis of Tako-tsubo syndrome is challenging in part due to similarities in presentation to an ACS [2]. The most utilized diagnostic criteria used is from the Mayo Clinic and requires that patients have echocardiographic findings of temporary hypokinesis, dyskinesis, or akinesis of the left ventricle; lack of coronary artery disease (CAD); acute electrocardiographic (ECG) changes or elevations in cardiac troponins; and no presence of pheochromocytoma or myocarditis [3]. Once identified, medical therapy with angiotensin-converting enzyme inhibitors and beta blockers is recommended [4].

In rare instances, serotonin syndrome also known as serotonin toxicity is a cause of Tako-tsubo syndrome. It is a potentially life-threating drug-induced toxidrome caused by medications which affect serotonin and ultimately leads to increased serotonergic activity in the peripheral and central nervous systems [5]. Several drug classes have been associated with a condition including selective serotonin reuptake inhibitors, serotonin norepinephrine reuptake inhibitors, serotonin modulators, and tricyclic antidepressants [5]. The clinical presentation of serotonin syndrome is variable with varying symptoms as well as differing levels of symptom severity [6]. The typical triad of clinical features is altered mental status (i.e., agitation and anxiety to confusion), autonomic hyperactivity (i.e., diaphoresis, tachycardia, hyperthermia, and diarrhea), and neuromuscular hyperactivity (i.e., myoclonus, hyperreflexia, and muscle rigidity) [6]. Included within the wide-ranging effects of excess serotonin are arterial vasoconstriction, bronchoconstriction, platelet aggregation, increased GI motility, altered wakefulness, decreased attention, altered affective behavior, altered thermoregulation, increased motor tone, and aggression [7]. Ultimately, this leads to a hyperadrenergic state leading to an increased release of catecholamines [8].

In this case report, we discuss the case of a 26-year-old female who was found to have Tako-tsubo syndrome following a generalized tonic-clonic seizure secondary to serotonin syndrome. We will discuss the proposed pathophysiologic mechanisms, diagnostic criteria, and treatment of Tako-tsubo syndrome.

2. Case Presentation

A 26-year-old Caucasian female with a past medical history of autism spectrum disorder, epilepsy, and depression presented following a seizure. From the emergency medical services (EMS) report, she had a generalized tonic-clonic seizure of unknown duration shortly before arrival and was encephalopathic during the initial evaluation. She was also noted to have urinary incontinence. While in the emergency department, the ECG showed anteroseptal ST-elevations (Figure 1) and the initial troponin was 1.10 ng/mL. Additionally, the creatine kinase (CK) on admission was 842 units/L. On physical exam, the patient was encephalopathic, myoclonus was present in the ankles, deep tendon reflexes in the upper and lower extremities were noted to be 3+ bilaterally, and the patient had an unremarkable cardiac exam. Cardiology and neurology were consulted, the patient was placed on a heparin drip and given full-dose aspirin, and a STAT transthoracic echocardiogram was ordered.

Reportedly, she was taking fluoxetine and buspirone for her anxiety and depression and zonisamide for her epilepsy as an outpatient. She had been adherent to her recommended psychiatric and antiepileptic regimens.

Additionally, at the time of admission, she was given a loading dose of levetiracetam and her home psychiatric medications were held. In addition to the heparin drip following admission, the troponins were trended and had reached a peak 6 hours after admission of 2.13 ng/mL. The troponin on 12-hour recheck was 1.51 ng/mL Also, her repeat ECG performed 6 hours after admission as well had subsequently changed from anteroseptal ST-segment elevations to normal sinus rhythm with no ST-segment elevations or depressions (Figure 1).

The STAT transthoracic echocardiography demonstrated reduced systolic function of the left ventricle with an ejection fraction of 25-30%. Additionally, the left ventricle was noted to have akinesis of the basal-mid anteroseptal walls and hypokinesis of the inferior wall (Figure 2). There were no abnormalities identified in the right atrium, left atrium, right ventricle, or heart valves.

The day following admission, the patient's encephalopathy had resolved though her CK had continued rise to 1143 units/L. She was continued on the heparin drip until the ischemic evaluation could be completed, her intravenous fluids were continued cautiously given the rising CK, and she was otherwise managed supportively. The patient was then evaluated by neurology who suspected the patient had developed serotonin syndrome due to her home use of fluoxetine and buspirone, acute metabolic encephalopathy, myoclonus, urinary incontinence, and hyperreflexia. As a result, it was recommended that her home psychiatric medications be held indefinitely and levetiracetam be continued for antiepileptic medication.

On hospital day 2, the patient's CK had reached its peak of 2155 units/L and later downtrended to 1918 units/L later that day. As her renal function had remained within normal limits with a creatinine of 0.53 mg/dL, a CTA of the coronary vessels was ordered to evaluate for possible ischemic heart disease. The study had demonstrated no significant areas of atherosclerosis or stenosis. No abnormalities of the coronary vessels were identified (Figure 3).

Following the results of the CTA of the coronary vessels, the heparin drip and aspirin were discontinued. Her antiepileptic medication was switched to levetiracetam and her zonisamide. Following continued holding of her psychiatric medication, her myoclonus and hyperreflexia had resolved as well. On hospital day 3, her intravenous fluids were discontinued. Lastly, she was started on metoprolol succinate and lisinopril for treatment of her new nonischemic cardiomyopathy. As she was hemodynamically stable, the patient was deemed appropriate for hospital discharge with instructions to follow up with an outpatient cardiologist in three to four weeks with a repeat echocardiogram to be performed at that time. Lastly, she desired to remain off of anticoagulation at the time of hospital discharge though understood that this would need to be reevaluated as an outpatient.

3. Discussion

The exact cause, etiology, and pathophysiologic mechanisms responsible for Tako-tsubo syndrome are unknown. The more accepted theories include catecholamine-induced cardiotoxicity, microvascular dysfunction, and complex integration of neuroendocrine physiology [1]. In most cases, there is believed to be an emotional or physiologic trigger initiating a stress response. Studies have shown that catecholamine concentrations are two to three times higher in Tako-tsubo syndrome in comparison to myocardial infarction. The excessive levels of catecholamines result in intracellular calcium overload consequently leading to myocardial cell injury and dysfunction [9]. This ultimately leads to the development of band necrosis, inflammatory cell infiltration, and fibrosis [10]. The microvascular dysfunction features include the development of endothelium dependent vasodilation, excess vasoconstriction, and abnormal myocardial perfusion which result in myocardial cell apoptosis [11]. In this patient's case of Tako-tsubo syndrome, the source of the excessive catecholamine release is believed to have been due to serotonin syndrome. In serotonin syndrome, the excess release of serotonin can lead to a hyperadrenergic state which may serve as a trigger for Tako-tsubo syndrome [8]. For this patient, her concurrent use of the medications fluoxetine and buspirone likely led to her case of serotonin syndrome.

Upon presentation to the emergency department, not only did the patient have a fever, seizure with postictal confusion, and myoclonus concerning for serotonin; she also had an elevated troponin and anteroseptal ST-segment elevations concerning both ACS and Tako-tsubo syndrome. When considering a case of Tako-tsubo syndrome, the clinical criteria most commonly used to identify a case were developed at Mayo Clinic and consist of four components: (1) temporary hypokinesis, dyskinesis, or akinesis in left ventricular segments with or without apical involvement; aberration in regional wall motion exceeding past a single vascular distribution; and the existence of stress elicitation; (2) the lack of significant coronary artery disease; (3) recent changes detected in the ECG (ST-segment elevation and/or T-wave inversion) or significant elevation of serum cardiac troponins; and (4) nonexistence of pheochromocytoma or myocarditis [3]. In this patient's case, she had anteroseptal ST-segment elevations with a negative coronary CT angiogram, no evidence of a pheochromocytoma or myocarditis, and a left ventricle with akinesis of the basal-mid anteroseptal wall and hypokinesis of the entire inferior wall. To rule out an ACS, the use of coronary vascular imaging, usually with coronary angiography or coronary CT scan, is typically employed to rule out coronary artery disease. Additionally, when the

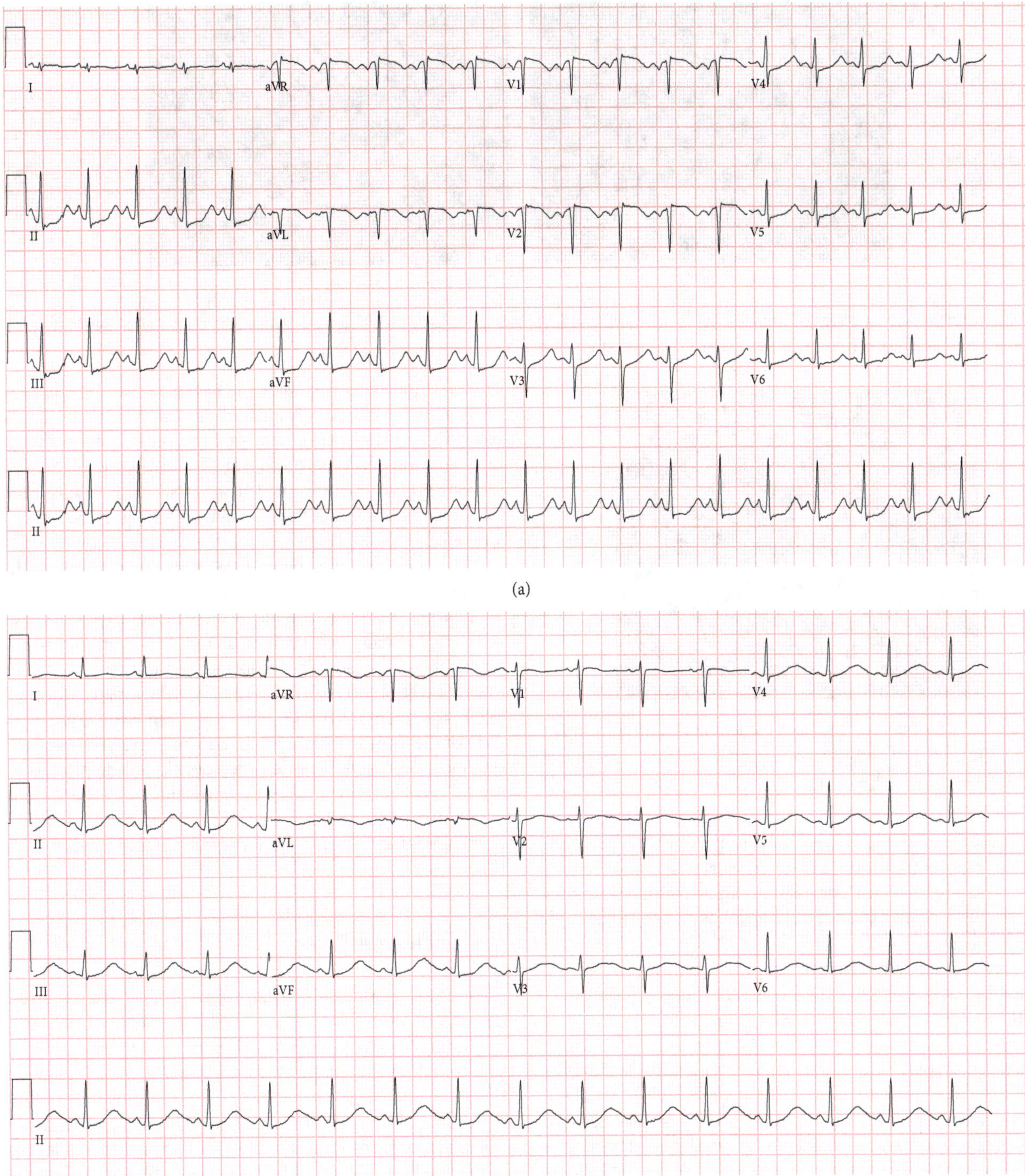

FIGURE 1: ECG (a): ECG on presentation. Sinus tachycardia with biatrial enlargement, rightward axis deviation, and septal infarction of indeterminate age with diffuse ST segment depressions in leads II, III, aVF, and V3-V6. ECG (b): repeat ECG, 6 hours after admission. Normal sinus rhythm with a prolonged QTc of 631.

diagnosis of Tako-tsubo syndrome is in doubt, cardiac magnetic resonance imaging can be used to evaluate right ventricular involvement as well as differentiate it from other cardiomyopathies [12]. In this patient's case, her diagnosis of Tako-tsubo syndrome was not in doubt so cardiac MRI was not utilized.

Until an ACS has been ruled out, treatment of Tako-tsubo syndrome typically mimics the treatment of CAD. This typically involves administration of oxygen, heparin, aspirin, and beta blockers [4]. Once Tako-tsubo syndrome is confirmed, it is reasonable to discontinue aspirin and continue beta blocker therapy due to the possible high catecholamine state and

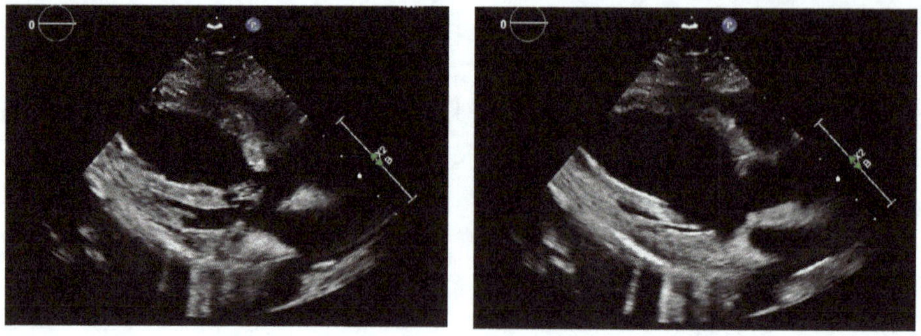

(a) (b)

Figure 2: (a) Systole and (b) diastole: transthoracic echocardiogram: left ventricular ejection fraction of 25-30% with reduced systolic function. Akinesis of the basal-mid anteroseptal wall and hypokinesis of the entire inferior wall.

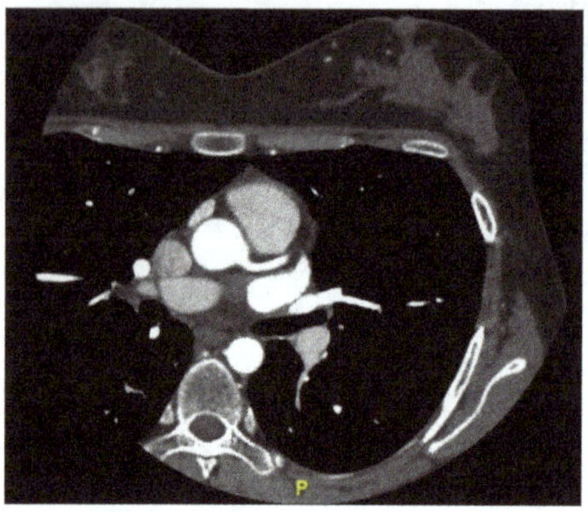

Figure 3: CTA of the coronary vessels demonstrates a patient left main and proximal segment of the left anterior descending branching off of the aorta.

angiotensin-converting enzyme inhibitor (ACE-I)/angiotensin receptor blocker (ARB) therapy for regional wall motion abnormality treatment [4]. Anticoagulation can be considered to prevent the development of an apical thrombus and reduce the risk of embolic events [4].

Even though Tako-tsubo syndrome is a transient condition, patients are at a substantial risk of complication, including during the initial hospitalization in which one in five patients is at risk of a significant adverse event [4]. Interestingly, the rates of in-hospital complications for Tako-tsubo syndrome are comparable to patients with an ACS (21% verses 19%) [4]. These adverse events are a result of both acute complications of Tako-tsubo syndrome itself, including cardiogenic shock, and cardiac arrest as well the result of a critical underlying illness [4, 13]. The most common adverse event is hypotension which can vary in severity, and it is usually the consequence of the left ventricular dysfunction [14]. Also of note, left ventricular outflow obstruction can occur and lead to worsening of the apical ballooning as it exposes the cardiac apex to higher wall stress in comparison to the basal myocardium of the left ventricle [15]. Further, both atrial and ventricular arrhythmias may be seen with atrial fibrillation being the most common, approximately 3%, though life-threatening arrhythmias such as torsade de pointes and polymorphic ventricular tachycardia can occur [4, 16]. Lastly, as previously alluded to, systemic thromboembolism is an important complication which can arise and increases the risk of ischemic stroke [2]. The most likely embolic source is from the left ventricle due to stasis of blood due to the wall motion dysfunction leading to the risk of developing a left ventricular mural thrombus [2]. The spontaneous improvement in the left ventricular function can then lead to embolization of the thrombus resulting in the ischemic stroke [2].

The majority of patients have a great prognosis with a recovery rate of 96% [17]. In-hospital mortality rates vary but are typically below 8%, and the recurrence rate is typically under 15% [18]. Usually, left ventricular function begins to recover within days and can fully recuperate within two months [19]. Patients with Tako-tsubo syndrome usually continue on heart failure treatment for twelve months and can be on anticoagulation for the same duration. In this patient's case, she was started on guideline-directed medical therapy with a beta blocker and an ACE-I. She had initially declined anticoagulation though acknowledged that this would be revisited at her follow-up appointment in 1 month with a repeat echocardiogram at that time as well.

4. Conclusion

Tako-tsubo syndrome is a temporary and reversible systolic dysfunction of the left ventricle's apical area, typically in the setting of an emotional or physical trigger [1]. In rare instances, this condition may be caused by serotonin syndrome due to the hyperadrenergic state leading to catecholamine release which leads to the development of band necrosis, inflammatory cell infiltration, and fibrosis within cardiac myocytes. Diagnosis of the condition is typically done utilizing the Mayo Clinic Criteria which includes motion abnormalities of the left ventricle, lack coronary artery disease, cardiac troponin or ECG changes, and the nonexistence myocarditis or pheochromocytoma. Initial evaluation of Tako-tsubo includes an ischemic evaluation for rule out of coronary artery disease. Once an ischemic etiology is ruled out, treatment is initiated with a beta blocker and angiotensin-converting enzyme inhibitor or an angiotensin receptor blocker. This treatment should be continued for at least twelve months, and a repeat echocardiogram should be completed 1 month after the identification suspected Tako-tsubo syndrome to ensure recovery of the left ventricular ejection fraction.

Disclosure

The views expressed in this publication represent those of the authors and do not necessarily represent the official views of HCA Healthcare or any of its affiliated entities.

Acknowledgments

This research was supported (in whole or in part) by HCA Healthcare and/or an HCA Healthcare-affiliated entity.

References

[1] K. Komamura, M. Fukui, T. Iwasaku, S. Hirorani, and T. Masuyama, "Takotsubo cardiomyopathy: pathophysiology, diagnosis, and treatment," *World Journal of Cardiology*, vol. 6, no. 7, pp. 602–609, 2014.

[2] T. Singh, H. Khan, D. T. Gamble, C. Scally, D. E. Newby, and D. Dawson, "Takotsubo syndrome: pathophysiology, emerging concepts, and clinical implications," *Circulation*, vol. 145, no. 13, pp. 1002–1019, 2022.

[3] A. Frustaci, F. Loperfido, N. Gentiloni, M. Caldarulo, E. Morgante, and M. A. Russo, "Catecholamine-induced cardiomyopathy in multiple endocrine neoplasia: a histologic, ultrastructural, and biochemical study," *Chest*, vol. 99, no. 2, pp. 382–385, 1991.

[4] C. Templin, J. R. Ghadri, J. Diekmann et al., "Clinical features and outcomes of Takotsubo (stress) cardiomyopathy," *The New England Journal of Medicine*, vol. 373, no. 10, pp. 929–938, 2015.

[5] L. V. Simon and M. Keenaghan, *Serotonin syndrome*, StatPearls Publishing, Treasure Island (FL), 2022.

[6] P. J. Mason, V. A. Morris, and T. J. Balcezak, "Serotonin syndrome. Presentation of 2 cases and review of the literature," *Medicine (Baltimore)*, vol. 79, no. 4, pp. 201–209, 2000.

[7] E. W. Boyer and M. Shannon, "The serotonin syndrome," *New England Journal of Medicine*, vol. 352, no. 11, pp. 1112–1120, 2005.

[8] A. A. Kohan, E. L. Yeyati, L. De Stefano et al., "Usefulness of MRI in takotsubo cardiomyopathy: a review of the literature," *Cardiovascular diagnosis and therapy*, vol. 4, no. 2, pp. 138–146, 2014.

[9] E. A. Martin, A. Prasad, C. S. Rihal, L. O. Lerman, and A. Lerman, "Endothelial function and vascular response to mental stress are impaired in patients with apical ballooning syndrome," *Journal of the American College of Cardiology*, vol. 56, no. 22, pp. 1840–1846, 2010.

[10] I. S. Wittstein, D. R. Thiemann, J. A. Lima et al., "Neurohumoral features of myocardial stunning due to sudden emotional stress," *The New England Journal of Medicine*, vol. 352, no. 6, pp. 539–548, 2005.

[11] A. Prasad, A. Lerman, and C. S. Rihal, "Apical ballooning syndrome (Tako-Tsubo or stress cardiomyopathy): a mimic of acute myocardial infarction," *American Heart Journal*, vol. 155, no. 3, pp. 408–417, 2008.

[12] S. Kurisu and Y. Kihara, "Clinical management of takotsubo cardiomyopathy," *Circulation Journal*, vol. 78, no. 7, pp. 1559–1566, 2014.

[13] A. Uribarri, I. J. Núñez-Gil, D. A. Conty et al., "Short- and long-term prognosis of patients with takotsubo syndrome based on different triggers: importance of the physical nature," *Journal of the American Heart Association*, vol. 8, no. 24, article e013701, 2019.

[14] D. Di Vece, R. Citro, V. L. Cammann et al., "Outcomes associated with cardiogenic shock in takotsubo syndrome," *Circulation*, vol. 139, no. 3, pp. 413–415, 2019.

[15] B. J. Maron, J. A. Towbin, G. Thiene et al., "Contemporary definitions and classification of the cardiomyopathies: an American Heart Association scientific statement from the Council on Clinical Cardiology, Heart Failure and Transplantation Committee; Quality of Care and Outcomes Research and Functional Genomics and Translational Biology Interdisciplinary Working Groups; and Council on Epidemiology and Prevention," *Circulation*, vol. 113, no. 14, pp. 1807–1816, 2006.

[16] B. Redfors, S. Jha, S. Thorleifsson et al., "Short- and long-term clinical outcomes for patients with Takotsubo syndrome and patients with myocardial infarction: a report from the Swedish Coronary Angiography and Angioplasty Registry," *Journal of the American Heart Association*, vol. 10, no. 17, article e017290, 2021.

[17] S. Kurisu, H. Sato, T. Kawagoe et al., "Tako-tsubo-like left ventricular dysfunction with ST-segment elevation: a novel cardiac syndrome mimicking acute myocardial infarction," *American Heart Journal*, vol. 143, no. 3, pp. 448–455, 2002.

[18] S. W. Sharkey and B. J. Maron, "Epidemiology and clinical profile of takotsubo cardiomyopathy," *Circulation Journal*, vol. 78, no. 9, pp. 2119–2128, 2014.

[19] S. Roshanzamir and R. Showkathali, "Takotsubo cardiomyopathy a short review," *Current Cardiology Reviews*, vol. 9, no. 3, pp. 191–196, 2013.

Complete Heart Block: A Rare Complication of Takotsubo Syndrome

N. F. N. Sakul,[1] **Srijan Shrestha**,[2] **Nikhita Balabbigari**,[1] **and Sapan Talati**[2]

[1]*Department of Internal Medicine, Overlook Medical Center, Summit, NJ 07901, USA*
[2]*Department of Cardiology, Morristown Medical Center, Morristown, NJ 07960, USA*

Correspondence should be addressed to N. F. N. Sakul; sakul68@gmail.com
Academic Editor: Man-Hong Jim

Takotsubo syndrome was believed to be a rare acute cardiac event until recently with takotsubo cardiomyopathy being its most commonly recognized and often the diagnostic feature. Its diagnosis is becoming increasingly common with varied clinical manifestations most of whom have favorable clinical outcomes, yet it can be associated with life-threatening complications. We report a case of takotsubo syndrome leading to complete heart block which is a unique complication of an otherwise self-resolving disease.

1. Introduction

Takotsubo syndrome as a cardiomyopathy is a distinct form of nonischemic cardiomyopathy characterized by abrupt onset transient regional dysfunction [1]. It is usually precipitated by an identifiable stressor and frequently presents with chest pain. The presence of arrhythmias is rare and the most common EKG abnormalities include ST segment elevation and T-wave inversions [2]. In recent years, some case reports have emerged regarding an uncommon association of AV blocks in takotsubo cardiomyopathy. While in this syndrome, the cardiomyopathy usually reverses itself, the AV blocks may not. This poses a therapeutic dilemma with respect to a possible need for intervention, such as pacemaker [3], for what was thought to be a relatively benign condition.

2. Case Presentation

This is a 73-year-old Caucasian female with history of hypertension and irritable bowel syndrome who presented to the hospital due to sudden onset retrosternal, squeezing, nonradiating chest heaviness during an episode of diarrhea. The pain was associated with minimal shortness of breath. She received aspirin 325 mg by EMS along with sublingual nitroglycerin. On examination in the emergency room, she had a blood pressure of 115/64 mm Hg, a regular heart rate of 67 beats per minute, a respiratory rate of 18 breaths per minute, and saturating 97% on room air. She had normal breath sounds and heart sounds on examination. She was started on nitroglycerin infusion, after which her chest heaviness partially improved but persisted. Initial EKG showed no acute changes but prolonged PR interval of 324 milliseconds (Figure 1).

The patient was known to have a history of prolonged PR interval noted on prior EKGs. Initial labs showed serum sodium 136 mmol/L, potassium 4.1 mmol/L, bicarbonate 22 mmol/L, chloride 102 mmol/L, BUN 42 mg/dL, creatinine 1 mg/dL, glucose 118 mg/dL, calcium 8.7 mg/dL, white cell count 7.3/nL, hemoglobin 12.1 g/dL, and platelet count 219/nL. Coagulation profile and hepatic function panel were also within normal limits. Initial troponin was 0.46 ng/dL which increased to 3.06 ng/dL after five hours. An initial diagnosis of NSTEMI was made, and the patient was started on a heparin infusion. Urgent coronary catheterization was organized.

Coronary angiogram demonstrated a nonobstructive coronary artery disease (Figures 2 and 3) with a ventriculogram showing apical ballooning and ejection fraction of 40% suggestive of takotsubo cardiomyopathy (Figures 4 and 5). The patient was admitted to the CCU, and a

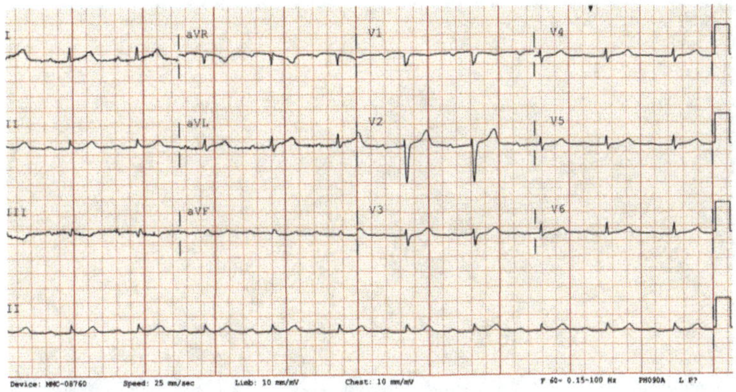

FIGURE 1: EKG on presentation showing sinus rhythm with prolonged PR interval.

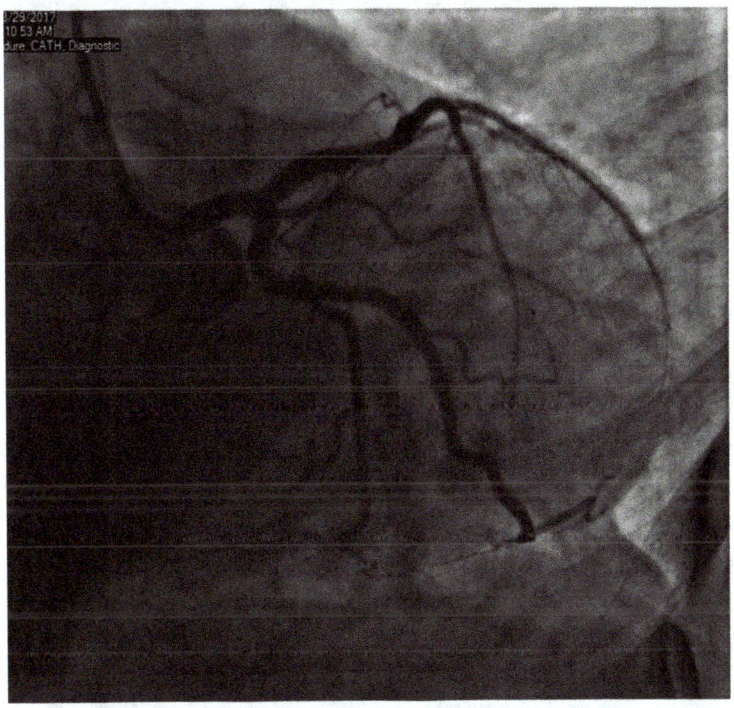

FIGURE 2: Coronary angiogram showing LAD caudal view.

transthoracic echo was done and consistent with the findings of coronary catheterization: it showed an ejection fraction of 45% with hyperdynamic inferobasal and anterior basal walls with apical ballooning indicative of takotsubo cardiomyopathy (Figure 6). She was diagnosed as having takotsubo syndrome, and her heparin infusion was discontinued. Her hospitalization was complicated by Mobitz 1 AV block (Figure 7), wide complex escape rhythms, and subsequent complete heart block (Figure 8). Because of her baseline prolonged PR interval and very high projected pacing burden, biventricular pacer was inserted. The patient remained hemodynamically stable and was discharged home after a couple of days.

A repeat echocardiogram was done outpatient, two months after hospitalization, and showed improvement: she had an ejection fraction of 55-60% with resolution of the apical ballooning and hyperdynamic wall motion changes, which were initially noted during hospitalization (Figure 6). Pacemaker interrogation revealed 100% ventricular pacing and continues to show 100% ventricular pacing even twenty months after hospital discharge. This signifies the persistence and chronicity of the AV block even after her hospitalization and after the resolution of her cardiomyopathy.

3. Discussion

Takotsubo syndrome is deemed clinically benign with most characteristic features reversing with supportive therapy within months. The wall motion abnormalities characteristic of takotsubo cardiomyopathy usually reverse completely. High-degree AV blocks and complete heart block accompanying takotsubo cardiomyopathy are a rare phenomenon [4]. However, unlike some other features associated with takotsubo cardiomyopathy, AV blocks may persist despite

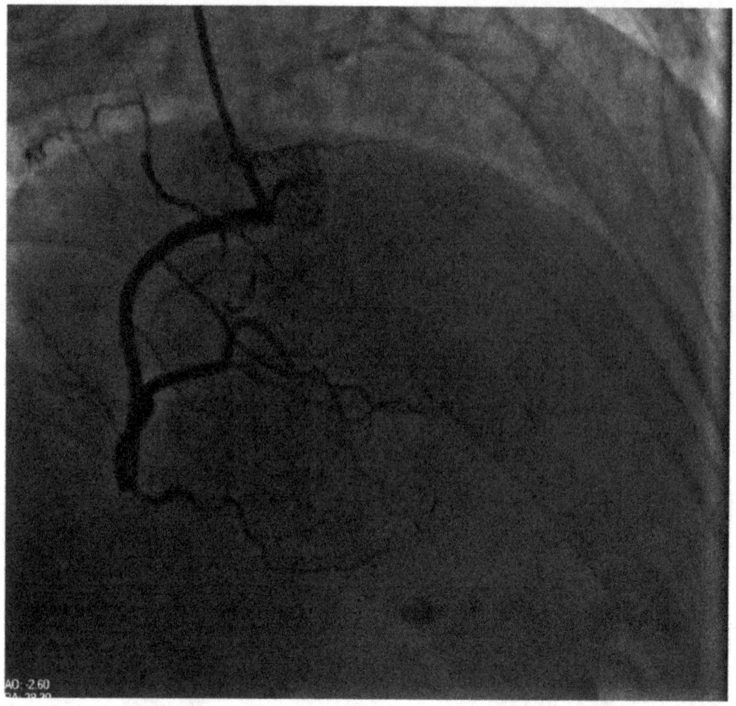

FIGURE 3: Coronary angiogram showing a view of the right coronary artery.

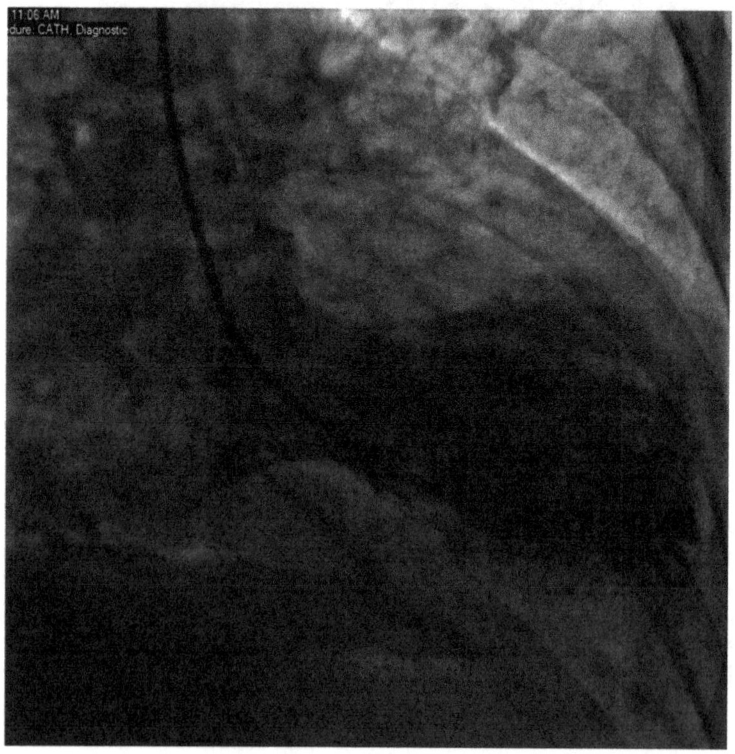

FIGURE 4: Left ventriculogram in systole.

optimal medical therapy and complete clinical recovery from other features. This may indicate that the recovery of the contractile system in takotsubo cardiomyopathy is faster than the recovery of the cardiac conduction system. Baranchuk et al. demonstrated a case in which high-degree AV block was present even after one year of initial takotsubo cardiomyopathy event but eventually resolved after 2 years of follow-up [5]. In our patient, pacemaker interrogation after 20 months of inciting event still suggested persistence of high AV block. The pathogenesis of takotsubo syndrome is not well understood, but catecholamine excess has been postulated as being central to the cause [2]. Some studies

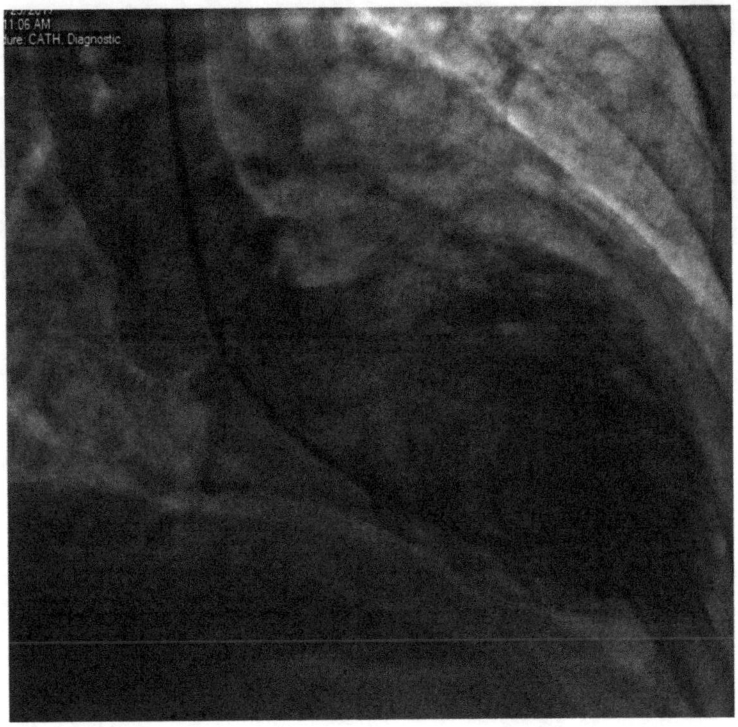

Figure 5: Left ventriculogram in diastole.

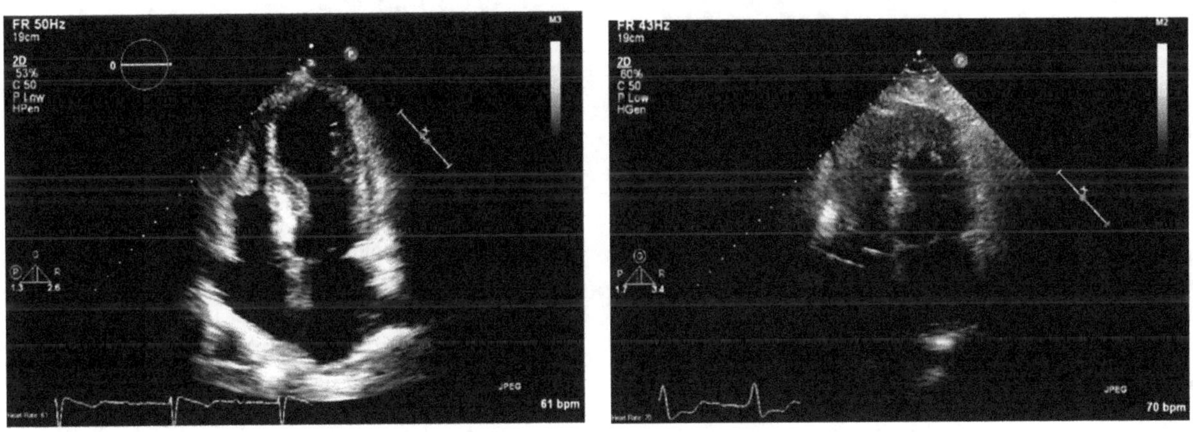

(a) (b)

Figure 6: Apical 4 chamber ECHO view (a) on presentation suggestive of takotsubo cardiomyopathy followed by repeat apical 4 chamber view (b) two months later showing recovery of previously noted wall motion abnormalities.

have even demonstrated higher circulating levels of epinephrine and norepinephrine levels in patients with takotsubo syndrome compared to patients diagnosed with myocardial infarction. Although conventional coronary angiogram does not show any obstructive lesions, some researchers suggest diffuse spasm of small branches of coronary arteries which may cause ischemia as an alternate mechanism of takotsubo cardiomyopathy [6, 7]. The latter mechanism may also explain the presence of AV conduction defects in takotsubo cardiomyopathy. There have been case reports in which AV block was shown to be the cause of takotsubo Syndrome, and the persistence of AV block in our patient despite improvement in her ventricular function raises the possibility of AV block with its subsequent symptoms as physical trigger for takotsubo syndrome. The absence of involvement of the basal segment of the left ventricle which is adjacent to the AV node also raises doubts about takotsubo syndrome causing AV block in our patient. But our patient was diagnosed as having takotsubo syndrome almost a day before continuous telemetry revealed her to be developing Mobitz type 1 block and ultimately complete heart block thus ruling out AV block as the cause of takotsubo syndrome in our patient.

4. Conclusion

Despite increasing knowledge and awareness of the historically enigmatic takotsubo syndrome, it is still believed to be

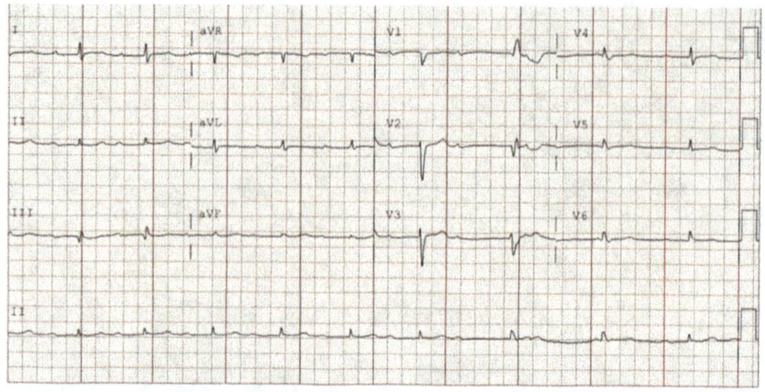

FIGURE 7: EKG showing Mobitz type 1 AV block.

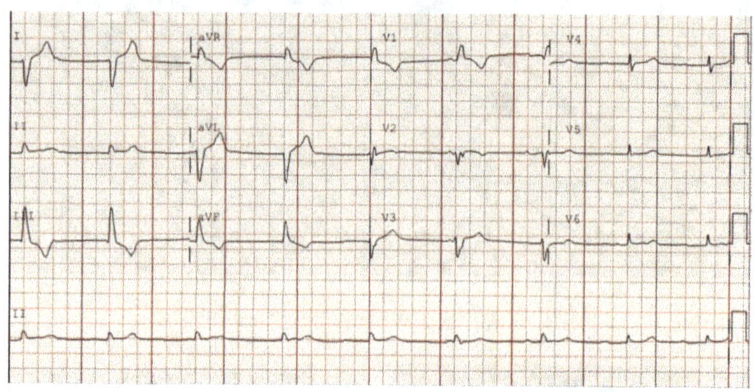

FIGURE 8: EKG showing third degree complete AV block.

a relatively benign and self-resolving entity. The recognition of AV conduction defects along with conventional and more common features is important as they may not resolve along with other features and may need intervention such as pacemaker implantation. Such situations are under recognized but are potentially life threatening and need timely management for patient safety.

Supplementary Materials

This is a four-chamber apical view on a transthoracic echocardiogram of the patient during her index hospitalization which shows the hyperdynamic inferobasal and anterobasal walls with apical ballooning consistent with Takotsubo cardiomyopathy. It also shows her EF to be around 40% with normal biatrial size, normal valvular function, and no pericardial effusion. *(Supplementary Materials)*

References

[1] K. Tsuchihashi, K. Ueshima, T. Uchida et al., "Transient left ventricular apical ballooning without coronary artery stenosis: a novel heart syndrome mimicking acute myocardial infarction," *Journal of the American College of Cardiology*, vol. 38, no. 1, pp. 11–18, 2001.

[2] K. H. Brown, R. G. Trohman, and C. Madias, "Arrhythmias in takotsubo cardiomyopathy," *Cardiac Electrophysiology Clinics*, vol. 7, no. 2, pp. 331–340, 2015.

[3] J. E. Madias, "Delving into the issue of life-threatening arrhythmias in patients with takotsubo syndrome," *International Journal of Cardiology*, vol. 195, p. 215, 2015.

[4] F. F. Syed, S. J. Asirvatham, and J. Francis, "Arrhythmia occurrence with takotsubo cardiomyopathy: a literature review," *Europace*, vol. 13, no. 6, pp. 780–788, 2011.

[5] A. Baranchuk, M. Nault, D. Redfearn, K. Bally, and C. Simpson, "A novel "proarrhythmic" disease: takotsubo cardiomyopathy," *Journal of Electrocardiology*, vol. 40, no. 4, pp. S13–S14, 2007.

[6] K. Dote, H. Sato, H. Tateishi, T. Uchida, and M. Ishihara, "Myocardial stunning due to simultaneous multivessel coronary spasms: a review of 5 cases," *Journal of Cardiology*, vol. 21, no. 2, pp. 203–214, 1991.

[7] S. Kurisu, H. Sato, T. Kawagoe et al., "Tako-tsubo-like left ventricular dysfunction with ST-segment elevation: a novel cardiac syndrome mimicking acute myocardial infarction," *American Heart Journal*, vol. 143, no. 3, pp. 448–455, 2002.

35

Clinical and Laboratory Improvement in Hyperadrenergic Postural Orthostatic Tachycardia Syndrome (POTS) after COVID-19 Infection

Rebecca A. Ocher,[1] **Erika Padilla**,[2] **Jonathan C. Hsu**,[2] **and Pam R. Taub**[2]

[1]*Department of Medicine, University of California, Los Angeles, Los Angeles, California, USA*
[2]*Division of Cardiovascular Medicine, Department of Medicine, University of California, San Diego, California, USA*

Correspondence should be addressed to Pam R. Taub; ptaub@health.ucsd.edu

Academic Editor: Ertugurul Ercan

A 32-year-old woman with a history of symptomatic supraventricular tachycardia, inappropriate sinus tachycardia, and hyperadrenergic POTS was treated with ivabradine and metoprolol. She then presented with bradycardia and Mobitz II second-degree AV block on event monitoring six weeks after COVID-19 infection. Her post-viral workup revealed normalization of catecholamine levels and significant symptomatic improvement in heart rate. To the authors' knowledge, this is the first reported case of improvement in POTS after COVID-19 infection. As our understanding of COVID-19 continues to improve, it will be vital to better understand the impact of COVID-19 dysautonomia on cardiac patients.

1. Introduction

POTS is a multifactorial disorder that most commonly affects young women [1]. POTS is a form of dysautonomia, a term that encompasses abnormal function of the autonomic nervous system [2]. Dysautonomia can more specifically be defined as either an overactivity or a failure of the sympathetic or parasympathetic components of the autonomic nervous system [3]. The pathophysiology of POTS is complex and variable, with five primary subtypes of disease (neuropathic, hypovolemic, primary hyperadrenergic, joint hypermobility-related, and immune-related) [1]. The presentations of POTS are heterogeneous, and, although the patient described was diagnosed with hyperadrenergic POTS, the pathophysiology of her POTS was most likely multifactorial [4]. The precise etiology of POTS is unknown, but there are several known stressors that may precipitate POTS—viral infection, pregnancy, vaccination, trauma, and psychosocial stress [1]. It is not surprising, therefore, that many cases of post-COVID-19 POTS/dysautonomia have been reported [5]. As our understanding of COVID-19 continues to grow, it will be important to assess how this viral infection can affect both the incidence of POTS and the impact of viral infection on patients previously diagnosed with POTS.

2. Case Presentation

A 32-year-old woman with history of Hashimoto's thyroiditis and migraines presented in September 2019 with complaints of elevated heart rate. An episode of supraventricular tachycardia was captured on electrocardiogram, and she was referred to electrophysiology for ablation. She underwent a slow pathway ablation for AV node reentrant tachycardia in January 2020. Post ablation, there were no inducible arrhythmias. However, post ablation, she complained of elevated heart rate into the 150s. In April 2020, she underwent slow pathway ablation once more and an implantable cardiac monitor was placed. This implanted monitor revealed inappropriate sinus tachycardia, for which she was symptomatic. There was no workup done to assess for POTS. She was then prescribed ivabradine for inappropriate sinus tachycardia, which improved her symptoms. Unfortunately, she also experienced blurred vision associated with ivabradine, a side effect

Table 1: Supine and standing vital signs and norepinephrine levels before and after COVID-19 infection.

	Before COVID-19 infection 9/21/2020	After COVID-19 infection 11/13/2020
Blood pressure: supine	118/84 mmHg	122/75 mmHg
Blood pressure: standing	127/84 mmHg	122/88 mmHg
Heart rate: supine	108 bpm	86 bpm
Heart rate: standing	125 bpm	97 bpm
Norepinephrine: supine	677 pg/mL	203 pg/mL
Norepinephrine: standing	855 pg/mL	419 pg/mL

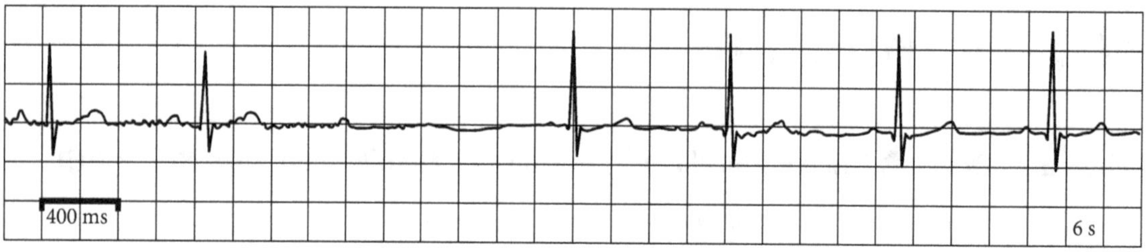

Figure 1: Zio XT Final Report 10/06/2020-10/19/2020 demonstrating Mobitz II second-degree AV block. 92 episodes of Mobitz II second-degree AV block were recorded.

that she could not tolerate due to her work demands as an airfield controller.

In July 2020, she underwent a partial sinus node ablation, after her two slow pathway ablations. She remained symptomatic with an elevated heart rate. It was then recommended by her electrophysiologist that she undergo a complete sinus node ablation with pacemaker placement due to the nature of her vocation (which prohibits her from taking medications that could impair her performance).

She sought a second opinion from a general cardiologist on September 21, 2020. On evaluation, the increase in her heart rate from 108 bpm while supine to 125 bpm while standing was suggestive of a POTS diagnosis [1]. Furthermore, her supine norepinephrine was 677 pg/mL and her standing norepinephrine level was 855 pg/mL, suggestive of hyperadrenergic POTS (Table 1). After shared decision making, the patient elected to maximize medical management once more with metoprolol and ivabradine, as well as a supervised exercise program. She took a leave of absence from her work while on these medications and was monitored via a non-real-time heart monitor for two weeks.

Of note, the patient tested positive for SARS-CoV-2 by PCR on September 24, 2020. She wore her heart monitor from October 6 through October 19, 2020. The results of her non-real-time heart monitor became available on November 10, 2020, and demonstrated bradycardia as low as 31 beats per minute and Mobitz II second-degree AV block (Figure 1). Given this reading, she was advised to present to the emergency department, and she was subsequently admitted to the cardiology service.

At the time of admission, the patient reported poor compliance with ivabradine and metoprolol, only taking these medications occasionally in the four weeks prior to her admission. Her event monitor reported 92 episodes of Mobitz II second-degree AV block lasting a total of 6 minutes and 32 seconds over the course of two weeks (Figure 1).

During her admission, the patient was evaluated by the electrophysiology service and was noted to have dropped beats on telemetry but was asymptomatic during these. Because she had two slow pathway AVNRT ablations, her fast pathway likely had a longer refractory period and the dropped beats were likely secondary to transient AV block. Because she had normal PR and QRS intervals, malignant AV nodal and infranodal pathology was thought to be unlikely. Pacemaker placement was deemed unnecessary. Metoprolol and ivabradine were not felt to be the cause of her bradycardia as she reported poor compliance with these medications prior to her admission.

After discharge, she was seen in the outpatient cardiology clinic on November 13, 2020, and her POTS was reevaluated. Her heart rate was 86 bpm while supine and 97 bpm standing. Further, her supine and standing norepinephrine levels had markedly decreased to 203 pg/mL and 419 pg/mL, respectively. The patient also reported subjectively feeling better since discharge. Heart monitoring in November 2020 recorded mostly sinus rhythm, with occasional periods of Type II AV Block, both Mobitz I and Mobitz II second-degree AV block. Since discharge, the patient has remained stable from a cardiac standpoint without requiring any chronotropic medications.

3. Discussion

While there have been reported cases of reversible POTS [6], to the authors' knowledge, this is the first reported case of both clinical and laboratory improvement in a patient with POTS after COVID-19 infection. It is important to note that there has been a broad range of COVID-19 dysautonomia reported in the literature, ranging from labile pressor requirements in the ICU to dizziness and palpitations after discharge [3, 7, 8]. The precise pathophysiology of this postviral dysautonomia has not been identified to date, but both the cytokine storm and an autoimmune response have been postulated as possible mechanisms of this autonomic dysfunction [3, 7]. Even patients that experience a mild form of COVID-19 infection may be susceptible to the long-term effects of COVID-19 dysautonomia [9]. Additionally, sympathetic overactivation may play an important role in the pathophysiology of COVID-19 infection, becoming an important variable in baseline hyperadrenergic patients [10]. All of these factors may contribute to long-term sympathetic dysregulation and immune dysregulation in recovered patients.

In this patient, we postulate that the COVID-19 infection could have "reset" her sympathetic nervous system. To this end, her previously diagnosed POTS clinically improved. Many patients anecdotally have reported both improvements and flares of POTS with viral infection. It will be important to follow this patient over time and monitor symptoms, vitals, and laboratory values, as there is no data to suggest how long these postviral effects may last. As we continue to better understand COVID-19 dysautonomia, it will be important to assess the impact on patients who may develop POTS, as well as patients with previously diagnosed POTS. Regardless of the etiology of POTS, it is important to educate patients that this is a dynamic disease and may evolve over time and that infections can significantly impact the disease trajectory.

Consent

Written informed consent was obtained from the patient.

References

[1] A. Zadourian, T. A. Doherty, I. Swiatkiewicz, and P. R. Taub, "Postural orthostatic tachycardia syndrome: prevalence, pathophysiology, and management," *Drugs*, vol. 78, no. 10, pp. 983–994, 2018.

[2] M. Bryarly, L. T. Phillips, Q. Fu, S. Vernino, and B. D. Levine, "Postural Orthostatic Tachycardia Syndrome:," *Journal of the American College of Cardiology*, vol. 73, no. 10, pp. 1207–1228, 2019.

[3] N. Eshak, M. Abdelnabi, S. Ball et al., "Dysautonomia: an overlooked neurological manifestation in a critically ill COVID-19 patient," *The American Journal of the Medical Sciences*, vol. 360, no. 4, pp. 427–429, 2020.

[4] P. R. Taub, A. Zadourian, H. Lo, C. Ormiston, S. Golshan, and J. C. Hus, "Randomized trial of ivabradine in patients with hyperadrenergic postural orthostatic tachycardia syndrome," *Journal of the American College of Cardiology*, vol. 77, no. 7, pp. 861–871, 2021.

[5] K. Kanjwal, S. Jamal, A. Kichloo, and B. P. Grubb, "New-onset postural orthostatic tachycardia syndrome following coronavirus disease 2019 infection," *The Journal of innovations in cardiac rhythm management*, vol. 11, no. 11, pp. 4302–4304, 2020.

[6] T. R. Aza Abdulla, "Reversible postural orthostatic tachycardia syndrome," *World Journal of Clinical Cases*, vol. 3, no. 7, 2015.

[7] M. Dani, A. Dirksen, P. Taraborrelli et al., "Autonomic dysfunction in long COVID: rationale, physiology and management strategies," *Clinical Medicine*, vol. 21, 2020.

[8] M. Puccioni-Sohler, A. R. Poton, M. Franklin, S. J. da Silva, R. Brindeiro, and A. Tanuri, "Current evidence of neurological features, diagnosis, and neuropathogenesis associated with COVID-19," *Revista da Sociedade Brasileira de Medicina Tropical*, vol. 53, 2020.

[9] P. Brodin, "Immune determinants of COVID-19 disease presentation and severity," *Nature Medicine*, vol. 27, no. 1, pp. 28–33, 2021.

[10] A. Porzionato, A. Emmi, S. Barbon et al., "Sympathetic activation: a potential link between comorbidities and COVID-19," *The FEBS Journal*, vol. 287, 2021.

Bidirectional Ventricular Tachycardia with Stress-Induced Cardiomyopathy

Ariyon Schreiber,[1] **Michael Gardner**,[2] **Chris Sossou**,[2] **Natasha Greene**,[2] **and Chowdhury Ahsan**[2]

[1]*University of Nevada Las Vegas School of Medicine, Department of Medicine, USA*
[2]*Department of Cardiology, University of Nevada, Las Vegas, Las Vegas, USA*

Correspondence should be addressed to Ariyon Schreiber; ariyon.schreiber@unlv.edu

Academic Editor: Luigi Sciarra

Bidirectional ventricular tachycardia (BDVT) is a rare electrocardiographic finding characterized by rapid, wide complex, alternating QRS morphology with 180-degree swings in the frontal plane axis or, less commonly, alternating right bundle branch and left bundle branch block morphology. The most proposed mechanisms for BDVT involve triggered activity or enhanced automaticity resulting from calcium dysregulation. Catecholamine surge can cause myocardial injury as well as calcium dysregulation resulting in enhanced automaticity that can lead to arrhythmias such as BDVT. This case report stands to describe a unique presentation of BDVT and stress-induced cardiomyopathy, resulting from catecholamine surge following multiple traumatic gunshot wounds in the setting of methamphetamine use.

1. Introduction

Bidirectional ventricular tachycardia (BDVT) is a unique phenomenon that has fascinated electrophysiologists since its first description in 1922 [1]. Characterization of BDVT on electrocardiogram (ECG) most commonly includes rapid, wide complex, and alternating QRS morphology with 180-degree swings in the frontal plane axis, and less commonly includes alternations of right bundle branch and left bundle branch forms [2]. Various etiologies for BDVT have been proposed, including digitalis toxicity, hypokalemia, Andersen-Tawil syndrome, acute myocarditis, and catecholaminergic polymorphic ventricular tachycardia (CPVT). Most of the proposed mechanisms involve triggered activity or enhanced automaticity resulting from calcium dysregulation [2]. We describe a unique case of BDVT, resulting from a catecholamine surge following multiple traumatic injuries in the setting of methamphetamine use. Furthermore, the BDVT described in this case was associated with a stress-induced cardiomyopathy, suggestive of Takotsubo's cardiomyopathy, which resolved within days.

2. Case Report

A 22-year-old male with no significant past medical history, including no history of arrhythmia or syncope, presented with multiple gunshot wounds to the face and bilateral upper extremities. The patient was intubated en route for airway protection.

Upon arrival to trauma resuscitation, the patient was noted to be tachycardic at 112-113 beats per minute, hypertensive with a systolic pressure > 200 mmHg (peak 241 mmHg), and saturating O_2 at 100%. Initial ECG demonstrated characteristics consistent with BDVT, including tachycardia with a left-axis deviation pattern alternating with a right-axis deviation pattern, as well as an alternating bundle branch block (Figure 1(a)). Repeat ECGs were found to be normal at both twenty minutes and four hours (Figure 1(b)).

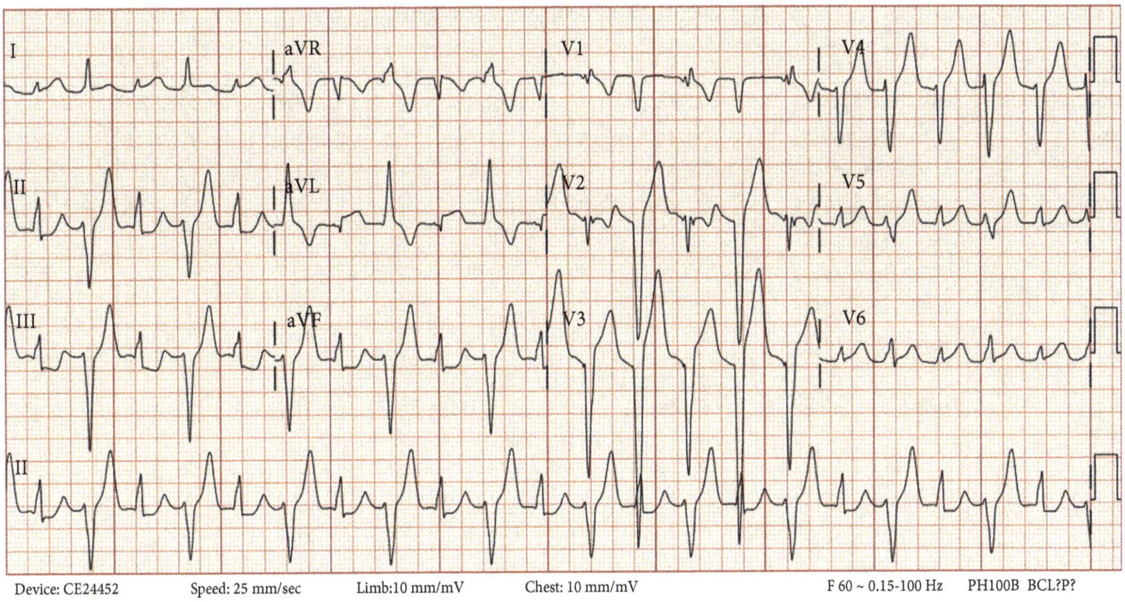

(a)

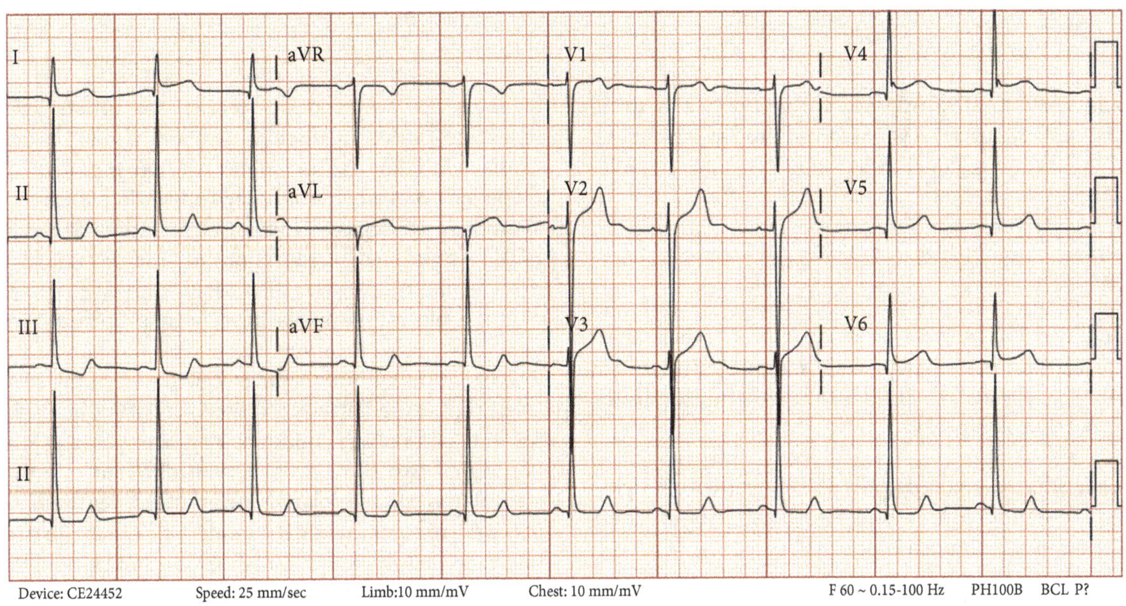

(b)

Figure 1: (a) ECG of patient upon presentation to the ED, demonstrating characteristics of BDVT. (b) 4 hours later: repeat ECG found to be normal.

Patient's labs were significant for mild hypokalemia, minimally elevated hs-troponin-I, and significant leukocytosis (Table 1). Urine drug screen demonstrated recent use of methamphetamine, benzodiazepines, and tetrahydrocannabinol.

Transthoracic echocardiography (TTE) demonstrated midleft ventricular (LV) apical hypokinesis and apical ballooning, basal LV hyperkinesis, and mildly reduced left ventricular systolic function (LVSF) consistent with stress-induced cardiomyopathy (Figure 2(a)). Recorded values included an end-diastolic volume (EDV) of 59.3 mL, an end-systolic volume (ESV) of 26.8 mL, and an ejection fraction (EF) of <55%.

Following numerous surgical interventions, the patient was successfully extubated and discharged on aggressive guideline-directed medical therapy (GDMT), per 2017 recommendations from the Journal of the American College of Cardiology (JACC) for mortality reduction in patients with reduced ejection fraction (EF) [3], including carvedilol 12.5 mg twice daily, lisinopril 5 mg once daily, and spironolactone 25 mg once daily. The patient was also instructed to follow up on an outpatient basis with cardiology. Due to patient's age and suspicion of prompt recovery, a repeat echo was performed 14 days later. Compared to the initial echocardiogram, LVSF improved to normal function, including

TABLE 1: Important laboratory values.

Laboratories	Reference	Day 1	Day 2	Day 3	Day 4	Day 5
White blood cell	3.10-10.20 K/mm^3	17.16 (H)	18.38 (H)	15.03 (H)	13.57 (H)	12.87 (H)
Hemoglobin	13.1-16.8 g/dL	8.1 (L)	7.4 (L)	7.1 (L)	9.6 (L)	9.9 (L)
Platelets	119-332 K/mm^3	173	179	169	240	275
Magnesium	1.60-2.60 mg/dL	1.80	1.72	1.74	1.61	1.61
Sodium	136-145 mmol/L	139	137	138	135	136
Potassium	3.5-5.1 mmol/L	3.2 (L)	4.5	4.0	4.6	4.1
Creatinine	0.55-1.3 mg/dL	0.91	0.86	0.86	0.72	.79
Calcium	8.4-10.2 mg/dL	7.7 (L)	8.3 (L)	8.3 (L)	7.2 (L)	8.2
Troponin I	0.020-0.040 ng/mL	10.669 (H) 9.168 (H) 7.467 (H)	6.224 (H) 3.798 (H) 2.072 (H)	1.753 (H) 1.807 (H)	—	—
pH, arterial	7.350-7.450	7.404	7.385	7.440	—	—
pCO_2, arterial	35.0-45.0 mmHg	40.5	47.1 (H)	37.6	—	—
pO_2, arterial	80.0-100 mmHg	465 (H)	148 (H)	190 (H)	—	—
O_2 Sat, arterial	90.0-100.0%	>100.5 (>)	99.9	100.0 (H)	—	—
PEEP	cmH_2O	5	5	—	—	—
FIO_2	%	100.0	40.0	46.0	—	—

increases in EDV to 109.6 mL, ESV to 40.6 mL, and EF to >55%. The left ventricle was visualized to be normal in size and without regional wall motion abnormalities (Figure 2(b)).

3. Discussion

BDVT is defined as a tachycardia showing beat-to-beat alternations in the QRS axis of ventricular complexes in at least some of the ECG leads [4]. Similar to cases reported in the literature, our ECG displays

(1) a left-axis deviation pattern alternating with a right-axis deviation pattern and visualization of an alternating bundle branch block [4]

(2) tachycardia occurring in a short burst, lasting only a few minutes, and resolving spontaneously

(3) wide QRS complexes [4]

(4) a regular rhythm despite an underlying rhythm of atrial fibrillation [4]

The exact etiology of our patient's BDVT is ultimately unknown. Though digitalis toxicity is the most common cause of BDVT, our patient reported no cardiac history and denied past or present digoxin use. Further, our patient was not taking any known herbal supplementation, eliminating concern for aconite poisoning. He had no past history nor familial history of cardiac arrest, ryanodine receptor mutations (RYR2), and/or neurologic deficits, ruling out Andersen-Tawil syndrome and decreasing the likelihood of CPVT, though this differential cannot be completely eliminated due to the potential of sporadic RYR2 mutations and lack of genetic exploration and counseling. Finally, he had no signs nor symptoms of recent viral illness, myocardial infarction, valvular disease, left ventricular hypertrophy, cardiac sarcoidosis, ischemic cardiomyopathy, or acute coronary syndrome, ultimately winnowing out a number of alternative etiologies. This patient's unique presentation of BDVT prompted exploration of the literature to best describe the mechanism and etiology involved.

Multiple mechanisms have been proposed for BDVT. One of the most prominent proposed mechanisms includes dysregulation of intracellular calcium leading to elevated levels that cause delayed afterdepolarization in anatomically separate parts of the conducting system. Baher et al. [5] proposed that two separate foci, with different rate thresholds for delayed afterdepolarization-induced ventricular bigeminy, were present in a rabbit model [6]. When the ventricular rate exceeded the lower threshold, bigeminy would develop. This would effectively double the heart rate, increasing the overall ventricular rate above the second threshold. Once this has developed, the two competing sites would simply alternate on a beat-to-beat basis. This is likely the mechanism underlying BDVT observed with digitalis toxicity and CPVT.

Genetic investigators have demonstrated that most families with CPVT have mutations in genes regulating the level and/or function of proteins responsible for the balance of intracellular myocyte calcium [7]. In addition to autosomal dominant mutations in the ryanodine receptor (RYR2), mutations in calsequestrin-2 (CasQ2), Kir2.1-inward-rectifier potassium channel (KCNJ2), calmodulin (CALM1), and triadin (TRDN) have been identified in families with the clinical picture of CPVT [7]. Most models to explain the disease focus on RyR2 mutations, as they account for more than half of diagnosed cases and multiple mutations have been identified [7]. The mouse models of RyR2 mutations suggested that delayed afterdepolarizations are

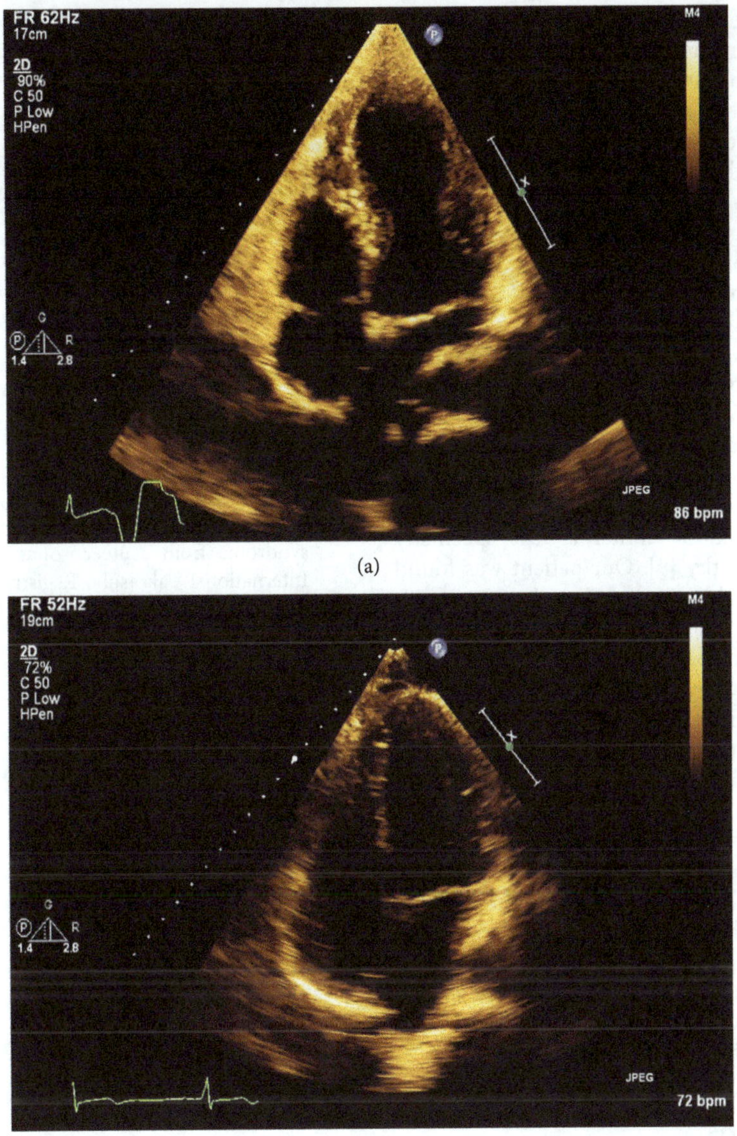

(a)

(b)

FIGURE 2: (a) TTE apical 4-chamber view in systole, demonstrating apical ballooning, suggestive of Takotsubo's stress-induced cardiomyopathy. (b) 14 days later: TTE apical 4-chamber view in systole, demonstrating resolution of patient's Takotsubo's stress-induced cardiomyopathy.

triggered in all myocytes when exposed to known stressors, such as caffeine and adrenaline, or spontaneously [6].

It is likely in our case that in the setting of multiple traumas and recent methamphetamine use, severe dysregulation of intracardiac calcium channels from catecholamine toxicity led to the manifestation of this unusual and rare arrhythmia. It is well known that methamphetamine use can lead to catecholamine toxicity by binding vesicular monoamine transporter 2, accumulating vesicles of dopamine in the synaptic cleft and norepinephrine in the cytosol, inhibiting enzyme monoamine oxidase to stabilize cytosolic catecholamine levels, inhibiting dopamine and norepinephrine transporters preventing catecholamine reuptake, and stimulating catecholamine release through exchange diffusion and modulation of receptor activity. This results in an acute upsurge in dopamine and norepinephrine, resulting in catecholamine toxicity and consequential calcium dysregulation.

Catecholamine toxicity explains not only the rare manifestation of BDVT but also our patient's stress-induced cardiomyopathy. It has been suggested that catecholamine surge can cause damage to cardiomyocytes by two primary mechanisms. The first mechanism is characterized by calcium overload, consecutive beta-adrenergic receptor-mediated activation of protein kinase A, and subsequent phosphorylation of multiple Ca^{2+}-cycling proteins, including sarcolemmal L-type Ca^{2+} channels, phospholamban, and sarcoplasmic reticulum ryanodine receptor Ca^{2+} release channels (RyR2) [7]. Increased intracellular calcium and calcium dysregulation lead to increased automaticity of the cardiac myocyte, resulting in this momentary manifestation of BDVT. The second mechanism is characterized by oxidative stress, primarily related to the transformation of catecholamines into "aminochromes." Aminochromes then undergo redox cycling in mitochondria to generate copious amounts of oxygen-derived free radicals [8]. This oxidative damage may have led to our patient's stress-induced cardiomyopathy and later reversal. Initiating aggressive GDMT likely played a role in this patient's spontaneous recovery. These two mechanisms can explain both our patient's manifested BDVT and his stress-induced cardiomyopathy.

With regard to the diagnosis of Takotsubo's cardiomyopathy, recent studies performed using the international Takotsubo registry have found a scoring system that can accurately differentiate Takotsubo syndrome from acute coronary syndrome without the use of coronary angiography with 89% sensitivity and 91% specificity [9]. Patients with scores of greater than 50 confer a 95% specificity for Takotsubo cardiomyopathy [9]. Our patient was found to have an underlying psychiatric disorder, absence of ST-segment changes on ECG, and physical and emotional triggers conferring a score of 61. Coronary angiography was deferred in his case due to several emergent surgical interventions, numerous comorbidities, and low suspicion for acute coronary syndrome. The patient was instructed to follow up outpatient with cardiology for angiography once stable; unfortunately, his records indicate that he has been, thus far, lost to follow up.

In conclusion, there is a great deal of data to explain the connection between BDVT, stress-induced cardiomyopathy, and catecholamine surge; however, there are no systematic studies to demonstrate evidence of connection. Herein, we provide the first-ever documented case of BDVT manifested alongside a stress-induced cardiomyopathy with apical morphology triggered by catecholamine surge.

Authors' Contributions

Ariyon Schreiber and Michael Gardner have equal authorship as first authors.

References

[1] C. Schwensen, "Ventricular tachycardia as the result of the administration of digitalis," *Heart*, vol. 9, pp. 199–204, 1922.

[2] S. A. Durrani, R. Sung, and M. Scheinman, "Bidirectional ventricular tachycardia due to a mixture of focal fascicular firing and reentry," *Cardiac Electrophysiology Clinics*, vol. 8, no. 4, pp. 753–764, 2016.

[3] C. W. Yancy, J. L. Januzzi, L. A. Allen et al., "2017 ACC expert consensus decision pathway for optimization of heart failure treatment: answers to 10 pivotal issues about heart failure with reduced ejection fraction: a report of the American College of Cardiology Task Force on Expert Consensus Decision Pathways," *Journal of the American College of Cardiology*, vol. 71, no. 2, pp. 201–230, 2018.

[4] S. Lévy and E. Aliot, "Bidirectional tachycardia: a new look on the mechanism," *Pacing and Clinical Electrophysiology*, vol. 12, no. 5, pp. 827–834, 1989.

[5] A. A. Baher, M. Uy, F. Xie, A. Garfinkel, Z. Qu, and J. N. Weiss, "Bidirectional ventricular tachycardia: ping pong in the His-Purkinje system," *Heart Rhythm*, vol. 8, no. 4, pp. 599–605, 2011.

[6] M. M. Benjamin, K. Hayes, M. E. Field, M. M. Scheinman, and K. S. Hoffmayer, "Bidirectional ventricular tachycardia in cardiac sarcoidosis," *Journal of Arrhythmia*, vol. 33, no. 1, pp. 69–72, 2017.

[7] M. Cerrone, B. Colombi, M. Santoro et al., "Bidirectional ventricular tachycardia and fibrillation elicited in a knock-in mouse model carrier of a mutation in the cardiac ryanodine receptor," *Circulation Research*, vol. 96, no. 10, pp. e77–e82, 2005.

[8] L. Liaudet, B. Calderari, and P. Pacher, "Pathophysiological mechanisms of catecholamine and cocaine-mediated cardiotoxicity," *Heart Failure Reviews*, vol. 19, no. 6, pp. 815–824, 2014.

[9] J. R. Ghadri, V. L. Cammann, S. Jurisic et al., "A novel clinical score (InterTAK Diagnostic Score) to differentiate takotsubo syndrome from acute coronary syndrome: results from the International Takotsubo Registry," *European Journal of Heart Failure*, vol. 19, no. 8, pp. 1036–1042, 2017.

37

Eosinophilic Myocarditis: An Often-Overlooked Diagnosis in Patients Presenting with Heart Failure

Young Min Cho,[1] **Abdullah Asreb**,[1] **Riaz Mahmood**,[1] **Ahmad Moaz**,[1] **and Ugochukwu Egolum**[2]

[1]*Internal Medicine Residency Program, Northeast Georgia Medical Center, Gainesville, Georgia, USA*
[2]*Georgia Heart Institute, Northeast Georgia Medical Center, Gainesville, Georgia, USA*

Correspondence should be addressed to Young Min Cho; mario.youngmin@gmail.com
Academic Editor: Yi Yan

Introduction. Hypereosinophilic syndrome (HES) is a rare disease characterized by unexplained peripheral eosinophilia along with evidence of end-organ damage. Cardiac involvement is the most life-threatening consequence and is frequently underreported with a prevalence of around 5%. The gold standard for diagnosis is myocardial biopsy, but less-invasive imaging such as cardiac MR (CMR) has been frequently used to help with the diagnosis. We are presenting a unique case of a patient diagnosed with Eosinophilic myocarditis (EM) supported by CMR with rapid improvement after starting steroid treatment. *Case Presentation.* A 67-year-old African American female with extensive cardiovascular disease history presenting with chest pain was diagnosed with EM secondary to hypereosinophilic syndrome (HES). Lab workup revealed absolute eosinophils of $4.70 \times 10^3/\mu L$ (normal $0 - 0.75 \times 10^3/\mu L$). Transthoracic echocardiography showed mild reduction in left ventricular function and a large obliterating thrombus in the right ventricular apex. CMR showed increased signal intensity at the left ventricular and right ventricular apex, consistent with myocardial edema. Subsequently, the patient was placed on dexamethasone 10 mg daily with significant symptomatic improvement. *Discussion.* EM is a rare complication of hypereosinophilic syndrome and can mimic common cardiovascular diseases such as acute exacerbation of heart failure or myocardial infarction. A high index of suspicion is essential especially in the setting of suggestive lab workup. CMR is a promising noninvasive and cost-effective alternative for myocardial biopsy in diagnosis.

1. Introduction

Hypereosinophilic syndrome (HES) is a rare disease characterized by unexplained peripheral eosinophilia along with evidence of end-organ damage. The estimated prevalence is between 0.36 and 6.3 per 100,000 [1]. It is defined as an absolute eosinophilic count (AEC) of $>1.5 \times 10^3$ cells/microL (μL) in the peripheral blood on two examinations separated in time by at least one month and/or pathologic evidence confirming tissue hypereosinophilia (HE) [2]. The persistent hypereosinophilia leads to eosinophilic-mediated organ dysfunction, and cardiac manifestations occur in only about 5% of the cases [3]. Earlier studies described much lower prevalence of cardiac involvement, but with the advancements in imaging and biopsy, the diagnosis rate is gradually increasing [4] [5]. As described by Loeffler in 1973, eosinophil-mediated heart disease has three stages [6]. The first stage is characterized by acute early necrosis due to eosinophilic and lymphocytic infiltration followed by subsequent eosinophil degranulation and microabscess formation within the myocardium [7]. In the second stage, thrombi formation occurs along the damaged endocardium of either or both ventricles and occasionally even within the atrium [8]. The final stage is the fibrotic stage, where the thrombus converts to fibrosis. This process leads to progressive tissue scarring and ultimately restrictive cardiomyopathy due to eosinophilic myocarditis (EM). Common clinical presentations are dyspnea, chest pain, signs of left-sided and/or right-sided congestive heart failure (CHF), mitral regurgitation, cardiomegaly, and T wave inversions.

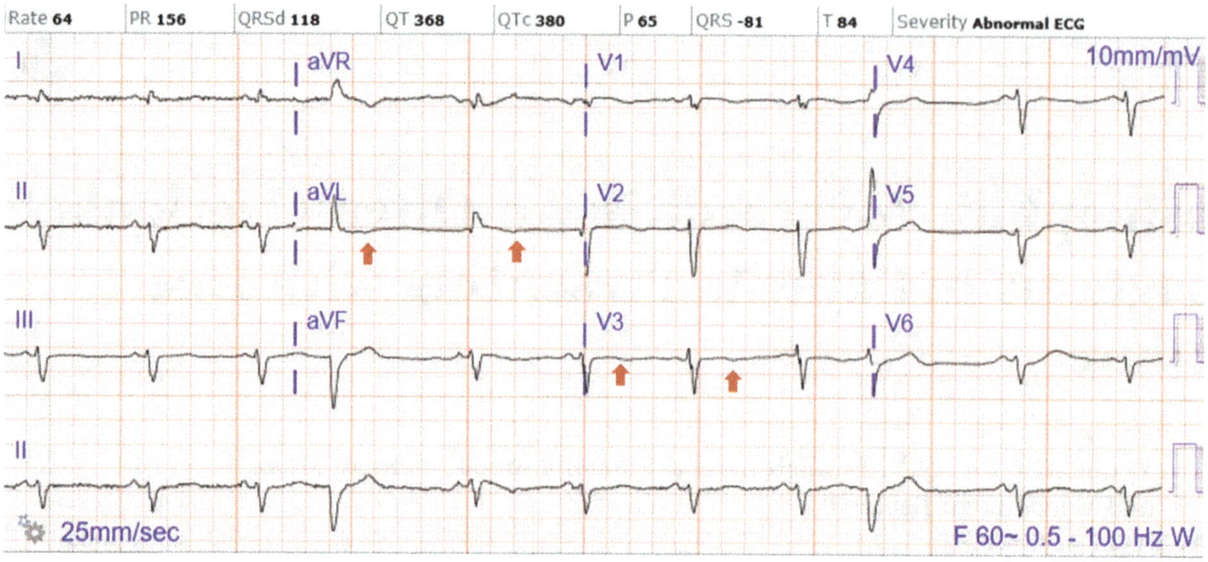

FIGURE 1: Electrocardiogram on a day of admission with sinus rhythm, left axis deviation, T wave inversion in aVL, and V3 and multiple premature ventricular contraction.

To this date, there are no standardized diagnostic criteria for EM, and typically, a multimodal imaging approach is utilized. Electrocardiogram (EKG) manifestations of myocarditis are ST-T changes, atrioventicular block (AV), bundle branch block, and ventricular arrhythmias, but the sensitivity and specificity are not enough to diagnose EM [9]. Transthoracic echocardiography (TTE) can detect intracardiac thrombi. The extent of fibrosis shows thickening of involved valve leaflets, and an increase in the intensity of endomyocardial echoes in areas of endomyocardial fibrosis. However, the accuracy of TTE to diagnosis is limited due to highly variable finding associated with myocarditis resulting false negative diagnosis [10]. Coronary angiography does not diagnose the EM, but it helps to rule out acute coronary disease. Cardiac magnetic resonance imaging (CMR) imaging plays a major role in the diagnosis as it reliably detects all aspects and stages of eosinophilic-mediated heart damage. The pattern of cardiac manifestations is variable and can include myocardial edema, fibrosis, and sedimentation of thrombotic material and reduced systolic or diastolic function [11]. Cardiac biopsy provides definitive evidence of eosinophil-associated cardiac disease by showing infiltration with eosinophils by staining of the biopsy for antibodies for eosinophil granule proteins [12]. Biopsy is usually reserved for cases where cardiac eosinophil involvement is uncertain. Cardiac MRI has high sensitivity for even the earliest stages of EM, and in this case report, we will highlight the role of CMR as a noninvasive tool for the early diagnosis of EM.

2. Case Presentation

A 67-year-old African American female with an extensive history of cardiovascular disease including heart failure with preserved ejection fraction (EF of 50-55%), hypertension, coronary artery disease treated with coronary artery bypass graft surgery, mitral valve repair, stage IV chronic kidney disease, and dyslipidemia presented to the ED with chest pain and interscapular back pain for four days. The chest pain was intermittent, sharp, and worsened with deep inspiration. On presentation, she was afebrile, with a blood pressure of 121/86 mmHg, a heart rate of 70 bpm, and a respiratory rate of 20 breaths per minute with SpO2 of 100% on room air. Physical examination was notable for jugular venous distension (JVD) at more than 10 cm H_2O at 90°. Laboratory workup was remarkable (creatinine level of 2.2 mg/dL (NR 0.6-1.00 mg/dL), BUN 31 mg/dL (NR 3.0-23.0 mg/dL), hemoglobin (Hgb) 9.8 g/dL (NR 12.0-16.0 g/dL), hematocrit 30.6% (NR 37.0-47.0%), absolute eosinophils $4.70 \times 10^3/\mu L$ (NR $0–0.75 \times 10^3/\mu L$), relative eosinophils 49% (NR 0-7%), D-dimer 3.118 μg/mL FEU (NR $\leq$ 0.400 μg/mL FEU), and B-type natriuretic peptide (BPEP) of 1,385.2 pg/mL (NR 0.0–100.0 pg/mL)). Cardiac panel was performed every 3 hours for ischemic evaluation and consistently remained within normal limits. Electrocardiogram (EKG) showed sinus rhythm, left axis deviation, T wave inversion in aVL, and V1, multiple premature ventricular complexes, and left anterior fascicular block (Figure 1). Her chest X-ray was unremarkable for acute finding. Chest

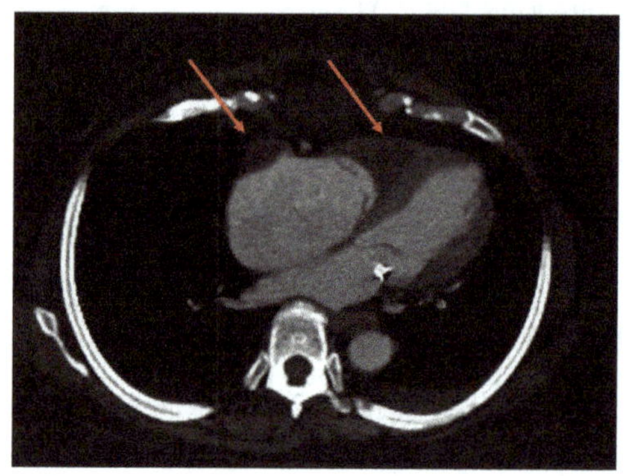

FIGURE 2: CTA showing evidence of right atrial and right ventricular apical thrombus (red arrows).

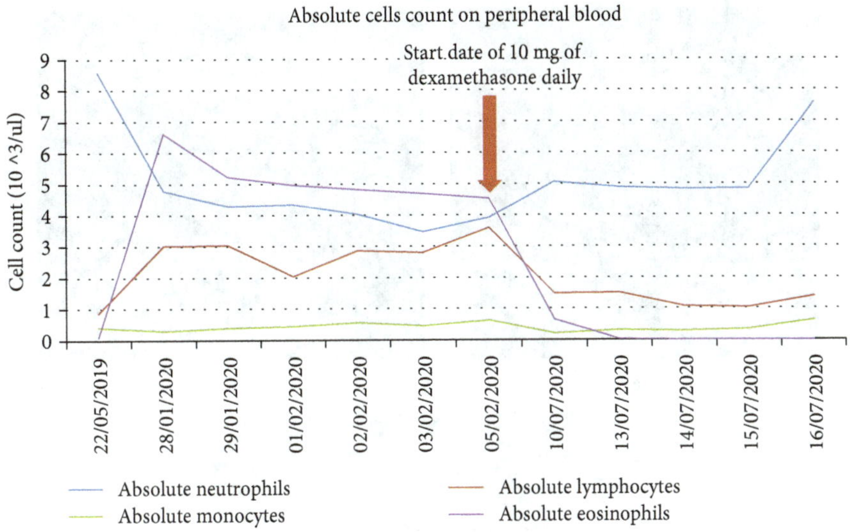

FIGURE 3: Trend of absolute eosinophil count from 5/22/19 to 7/16/2020 and start date of dexamethasone 10 mg daily.

computed tomography angiography (CTA) was negative for pulmonary embolism or aortic dissection; however, there was evidence of right atrial and right ventricular apical thrombus (Figure 2). Transthoracic echocardiography (TTE) demonstrated midrange left ventricular systolic function (estimated ejection fraction 45-50%). Right ventricular systolic function was moderately reduced. A homogeneous obliterative mass was detected at the right ventricular apex (video 1). Subsequently, the patient was placed on unfractionated heparin infusion. A review of her medical records revealed a high level of eosinophils for the past 3 months (Figure 3), qualifying her for a diagnosis of HES. Her eosinophilia in combination with the imaging findings was highly suggestive of eosinophilic myocarditis (EM). Cardiac MRI without gadolinium contrast infusion due to worsening renal function was subsequently performed. T2-weighted images showed increased signal intensity at the left ventricular and right ventricular apex, consistent with myocardial edema (MRI Figure 4(a)). T1-weighted images showed increased signal intensity in the same area (MRI Figure 4(b)). Balanced steady free precession images showed mildly reduced left ventricular systolic function with calculated EF of 44% with probable right ventricular apical and right atrial thrombus (MRI Figures 4(c)). Clinical history in combination with imaging data from echocardiography and CMR was highly suggestive of eosinophilic myocarditis. Further studies including SARS-COV-2 PCR and Stool ova/parasite studies were negative. Laboratory workup for antinuclear antibodies (ANA), anti-DNA, perinuclear antineutrophil cytoplasmic antibodies (p-ANCA), and antimyeloperoxidase (MPO) were also negative. Bone marrow biopsy was performed and showed hypereosinophilia. Fluorescence in situ hybridization (FISH) for factor interacting with PAPOLA and CPSF1 (FIP1L1) platelet-derived growth factor receptor α (PDGFRA) was negative for rearrangements. Given her presentation and workup suggestive of HES, the patient received the diagnosis of EM due to HES. The patient was started on corticosteroids with significant improvement in her symptoms. With the patient's improvement after steroids and highly suggestive findings on MRI, cardiac biopsy was deferred. She was discharged home on oral anticoagulation and steroids with close follow-up with cardiology.

3. Discussion

HES is a rare disease which must be suspected in individuals with persistent eosinophilia in peripheral blood on at least two occasions with a minimum time interval of 4 weeks [3]. The diagnosis of EM is challenging particularly due to the lack of specific diagnostic criteria and rarity of the condition. A high index of suspicion must be kept while working up patients with peripheral eosinophilia and heart failure. During the diagnostic workup, it is crucial also to identify secondary causes such as eosinophilic leukemia, eosinophilia from drug reactions, and parasitic infections. Regardless of the cause of eosinophilia, EM can be life-threatening if not diagnosed early and managed appropriately.

Endomyocardial biopsy is the gold standard for diagnosis of EM [1]. Noninvasive cardiovascular imaging, however, has gradually gained more recognition as an accepted initial alternative where cardiac biopsy is not feasible. Biopsy can also be of limited sensitivity if the sample was not sufficient and imposes greater risk on the patient. It is estimated that the sensitivity of biopsy is around 54% [7]. As demonstrated by Looi et al., the use of CMR assists in the early diagnosis of the disease and the initiation of appropriate therapy [13].

In our case, the diagnosis of EM was made based on the combination of history of presenting illness, physical examination, TTE findings, and CMR along with the finding of peripheral eosinophilia which was further supported by the bone marrow biopsy. The CMR on T1-weighted fat showed increased signal intensity in the myocardium and T2 with increased signaling intensity of myocardium in the appendix of left and right ventricles consistent with myocardial hyperemia, muscular inflammation, and myocardial edema, respectively. The patient did not receive a myocardial biopsy

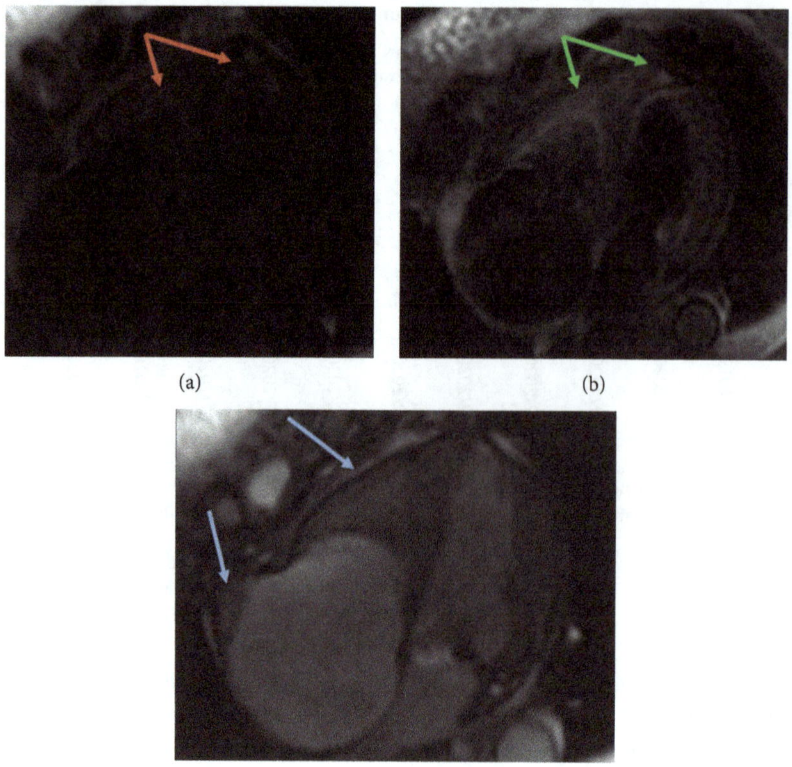

(c)

FIGURE 4: CMR. (a) Double inversion recovery (IR) T2-weighted axial imaging showing increased signal intensity of myocardium in the appendix of left and right ventricles consistent with myocardial edema (red arrows). (b) Tripe IR T1-weighted fat saturation axial image showing again signal intensity in the myocardium (green arrows). (c) Balanced steady state free precession (bSSFP) horizontal long axis still frame showing increase signaling with severe right atrial enlargement and possible thrombus (blue arrows).

prior to receiving treatment with steroids and had a subsequent rapid symptomatic improvement after a course of high-dose steroid therapy and was safely discharged home.

Findings that are suggestive of EM on CMR include hyperintesity on T1 (myocardial hyperemia) or T2- (tissue edema) weighted imaging with subendocardial late gadolinium enhancement and thickened fibrotic changes with inflammatory infiltrates [14, 15].

Often, there will be an associated intracardiac thrombus, which was the case in our patient as well.

Multiple limitations such as sampling errors, severe complications (perforation, tamponade), cost, and availability limit the use of endomyocardial biopsy, compromising patient safety. Therefore, a recent meeting by the International Consensus Group of Cardiovascular MR supports using CMR as a diagnosis method combined with clinical evidence [16].

Finally, another promising imaging modality is the use of PET-MRI scan as an alternative tool to assess treatment responsiveness. PET-MRI can show the gadolimium enhancement in the myopericardium and locate the inflammation [17]. However, there is no literature finding using the PET-MRI as a diagnosis tool for EM and clinical correlation, and other imaging might be necessary to support the diagnosis.

4. Conclusion

EM secondary to idiopathic HES remains a challenging diagnosis. The combination of clinical presentation, lab workup revealing eosinophilia, CMR findings, and TTE are helpful in the diagnosis and initiating treatment early. Findings on CMR that raise suspicion for EM include thickened fibrotic ventricles and edema of the ventricular wall.

Consent

Consent was obtained and saved at Northeast Georgia Medical Center.

Authors' Contributions

AA, YMC, and RM retrieved and corroborated the data. AA, YMC, and RM collaborated in the discussion. RM, AM, and UE collaborated in the internal review and proofreading. All authors contributed to manuscript revision and read and approved the submitted version. AA and YMC contributed equally to the work.

Acknowledgments

We thank Dr. Ioannis Parastatidis (Department of Cardiology at Northeast Georgia Medical Center) for reading the CMR and helping to develop the discussion.

References

[1] M. M. Crane, C. M. Chang, M. G. Kobayashi, and P. F. Weller, "Incidence of myeloproliferative hypereosinophilic syndrome in the United States and an estimate of all hypereosinophilic syndrome incidence," *Journal of Allergy and Clinical Immunology*, vol. 126, no. 1, pp. 179–181, 2010.

[2] P. Valent, A. D. Klion, H.-P. Horny et al., "Contemporary consensus proposal on criteria and classification of eosinophilic disorders and related syndromes," *Journal of Allergy and Clinical Immunology*, vol. 130, no. 3, pp. 607–612.e9, 2012.

[3] W. Shomali and J. Gotlib, "World Health Organization-defined eosinophilic disorders: 2019 update on diagnosis, risk stratification, and management," *American Journal of Hematology*, vol. 94, no. 10, pp. 1149–1167, 2019.

[4] P. U. Ogbogu, D. R. Rosing, and M. K. Horne, "Cardiovascular manifestations of hypereosinophilic syndromes," *Immunology and Allergy Clinics of North America*, vol. 27, no. 3, pp. 457–475, 2007.

[5] R. Mankad, C. Bonnichsen, and S. Mankad, "Hypereosinophilic syndrome: cardiac diagnosis and management," *Heart*, vol. 102, no. 2, pp. 100–106, 2016.

[6] I. F. Brockington and E. G. Olsen, "Loffler's endocarditis and Davies' endomyocardial fibrosis," *American Heart Journal*, vol. 85, no. 3, pp. 308–322, 1973.

[7] H. Sasano, R. Virmani, R. H. Patterson, M. Robinowitz, and J. G. Guccion, "Eosinophilic products lead to myocardial damage," *Human Pathology*, vol. 20, no. 9, pp. 850–857, 1989.

[8] M. Tanino, K. Kitamura, G. Ohta, Y. Yamamoto, and G. Sugioka, "Hypereosinophilic syndrome with extensive myocardial involvement and mitral valve thrombus instead of mural thrombi," *Pathology International*, vol. 33, no. 6, pp. 1233–1242, 1983.

[9] P. Kuchynka, T. Palecek, M. Masek et al., "Current diagnostic and therapeutic aspects of eosinophilic myocarditis," *BioMed Research International*, vol. 2016, Article ID 2829583, 6 pages, 2016.

[10] N. Tran, C. S. Kwok, S. Bennett, K. Ratib, G. Heatlie, and T. Phan, "Idiopathic eosinophilic myocarditis presenting with features of an acute coronary syndrome," *Echo Research and Practice*, vol. 7, no. 1, pp. K1–K6, 2020.

[11] C. Merten, H. Beurich, D. Zachow, F. Arndt, F. Moosig, and G. Richardt, "Cardiac involvement in hypereosinophilic syndromes detected by cardiac magnetic resonance imaging," *Journal of Cardiovascular Magnetic Resonance*, vol. 17, no. S1, pp. 1-2, 2015.

[12] B. L. Wright, K. M. Leiferman, and G. J. Gleich, "Eosinophil granule protein localization in eosinophilic endomyocardial disease," *New England Journal of Medicine*, vol. 365, no. 2, pp. 187-188, 2011.

[13] J. L. Looi, P. Ruygrok, G. Royle, Z. Raos, C. Hood, and A. J. Kerr, "Acute eosinophilic endomyocarditis: early diagnosis and localisation of the lesion by cardiac magnetic resonance imaging," *The International Journal of Cardiovascular Imaging*, vol. 26, no. S1, pp. 151–154, 2010.

[14] I. S. Syed, M. W. Martinez, D.-L. Feng, and J. F. Glockner, "Cardiac magnetic resonance imaging of eosinophilic endomyocardial disease," *International Journal of Cardiology*, vol. 126, no. 3, pp. e50–e52, 2008.

[15] E. Y. Kim, S.-A. Chang, Y.-K. Lee, J.-O. Choi, and Y. H. Choe, "Early non-invasive diagnosis and treatment of acute eosinophlic myopericarditis by cardiac magnetic resonance," *Journal of Korean Medical Science*, vol. 26, no. 11, pp. 1522–1526, 2011.

[16] M. G. Friedrich, U. Sechtem, J. Schulz-Menger et al., "Cardiovascular magnetic resonance in myocarditis: a JACC white paper," *Journal of the American College of Cardiology*, vol. 53, no. 17, pp. 1475–1487, 2009.

[17] A. Parikh, M. G. Trivieri, A. Lala et al., "PET/MRI: a novel imaging modality to guide tailored immunotherapy in eosinophilic myocarditis," *Journal of the American College of Cardiology*, vol. 73, no. 9, pp. 2891–2891, 2019.

38

Stress-Induced Cardiomyopathy Secondary to COVID-19

Aneesh Bapat, Abhishek Maan, and E. Kevin Heist

Cardiac Arrhythmia Service, Massachusetts General Hospital, Boston, MA 02114, USA

Correspondence should be addressed to E. Kevin Heist; kheist@partners.org

Academic Editor: Ertugrul Ercan

A 67-year-old female with prior medical history of HTN and asthma presented with acute-onset dyspnea and nausea for 4 days prior to admission. Upon initial encounter in the emergency room, she was found to have findings of abnormal pulmonary infiltrates and consequent workup revealed COVID-19. During further hospital course, the patient developed abnormal EKG and echocardiographic findings consistent with stress-induced cardiomyopathy.

1. Introduction

As the world deals with the ongoing SARS-CoV2 pandemic, there is growing recognition of its cardiovascular effects, which include myocarditis, arrhythmias, and thromboemboli. Given the degree to which the pandemic has affected daily life, it is associated with significant social and emotional stress in addition to its health-related effects. Herein, we describe a case of stress-related cardiomyopathy—first recognized via marked repolarization abnormalities on electrocardiogram—in a patient with SARS-CoV2 in the absence of ongoing competing cardiovascular issues. We discuss the typical electrocardiographic findings related to stress-induced cardiomyopathy and survey the literature for mechanistic insights. As the ongoing pandemic continues to take its course, it will be important to remain vigilant about the electrical findings of this entity, which are accompanied by an increased risk of arrhythmia.

2. Case Presentation

2.1. History of Present Illness. A 67-year-old female presented to the ER with approximately 4 days of exertional dyspnea. These symptoms were accompanied with significant nausea. Despite the use of rescue inhalers, her symptoms persisted and she sought further medical attention in the ER. On EMS arrival, she was found to have an oxygen saturation < 90% on room air and required oxygen supplementation with a nonrebreather.

2.2. Past Medical History. The patient's relevant past medical history was remarkable for asthma, HTN, and DM: all of these were well controlled. She did not have any prior structural heart disease history; however, a prior echocardiogram (which was done for evaluation of syncope) in 2006 had shown left ventricular ejection fraction of 65% without any regional wall motion abnormalities. In addition, a noncontrast chest CT done within a year of this admission incidentally showed mild to moderate coronary and aortic arch calcification.

2.3. Emergency Room Evaluation. On arrival to the ER, the patient was found to be tachycardic with a HR of 118 bpm (Figure 1(b)) and required 2-4 liters of supplemental oxygen. Chest XR revealed "bilateral predominantly peripherally distributed patchy opacities" (Figure 1(a)). Her initial laboratory investigation was remarkable for elevations in LDH, CK, and inflammatory markers, but with a normal high-sensitivity troponin T (Table 1). The polymerase chain reaction test for SARS-CoV2 was detected to be positive.

2.4. Initial Hospital Course. The patient was admitted to the inpatient non-ICU unit and was primarily managed with supportive care. She required 2-3 l/min of O_2 during the day and 4-6 l/min of O_2 overnight along with nocturnal proning. She did not require treatment with any investigational pharmacotherapy including hydroxychloroquine, remdesivir, or biologic monoclonal antibodies.

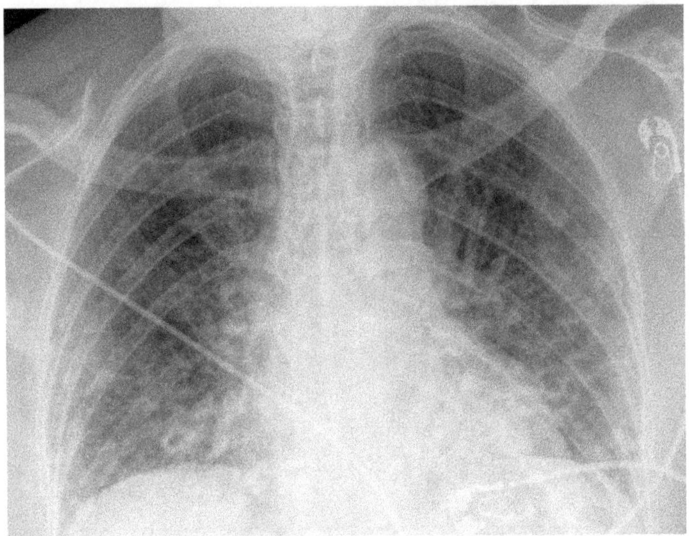

(a)

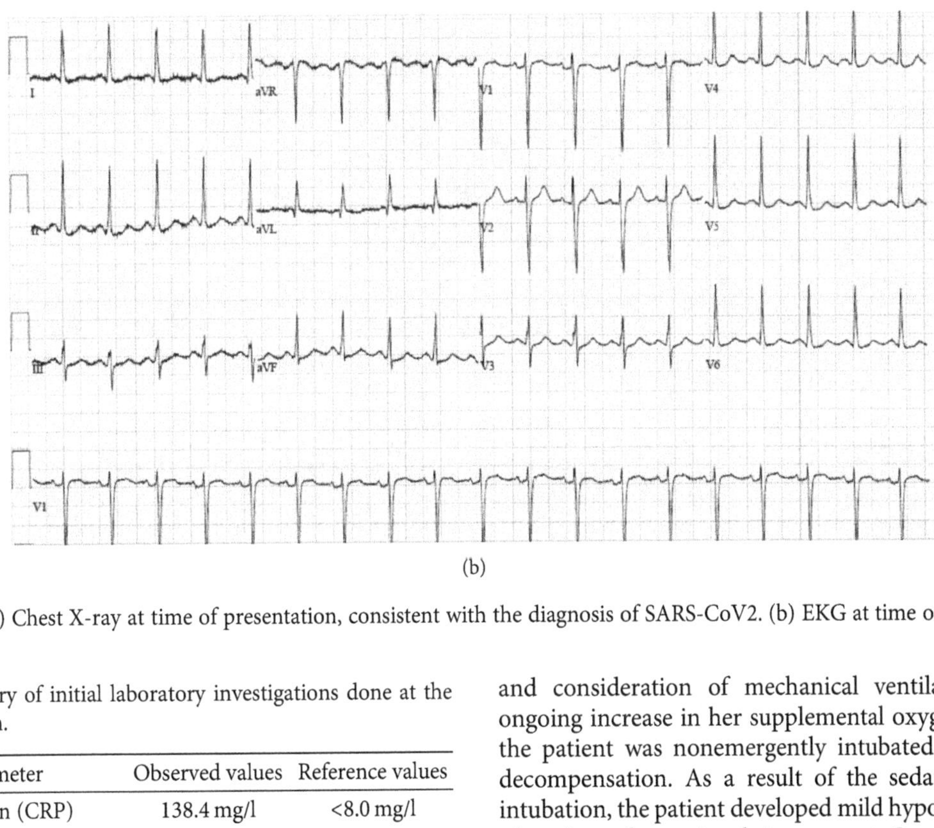

(b)

FIGURE 1: (a) Chest X-ray at time of presentation, consistent with the diagnosis of SARS-CoV2. (b) EKG at time of presentation.

TABLE 1: Summary of initial laboratory investigations done at the time of admission.

Laboratory parameter	Observed values	Reference values
C-reactive protein (CRP)	138.4 mg/l	<8.0 mg/l
Serum ferritin	328 μg/l	10-100 μg/l
Serum creatinine	0.76 mg/dl	0.60-1.50 mg/l
Lactate dehydrogenase (LDH)	318 U	110-210 U/l
NT-proBNP	474 ng/l	0-900 ng/l
hs-troponin	10 ng/l	0-9 ng/l

2.5. Clinical Decompensation and ICU Course. On the fourth day of her hospitalization, the patient ambulated to the restroom and on return had a desaturation to <85% oxygen. She required a rapid uptitration of supplemental oxygen via facemask, so she was transferred to the ICU for closer monitoring and consideration of mechanical ventilation. Given the ongoing increase in her supplemental oxygen requirements, the patient was nonemergently intubated to avoid further decompensation. As a result of the sedation required for intubation, the patient developed mild hypotension requiring a low dose of norepinephrine support. Over the course of the day, her pressor requirement remained unchanged, and her respiratory status was stable on minimal ventilation settings with a PaO_2/FiO_2 ratio of >150.

On the night of her respiratory decompensation and transfer to the ICU, a routine EKG was done and was remarkable for new repolarization abnormalities (Figure 2(a)). At that time, there was no clinical decompensation or change in her ventilatory or pressor support requirements. Over the following 48 hours, serial EKGs (Figures 2(b)–2(c)) showed continued persistence of T wave inversions and progressive prolongation in the QT interval. High-sensitivity troponin levels were checked at the time of the patient's initial

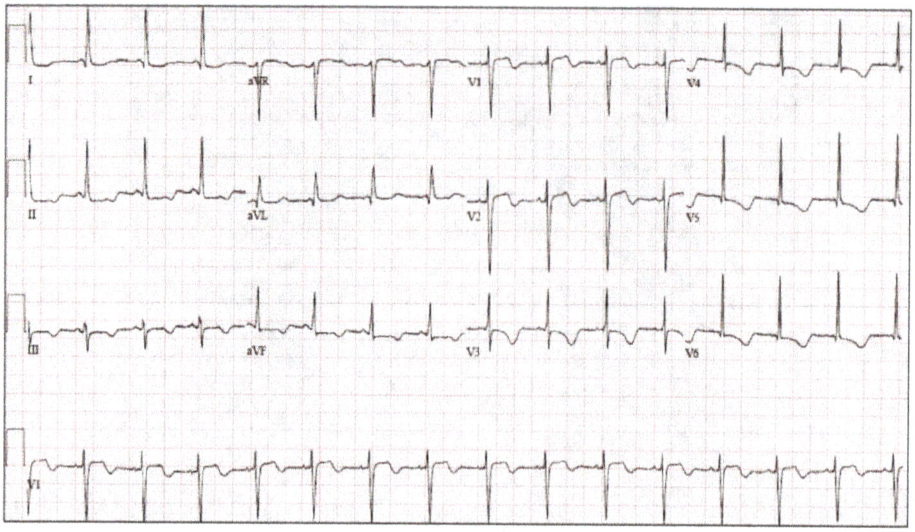

(a)

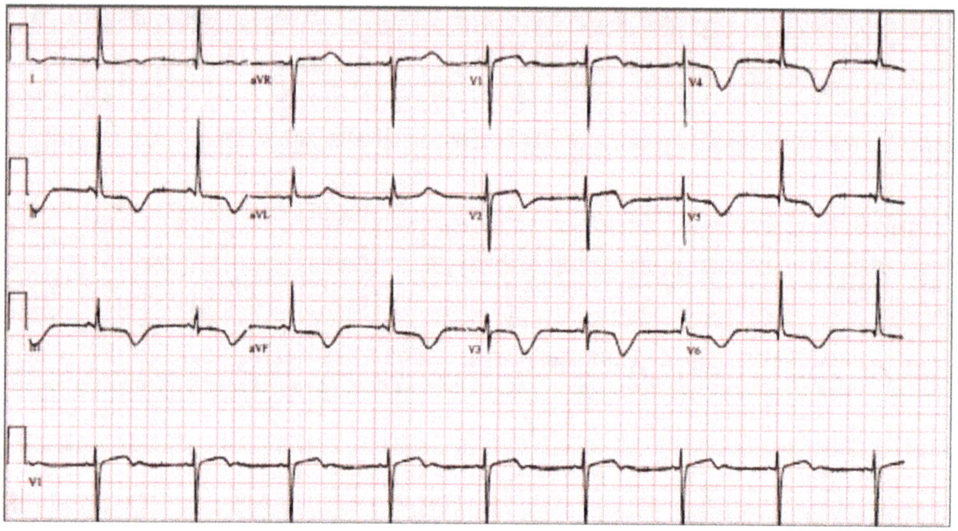

(b)

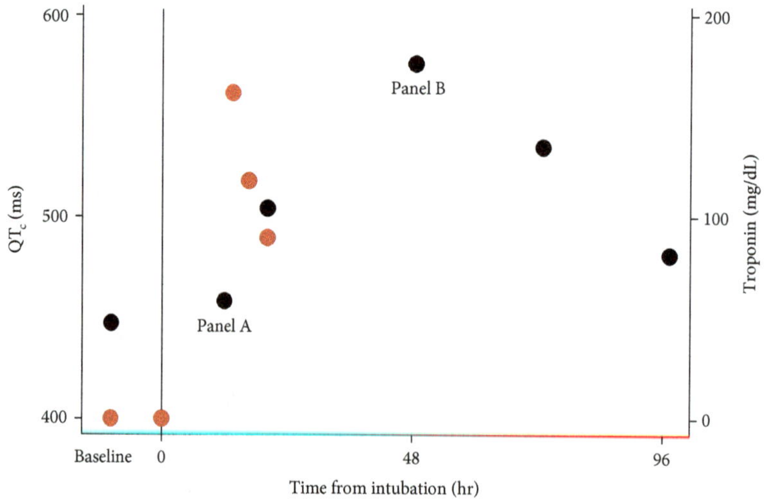

(c)

FIGURE 2: (a) EKG done approximately 12 hours after respiratory decompensation requiring intubation showing ST elevations and biphasic T waves. (b) EKG done approximately 48 hours after intubation showing marked QT prolongation. (c) Time course of QTc and hsTnT values after intubation.

respiratory decompensation and then again in the context of the EKG finding; there was biomarker evidence of cardiac injury which quickly resolved (Figure 2(c)). A TTE done approximately 24 hours after the patient's respiratory decompensation revealed preserved left ventricular ejection fraction of 61% but with new apical hypokinesis. (Figure 3, Supplemental Video #1).

2.6. Differential Diagnosis. We suspect that the patient's clinical decompensation was secondary to respiratory decompensation which has been well-reported in light of the current COVID-19 pandemic. Additionally, we suspect that the subsequent electrical and structural cardiac abnormalities resulted from a stress-induced cardiomyopathy. However, the differential diagnosis includes coronary ischemia, and an ischemic evaluation is warranted when clinically relevant. The remainder of the differential diagnosis includes a myocarditis perhaps related to viral infection, a drug-related QT prolongation, and repolarization changes related to metabolic disarray; there is no evidence to support any of these diagnoses.

2.7. Follow-Up. Over the subsequent 2 weeks, the patient was gradually weaned from ventilator and pressor support. She was managed conservatively without any specific antiviral medications including hydroxychloroquine. Given the concern for LV dysfunction, she was started on metoprolol, and this was continued at discharge. Her HTN treatment regimen included lisinopril, which was continued. Her EKG abnormalities gradually resolved, with progressive normalization of her QT interval. She was eventually discharged to rehabilitation and will follow up with a plan for an outpatient reassessment of her LV function.

3. Discussion

We describe a case of a young patient who had initially presented with acute respiratory illness secondary to COVID-19 which rapidly progressed to hypoxic respiratory failure and required mechanical ventilatory support on day 8 after symptom onset. Her course has been complicated by biomarker evidence of myocardial injury, marked repolarization abnormalities, and TTE showing apical hypokinesis with sparing of basal segment along with overall preserved LV function. Overall, these data are supportive of a diagnosis of a stress-induced cardiomyopathy resulting from COVID-19 infection and correlated temporally to the timing of intubation.

In general, this is considered a diagnosis of exclusion, and in this case, the most glaring differential diagnosis is a critical coronary lesion affecting her apex. Unfortunately, given the patient's continued respiratory recovery, an ischemic evaluation has not yet been pursued, but this would be appropriate at time of follow-up. However, the relatively mild elevation in hs-troponin in her case seemed to correlate very well with the timing of intubation. Furthermore, the troponin elevation quickly resolved while the EKG changes continued to be persistent (Figure 2(c)) in the context of typical wall motion abnormalities of Takotsubo cardiomyopathy.

COVID-19 has led to a rapid increase in hospital admissions and mortality across the globe. Based on the initial publications, the patients with COVID-19 infection presented with myriad of symptoms ranging from fever, upper respiratory infection, and acute kidney injury. Additionally, a significant proportion of patients have also been reported to have myocarditis and acute cardiac injury. Currently published reports have reported a correlation between acute cardiac injuries with an increased risk of overall mortality.

Stress cardiomyopathy, also known as Takotsubo cardiomyopathy (TCM), was first described in 1991 and initially thought to be the result of multivessel coronary spasm in the absence of fixed epicardial coronary disease [1]. Cardiovascular findings included a typical echocardiographic pattern of apical hypokinesis with basal hyperkinesis. This cardiomyopathy—later described as "broken heart syndrome"—was found to be associated with sudden emotional stress and elevated sympathetic stimulation [2]. Triggers can be emotional or physical stressors, and in some cases, the cardiomyopathy has also been reported in the context of ongoing treatment of another critical illness. Our patient presented with SARS-CoV2 infection and developed rapid-onset respiratory distress requiring intubation and so was certainly exposed to sufficient stressors which would contribute to the development of TCM. Short-term consequences may include fulminant heart failure and cardiogenic shock, outflow tract obstruction, arrhythmias, and systemic thromboembolism. Management is generally supportive with special care taken to be vigilant for and aggressively treat the complications. Recovery of LV function is gradual but generally occurs over the course of weeks to months [3].

The EKG changes seen in this patient are typical for Takotsubo cardiomyopathy, which tends to primarily affect ventricular repolarization [2]. An early description of the temporal evolution of EKG changes in patients with TCM was consistent with that in the patient presented here: initial ST-segment elevations as well as inverted T waves in V3-V6 with progressive deepening of the TWI over the subsequent 2-3 days associated with a prolongation in QTc [4]. Given the overlap in presentation as compared to an acute myocardial infarction, there are a number of EKG-based criteria that have been validated to differentiate TCM and acute myocardial infarction [5]. Although these changes in repolarization generally resolve in the long term [4], they carry an increased risk of potentially life-threatening ventricular arrhythmias [6].

The mechanisms underlying TCM have been elusive, but a catecholamine surge seems to be the unifying driver with consequent endothelial dysfunction—including vasospasm and SCAD—and inflammation [7–9]. Similarly, the etiology of the EKG changes and altered ventricular repolarization is yet to be defined and any explanation is speculative based on analogous model systems. Animal models of TCM generally involve an acute injection of isoproterenol in rats, which results in a transient apical akinesis associated with evidence of calcium- (Ca^{++}-) overload-induced contractile dysfunction as well as increased diastolic Ca^{++} leak from the sarcoplasmic reticulum [10, 11]. Although the latter may certainly be arrhythmogenic, it would not explain the QT prolongation. The effect of sympathetic tone on ventricular

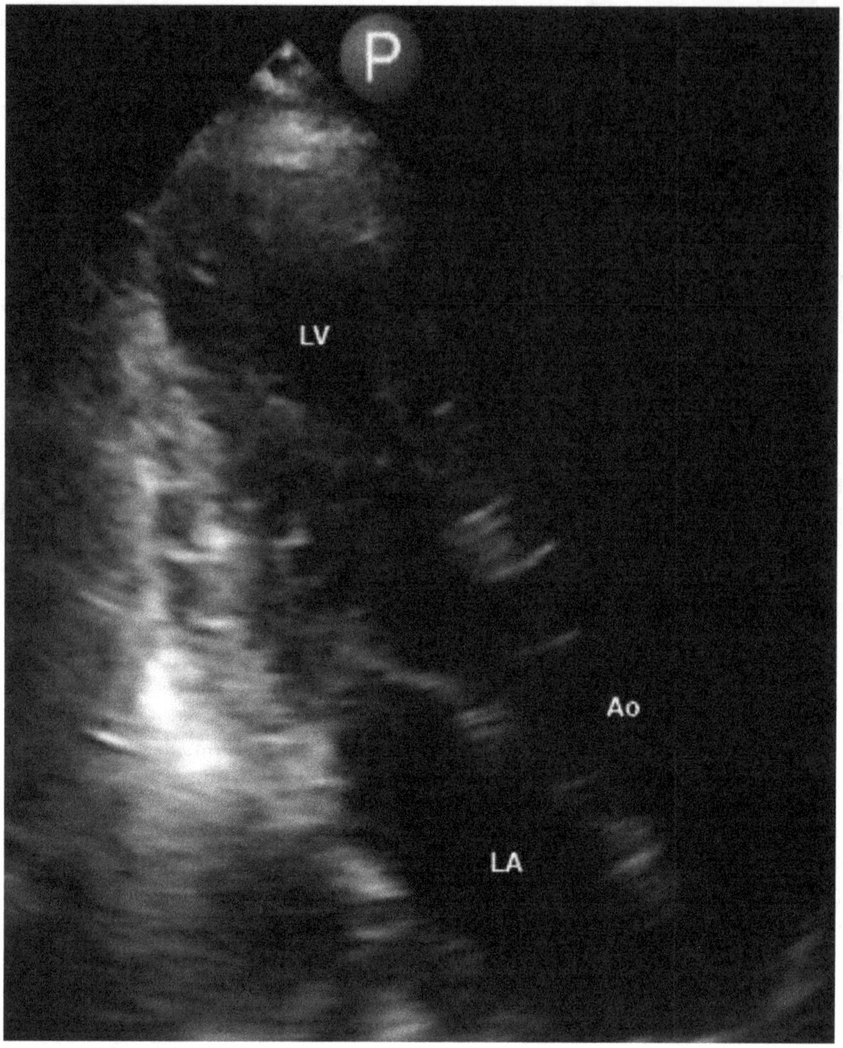

FIGURE 3: Image of the apical view of transthoracic echocardiogram showing apical hypokinesis.

repolarization is more complicated, as catecholamines such as epinephrine increase the flux through both repolarizing outward K^+ currents and depolarizing inward Ca^{++} currents; the net effects determine the overall effect on QT interval [12]. Interestingly, theoretical models as well as studies in isolated myocytes have suggested that the acute effects of catecholamines may preferentially affect calcium currents, leading to transient APD prolongation and early afterdepolarizations. These effects reflect differential kinetics, which only occur with acute exposure to catecholamines, and resolve in the steady state [13]. The dynamic effects described certainly mimic the clinical observation of transient QT prolongation seen with stress-induced cardiomyopathy.

Although the primary insults from SARS-CoV2 infection are respiratory, there has been a wide variety of diverse multi-organ manifestations. There are case reports of TCM in the context of a pericardial effusion [14] as well as a reverse TCM in the context of myocarditis [15]. Here, we present a case of TCM in the absence of any other cardiac insults. However, the SARS-CoV2 pandemic presents a myriad of potential triggers for TCM which include not only acute illness but also the social and emotional factors. The profound EKG findings are of special importance in this context. Although the use of hydroxychloroquine has fallen out of favor, treatment with azithromycin remains in the arsenal for most patients, both of which remain to be associated with the risk of QT prolongation. Additionally, early observations made during the pandemic have also suggested an increased risk of arrhythmia and sudden cardiac death associated with the virus. As the SARS-CoV2 pandemic continues to escalate, it would be prudent to remain vigilant towards the structural and electrical adverse effects which occur with TCM in the setting of acute illness.

4. Conclusions

We report a case of TCM with typical electrical and structural manifestations in the context of acute respiratory illness secondary to COVID-19 infection.

Abbreviations

HTN: Hypertension
COVID-19: Coronavirus disease 19

SARS-CoV2: Severe acute respiratory syndrome coronavirus 2
ER: Emergency room
EMS: Emergency medical services
DM: Diabetes mellitus
HR: Heart rate
CT: Computed tomography
LDH: Lactate dehydrogenase
CK: Creatine kinase
XR: X-ray
ICU: Intensive care unit
EKG: Electrocardiogram
TTE: Transthoracic echocardiogram
LV: Left ventricle
APD: Action potential duration.

Acknowledgments

AM received research grants from Medtronic, Biosense Webster, and Biotronik and research support for planned research, 07/2020, from Bardy Rx Inc EKH received research grants from Abbott, Biotronik, and Pfizer and honorarium from Medtronic, Biotronik, and Abbott.

References

[1] K. Dote, H. Sato, H. Tateishi, T. Uchida, and M. Ishihara, "Myocardial stunning due to simultaneous multivessel coronary spasms: a review of 5 cases," *Journal of Cardiology*, vol. 21, no. 2, pp. 203–214, 1991.

[2] I. S. Wittstein, D. R. Thiemann, J. A. C. Lima et al., "Neurohumoral features of myocardial stunning due to sudden emotional stress," *New England Journal of Medicine*, vol. 352, no. 6, pp. 539–548, 2005.

[3] S. W. Sharkey, "A clinical perspective of the takotsubo syndrome," *Heart Failure Clinics*, vol. 12, no. 4, pp. 507–520, 2016.

[4] S. Kurisu, I. Inoue, T. Kawagoe et al., "Time course of electrocardiographic changes in patients with tako-tsubo syndrome - comparison with acute myocardial infarction with minimal enzymatic release," *Circulation Journal*, vol. 68, no. 1, pp. 77–81, 2004.

[5] A. H. Frangieh, S. Obeid, J. R. Ghadri et al., "ECG criteria to differentiate between Takotsubo (stress) cardiomyopathy and myocardial infarction," *Journal of the American Heart Association*, vol. 5, no. 6, 2016.

[6] C. Madias, T. P. Fitzgibbons, A. A. Alsheikh-Ali et al., "Acquired long QT syndrome from stress cardiomyopathy is associated with ventricular arrhythmias and torsades de pointes," *Heart Rhythm*, vol. 8, no. 4, pp. 555–561, 2011.

[7] A. M. Ciutac and D. Dawson, "The role of inflammation in stress cardiomyopathy," *Trends in Cardiovascular Medicine*, vol. S1050-1738, no. 20, pp. 30042–30046, 2020.

[8] J. M. Duran, S. Naderi, M. Vidula et al., "Spontaneous coronary artery dissection and its association with takotsubo syndrome: novel insights from a tertiary center registry," *Catheterization and Cardiovascular Interventions*, vol. 95, no. 3, pp. 485–491, 2019.

[9] G. Gintant, "An evaluation of hERG current assay performance: translating preclinical safety studies to clinical QT prolongation," *Pharmacology & Therapeutics*, vol. 129, no. 2, pp. 109–119, 2011.

[10] G. M. Ellison, D. Torella, I. Karakikes et al., "Acute β-adrenergic overload produces myocyte damage through calcium leakage from the ryanodine receptor 2 but spares cardiac stem cells," *The Journal of Biological Chemistry*, vol. 282, no. 15, pp. 11397–11409, 2007.

[11] P. Pérez-Treviño, J. Sepúlveda-Leal, and J. Altamirano, "Simultaneous assessment of calcium handling and contractility dynamics in isolated ventricular myocytes of a rat model of post-acute isoproterenol-induced cardiomyopathy," *Cell Calcium*, vol. 86, article 102138, 2020.

[12] H. Vyas and M. J. Ackerman, "Epinephrine QT stress testing in congenital long QT syndrome," *Journal of Electrocardiology*, vol. 39, no. 4, pp. S107–S113, 2006.

[13] Y. Xie, E. Grandi, J. L. Puglisi, D. Sato, and D. M. Bers, "β-Adrenergic stimulation activates early afterdepolarizations transiently via kinetic mismatch of PKA targets," *Journal of Molecular and Cellular Cardiology*, vol. 58, pp. 153–161, 2013.

[14] M. F. Dabbagh, L. Aurora, P. D'Souza, A. J. Weinmann, P. Bhargava, and M. B. Basir, "Cardiac tamponade secondary to COVID-19," *JACC: Case Reports*, vol. 2, no. 9, pp. 1326–1330, 2020.

[15] S. Sala, G. Peretto, M. Gramegna et al., "Acute myocarditis presenting as a reverse Tako-Tsubo syndrome in a patient with SARS-CoV-2 respiratory infection," *European Heart Journal*, vol. 41, no. 19, pp. 1861-1862, 2020.

39

Concurrent Negative-Pressure Pulmonary Edema (NPPE) and Takotsubo Syndrome (TTS) after Upper Airway Obstruction

Evan Harmon[1] **Sebastian Estrada,**[1] **Ryan J. Koene,**[2] **Sula Mazimba,**[1] **and Younghoon Kwon**[1]

[1]*University of Virginia Health System, Charlottesville, VA, USA*
[2]*Cleveland Clinic Foundation, Cleveland, OH, USA*

Correspondence should be addressed to Evan Harmon; eharmon@virginia.edu

Academic Editor: Manabu Shirotani

Upper airway obstruction is a potentially life-threatening emergency often encountered in the acute care, perioperative, and critical care settings. One important complication of acute obstruction is negative-pressure pulmonary edema (NPPE). We describe two cases of acute upper airway obstruction, both of which resulted in flash pulmonary edema complicated by acute hypoxic respiratory failure. Though NPPE was suspected, these patients were also found to have Takotsubo syndrome (TTS). Neither patient had prior cardiac disease, and both subsequently had a negative ischemic workup. Because TTS is a condition triggered by hyperadrenergic states, the acute airway obstruction alone or in combination with NPPE was the likely explanation for TTS in each case. These cases highlight the importance of also considering cardiogenic causes of pulmonary edema in the setting of upper airway obstruction, which we suspect generates a profound catecholamine surge and places patients at increased risk of TTS development.

1. Introduction

NPPE is a rare but well-described complication of upper airway obstruction and has been of particular interest to clinicians and researchers alike as it represents one of the few noncardiogenic causes of flash pulmonary edema. However, acute obstruction may also place patients at higher risk of cardiac complications which can cause or exacerbate pulmonary edema. One such complication is the development of Takotsubo syndrome (TTS), which is underdiagnosed, particularly in the perioperative and critical care settings, given that it is commonly mistaken for an acute coronary syndrome with subsequent ischemic cardiomyopathy. Though both NPPE and TTS individually have been well-described, there is a paucity of reports describing the sudden, concurrent development of *both* NPPE and TTS in patients suffering acute upper airway obstruction.

2. Case Descriptions

2.1. Case 1. A 39-year-old woman with a history of borderline personality disorder, bipolar disorder, and depression presented to the emergency department (ED) intubated after a suicide attempt by hanging. Her partner at the bedside estimated the patient had been hanging for roughly ten minutes prior to being discovered and also suspected concurrent overdose on home alprazolam. Admission vital signs and exam were remarkable for HR 112 bpm, BP 90/60 mmHg, pupils 6 mm and reactive to light, GCS 3, and neck erythema.

The initial laboratory workup was notable for white blood cell (WBC) count 18.6 K/μL, troponin 0.24 ng/mL (peak of 1.78 ng/mL), and arterial blood gas (ABG) on FiO_2 100% demonstrating pH 7.201, pCO_2 36 mmHg, pO_2 231.6 mmHg, bicarbonate 13.8 mmol/L, anion gap 8 mmol/L, and lactate 0.86 mmol/L. Electrocardiogram demonstrated

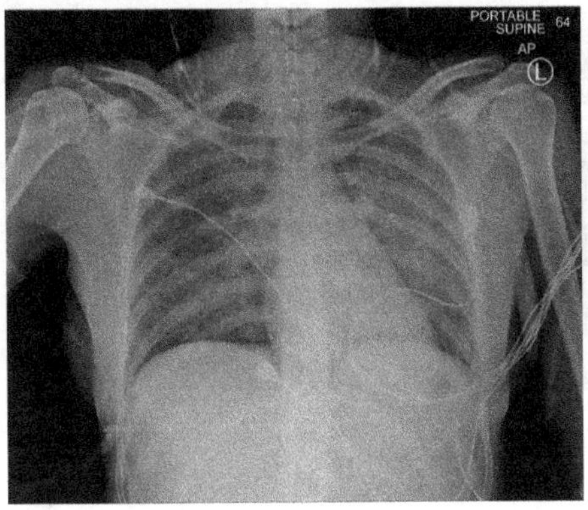

FIGURE 1: Chest radiograph demonstrating diffuse pulmonary edema upon admission to the emergency department.

sinus tachycardia with no ST-segment or T-wave changes. Trauma imaging in the ED included contrasted tomography (CT) of the head without contrast, CT cervical spine, and CT angiography of the neck, which were negative for cervical spine injury, cervical artery dissection, or brain hemorrhage or infarct. However, chest X-ray (CXR) demonstrated diffuse, bilateral pulmonary edema (Figure 1). The patient was also found to be hypotensive and required vasopressor support. She was transferred to the intensive care unit (ICU) for further management of NPPE complicated by acute hypoxic respiratory failure, severe nonanion gap metabolic acidosis, and presumed type II non-ST-segment elevation myocardial infarction (NSTEMI).

Shortly after arrival to the ICU, transthoracic echocardiogram (TTE) was obtained which demonstrated a left ventricular (LV) ejection fraction (LVEF) 40-45% and LV wall-motion abnormality consistent with midventricular form of Takotsubo syndrome (TTS, Figure 2). Intravenous diuresis with furosemide was administered with satisfactory response. Additionally, the patient's metabolic derangements corrected with supportive measures, sedation and vasopressor support were weaned, and she was successfully extubated within 48 hours of admission without any adverse neurologic sequelae. She was successfully started on metoprolol tartrate 25 mg twice daily with goal conversion to succinate formulation and uptitration to therapeutic effect as hemodynamically tolerated. The patient was transferred for continued inpatient psychiatric evaluation and management. Follow-up echocardiogram three months after initial TTE demonstrated full recovery of LV function.

2.2. Case 2. A 64-year-old man without history of cardiac disease was admitted for debridement of anterior mandibular osteomyelitis. Preoperative cardiopulmonary assessment was unremarkable, and the patient tolerated the procedure well. Shortly after extubation, he unexpectedly demonstrated labored breathing with inspiratory stridor. Laryngospasm was visualized by direct laryngoscopy, and the patient ultimately required reintubation. Appropriate endotracheal tube placement was confirmed by chest rise and CO_2 monitor, yet the patient was found to have oxygen saturation of 90% on 100% FiO_2. He subsequently became severely hypotensive requiring vasopressor support and ICU admission.

Upon arrival, pulmonary auscultation revealed bilateral rales, and frothy secretions were suctioned via the endotracheal tube. The initial workup was most significant for troponin elevated to 1.76 ng/mL (normal < 0.021 ng/mL), electrocardiogram with new, diffuse, deep T-wave inversions, CXR demonstrating flash pulmonary edema, and bedside TTE demonstrating severely reduced LVEF of 20% with diffuse akinesis involving the mid-to-apical segments of the LV with basal sparing. Right ventricular function was normal. Coronary angiogram was negative for acute coronary syndrome or any significant obstructive coronary artery disease.

These findings suggested TTS as the etiology of patient's acute cardiogenic shock. He responded well to intravenous diuretic therapy and was successfully extubated and weaned from all inotropic/vasopressor support within five days of ICU admission. This clinical improvement corresponded with radiographic resolution of his pulmonary edema. Seven days after initial presentation, repeat TTE demonstrated EF improvement to greater than 40% with distal anteroseptal periapical and distal inferoseptal hypokinesis and akinesis. At ambulatory follow-up appointment two months after hospital discharge, he was found to be asymptomatic with ECG normalization.

3. Discussion

Negative-pressure pulmonary edema (NPPE) is an increasingly described life-threatening emergency in the perioperative and critical care settings. Upper airway obstruction is the fundamental etiology of this phenomenon, with upper airway infection, tumor, and laryngospasm thought to be the most common causes [1]. Though a myriad of etiologies have been associated with NPPE since first reported in the pediatric literature over forty years ago [2], a unifying pathophysiological process has been elusive to date. Overall, it is thought that inspiratory effort against an obstructed glottis results in increased hydrostatic forces in the pulmonary microvasculature. This disruption of Starling forces, combined with profoundly negative intrathoracic airway pressures, results in fluid extravasation into the interstitium and subsequent flash pulmonary edema.

However, we describe two cases of NPPE, one due to asphyxiation and the other laryngospasm, which were further complicated by Takotsubo syndrome (TTS), an acute heart failure syndrome typically affecting women over the age of 50. It is characterized by apical or midventricular LV dysfunction with new ECG and/or serum cardiac biomarker abnormalities but without obstructive coronary disease and/or plaque rupture by coronary angiography [3]. To our knowledge, these cases represent two of only four total reports of concurrent NPPE and TTS [4, 5]. A number of pathophysiologic mechanisms of TTS have been proposed which typically revolve around a sudden and profound catecholamine release, including catecholamine-induced multivessel epicardial spasm and cyclic AMP-mediated intracellular calcium overload [6, 7]. Each of these mechanisms directly induce myocyte injury, though the role of the former in TTS propagation may be less relevant given that TTS may be precipitated by direct beta-agonism.

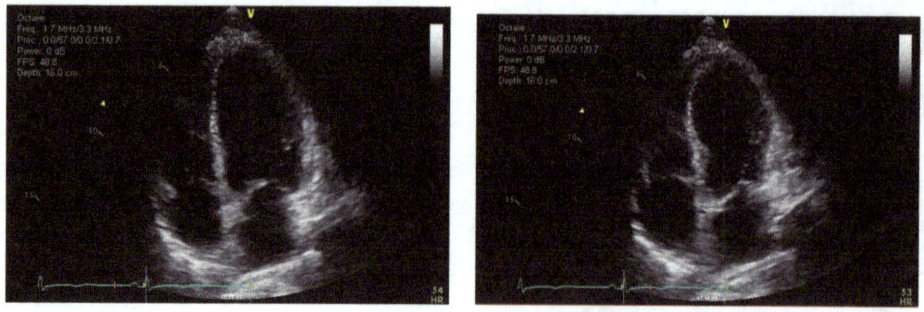

(a) (b)

Figure 2: Echocardiographic images demonstrating end-diastole (a) and end-systole (b). Basal and apical thickening with sparing of the midchamber segments indicates a midventricular variant of TTS.

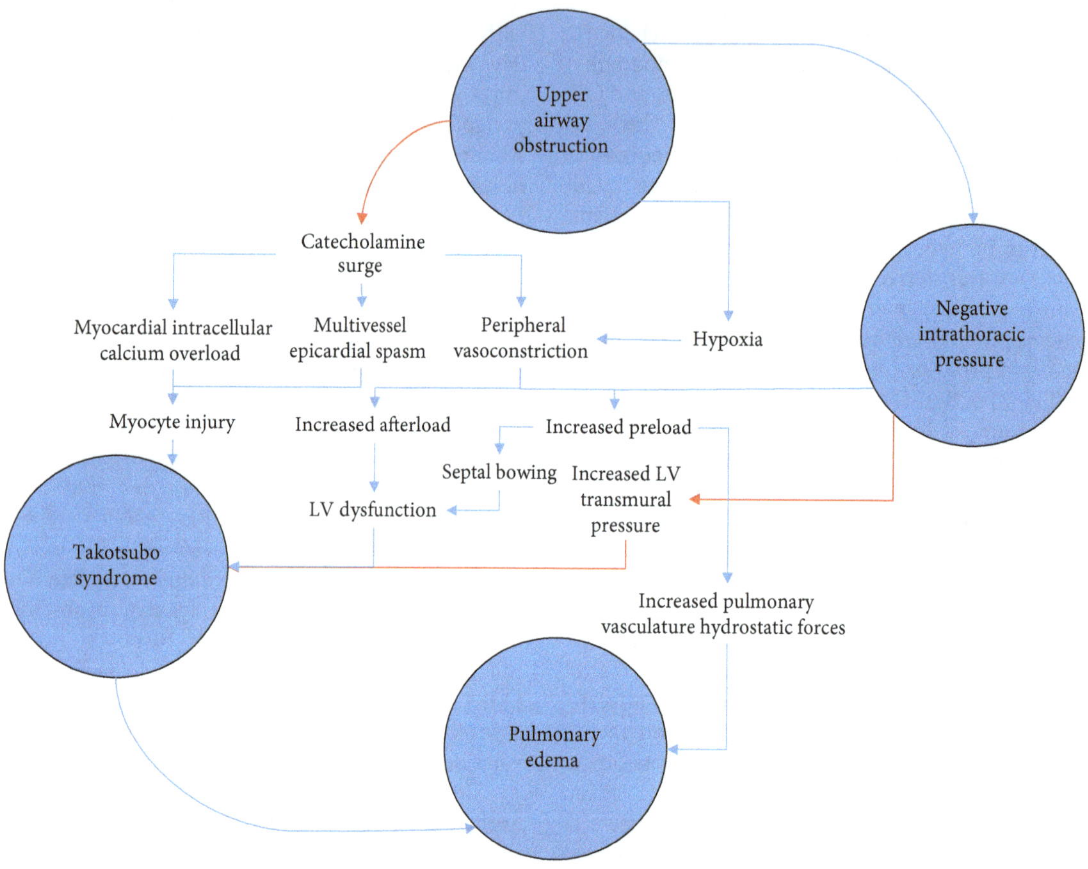

Figure 3: Proposed pathophysiologic diagram of NPPE and TTS. Notice multiple shared processes between the two which are thought to contribute to pulmonary edema following upper airway obstruction (note: red indicates proposed mechanisms).

Specifically, increasing evidence suggests elevated levels of peripheral epinephrine alter $\beta 2$-adrenergic receptor signaling by inducing a switch from stimulatory to inhibitory G protein subcellular signaling [8].

It is precisely this catecholaminergic surge which we suspect serves as the pathophysiologic link between NPPE and TTS (Figure 3). Attempted inhalation against a fixed obstruction in the form of a closed glottis results in both negative intrathoracic pressure *and* what is likely a dramatic catecholaminergic surge. This hyperadrenergic state not only contributes to both direct and indirect myocyte injuries as previously described but also results in peripheral vasoconstriction which serves to increase both preload and afterload. A sudden increase in right ventricular preload has two primary effects: first, pulmonary vasculature volume increases, contributing to increased hydrostatic forces. Second, greater venous return to the RV may result in septal bowing with resultant LV outflow tract obstruction, thereby diminishing LV EF. Additionally, elevated peripheral sympathetic activity results in arterial vasoconstriction, and this increased afterload places undue strain on the LV. Finally, negative intrathoracic airway pressure itself has been demonstrated to increase LV transmural pressure, further diminishing LV function.

Thus, upper airway obstruction may compromise LV function by at least four mechanisms: increased RV preload with resultant septal bowing, increased afterload via catecholamine-induced vasoconstriction, increased LV transmural pressure via the sudden generation of negative intrathoracic pressure, and rarely, as in the cases reported here, catecholamine-induced cardiomyocyte damage resulting in TTS. It should also be noted that increasing evidence has implicated the shedding of endovascular glycocalyx, an important regulator of vascular permeability, as a critical pathophysiologic mechanism at the cellular level by which TTS may induce pulmonary edema [10]. The summative effect of these physiologic insults is almost certain to be cardiogenic shock, which worsens pulmonary vasculature congestion and exacerbates NPPE. The final pathway of these processes is flash pulmonary edema with acute respiratory distress and often failure, which is accompanied by further catecholamine production, promoting a complex, life-threatening pathophysiologic cycle.

Therefore, flash pulmonary edema complicated by acute hypoxic respiratory failure encountered in the setting of upper airway obstruction may be due to both noncardiogenic *and* cardiogenic factors. This is especially important to remember in the perioperative period, when cardiac dysfunction due to TTS may be misattributed to infarction. We recommend emergent cardiac evaluation including troponin, ECG, and bedside TTE. In patients with troponinemia, newly reduced or worsened EF, wall-motion abnormalities, and/or ischemic changes on ECG, a more invasive workup including coronary angiogram should be considered. A profound elevation in BNP or NT-proBNP disproportionate to troponin elevation may also serve as an indicator of TTS rather than evolving myocardial infarction. If no ischemic etiology is identified, diagnosis may ultimately be confirmed by the visualization of diffuse, nonlocalizing ventricular edema on cardiac MRI. Management should focus on intravenous diuresis, positive-pressure ventilation, and hemodynamic support. Future research should determine what prognostic significance, if any, should be ascribed to the concurrent development of NPPE with TTS in patients with acute upper airway obstruction. Anecdotal evidence derived from the cases presented here and those reported elsewhere suggests that full recovery of LVEF can be expected with proper management, though the aforementioned pathophysiologic changes in LV structure may persist.

4. Conclusion

NPPE is a relatively rare but well-described life-threatening complication of upper airway obstruction. However, TTS is one of multiple cardiogenic etiologies which may also be contributing to flash pulmonary edema in this patient population. Though the precise mechanisms by which each of these pathologies occur have not been delineated, we suspect upper airway obstruction alone or in combination with NPPE generates a profound catecholamine surge which may be a key in triggering TTS. In select patients, ischemic evaluation may be warranted. Despite rapid and dramatic cardiopulmonary compromise, these patients appear to quickly achieve full recovery with proper management, though further research is necessary to definitively determine long-term prognosis.

References

[1] M. Bhattacharya, R. H. Kallet, L. B. Ware, and M. A. Matthay, "Negative-pressure pulmonary edema," *Chest*, vol. 150, no. 4, pp. 927–933, 2016.

[2] M. A. Capitanio and J. A. Kirkpatrick, "Obstructions of the upper airway in children as reflected on the chest radiograph," *Radiology*, vol. 107, no. 1, pp. 159–161, 1973.

[3] K. A. Bybee, T. Kara, A. Prasad et al., "Systematic review: transient left ventricular apical ballooning: a syndrome that mimics ST-segment elevation myocardial infarction," *Annals of Internal Medicine*, vol. 141, no. 11, pp. 858–865, 2004.

[4] S. H. Lee, C. H. Chang, J. S. Park, and S. B. Nam, "Stress-induced cardiomyopathy after negative pressure pulmonary edema during emergence from anesthesia -A case report-," *Korean Journal of Anesthesiology*, vol. 62, no. 1, pp. 79–82, 2012.

[5] K. S. Bharathi, S. Kulkarni, K. S. Sadananda, and C. L. Gurudatt, "Takotsubo cardiomyopathy precipitated by negative pressure pulmonary oedema following total thyroidectomy," *Indian Journal of Anaesthesia*, vol. 60, no. 3, pp. 202–205, 2016.

[6] M. Gianni, F. Dentali, A. M. Grandi, G. Sumner, R. Hiralal, and E. Lonn, "Apical ballooning syndrome or takotsubo cardiomyopathy: a systematic review," *European Heart Journal*, vol. 27, no. 13, pp. 1523–1529, 2006.

[7] D. L. Mann, R. L. Kent, B. Parsons, and G. Cooper 4th, "Adrenergic effects on the biology of the adult mammalian cardiocyte," *Circulation*, vol. 85, no. 2, pp. 790–804, 1992.

[8] H. Paur, P. T. Wright, M. B. Sikkel et al., "High Levels of Circulating Epinephrine Trigger Apical Cardiodepression in a β2-Adrenergic Receptor/Gi-Dependent Manner," *Circulation*, vol. 126, no. 6, pp. 697–706, 2012.

[9] T. H. Nguyen, S. Liu, G. J. Ong, I. Stafford, M. P. Frenneaux, and J. D. Horowitz, "Glycocalyx shedding is markedly increased during the acute phase of Takotsubo cardiomyopathy," *International Journal of Cardiology*, vol. 243, pp. 296–299, 2017.

Antepartum Diagnosis and Management of Lamin A/C Disease

Nosheen Reza,[1] Jessica L. Chowns,[1] Amy Marzolf,[1] Jessica Kim,[1] Lisa D. Levine,[2] Gregory Supple,[3] and Anjali Tiku Owens[1]

[1]*Center for Inherited Cardiovascular Disease, Division of Cardiovascular Medicine, Perelman School of Medicine, University of Pennsylvania, Philadelphia, PA, USA*
[2]*Maternal and Child Health Research Center, Department of Obstetrics and Gynecology, Perelman School of Medicine, University of Pennsylvania, Philadelphia, PA, USA*
[3]*Cardiac Electrophysiology Section, Division of Cardiovascular Medicine, Perelman School of Medicine, University of Pennsylvania, Philadelphia, PA, USA*

Correspondence should be addressed to Nosheen Reza; nosheen.reza@pennmedicine.upenn.edu

Academic Editor: Hajime Kataoka

Lamin A/C cardiac disease is a genetic cardiomyopathy and arrhythmia syndrome caused by alterations in the function of the nuclear lamin A and C proteins. It is inherited in an autosomal dominant manner and usually presents in mid- to late adulthood with atrioventricular conduction abnormalities, atrial and ventricular arrhythmias, biventricular dysfunction, and advanced heart failure. While rare, women of childbearing age can exhibit an aggressive disease course, and appropriate risk stratification and management are critical. Here, we present a case of newly diagnosed lamin A/C cardiac disease in a pregnant woman.

1. Introduction

The majority of arrhythmias in pregnancy are benign, but the recognition of arrhythmias with high-risk features is critical to the avoidance of adverse maternal and fetal outcomes. We report this rare case of the antepartum diagnosis and management of lamin A/C disease.

2. Case Report

A 33-year-old woman presented to our electrophysiology clinic for evaluation of 1st degree atrioventricular (AV) delay. She had been diagnosed with this finding 2 years prior while undergoing biannual fitness testing in the Navy. At that time, she had undergone Holter monitoring and treadmill stress echocardiography that did not show malignant conduction disease, arrhythmias, or structural heart disease.

At this electrophysiology clinic visit, she reported mild exercise intolerance and a sense that her "heart was not keeping up," which she attributed to physical deconditioning. Her electrocardiogram (ECG) was notable for sinus rhythm at 71 beats per minute with a PR interval of 214 milliseconds and was otherwise unremarkable (Figure 1(a)). She underwent repeat treadmill stress testing to assess her heart rate response and AV conduction; she achieved 78% of the maximum predicted heart rate and had superiorly directed premature ventricular contractions (PVCs) and slow accelerated idioventricular rhythm during recovery. Cardiac magnetic resonance imaging, performed to evaluate for infiltrative disease, showed normal biventricular function, normal chamber structure and dimensions, and no late gadolinium enhancement. She was diagnosed with high vagal tone.

At her next follow-up two years later at age 35, she was 22 weeks pregnant with her first child. She reported becoming easily dyspneic with exercise in the context of a 10-15-pound weight gain and intermittent palpitations. Her ECG showed sinus bradycardia, a competing junctional rhythm, occasional PVCs, and poor R wave progression—all of which were new (Figure 1(c)). Review of her family history revealed

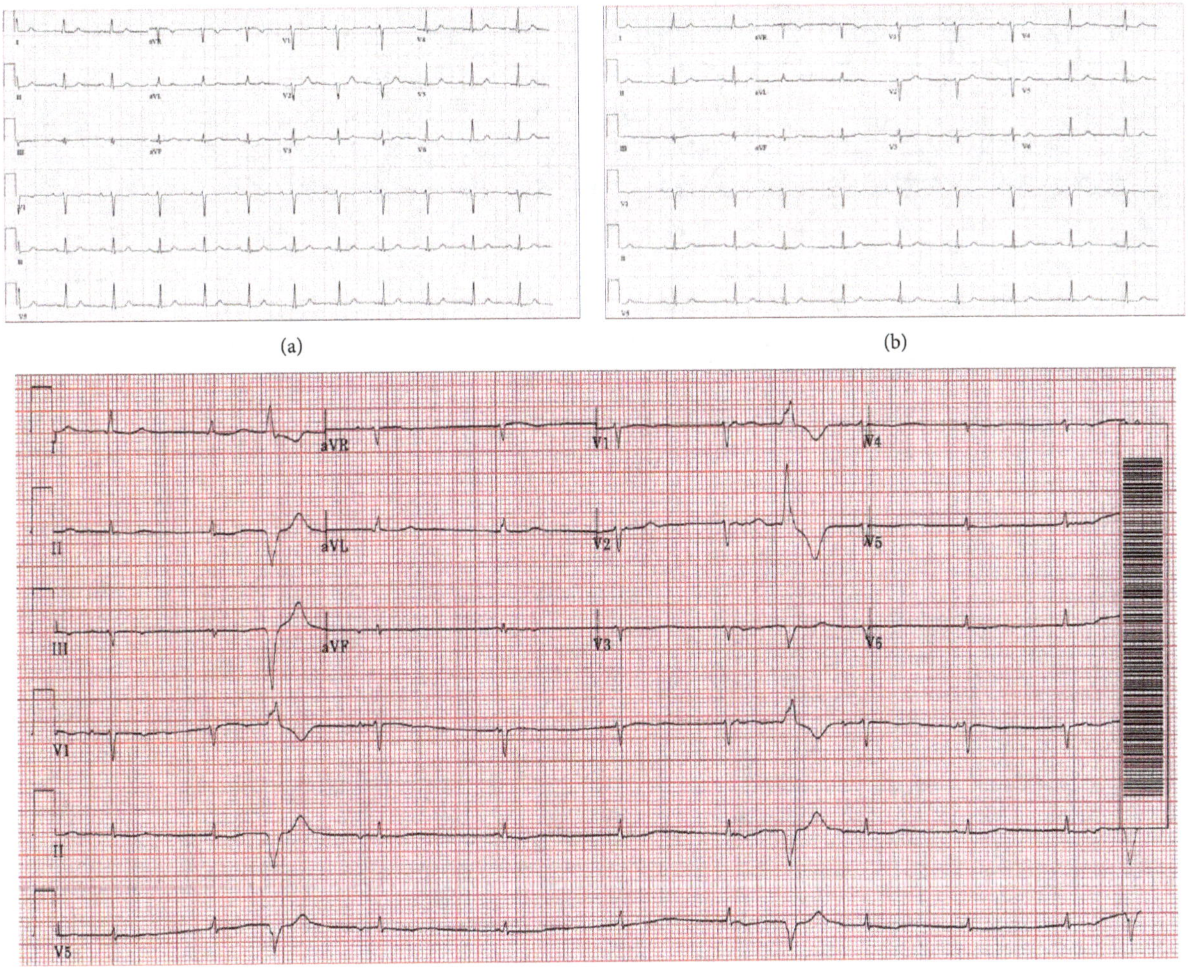

(a) (b) (c)

Figure 1: Serial ECGs: initial ECG performed at age 33 (a) with sinus rhythm and prolonged PR interval. Surveillance ECG performed one year later at age 34 (b) with slowing of the sinus rate and prolonged PR interval. First ECG during pregnancy performed at age 35 (c) showed new sinus bradycardia with competing junctional rhythm, occasional PVCs (RBS axis), and lower voltage QRS and poor R wave progression. Paper speed and amplification: 25 mm/s and 1 mV/10 mm.

that her father died at age 47 while awaiting heart transplantation for presumed end-stage ischemic cardiomyopathy. Given these findings, a 30-day ambulatory arrhythmia monitor was ordered, and within the first two weeks, sinus node dysfunction and frequent multifocal ventricular arrhythmias were captured (Figure 2). In the setting of both her tachy- and bradyarrhythmias and concerning family history, a genetic disorder was suspected. She underwent urgent and successful dual-chamber implantable cardioverter defibrillator (ICD) implantation at 25 weeks gestation, was started on metoprolol, and established care with our Maternal-Fetal Medicine program.

She was referred to our inherited cardiovascular disease center for genetic counseling and testing. Her three-generation family history was notable for cardiomyopathy in her father and heart issues in her paternal grandfather (Figure 3). She underwent genetic sequencing of 121 genes associated with cardiomyopathy and arrhythmia through GeneDx (Gaithersburg, Maryland) and was found to be heterozygous for two different pathogenic variants—a frameshift variant in *LMNA* (c.1174_1178delAGCCC; p.Ser392-TyrfsX32) and a missense variant in *MYBPC3* (c.1504C>T; p.Arg502Trp). This specific *LMNA* variant had not previously been reported but was predicted to result in either protein truncation or loss of protein product through nonsense-mediated mRNA decay and was therefore felt to be the likely cause of her arrhythmias. The *MYBPC3* (c.1504C>T) variant had previously been reported in multiple individuals in association with hypertrophic cardiomyopathy. Cascade screening of first-degree relatives was recommended.

At 32 weeks gestation, device interrogation and manual review of reported events showed several prolonged episodes of atrial fibrillation. After extensive discussion regarding the risks and benefits of therapeutic anticoagulation, she was started on prophylactic enoxaparin with the plan to undergo induction of labor at term (37 weeks gestation). She underwent an uncomplicated low transverse cesarean section due to nonreassuring fetal heart tones during her induction. She

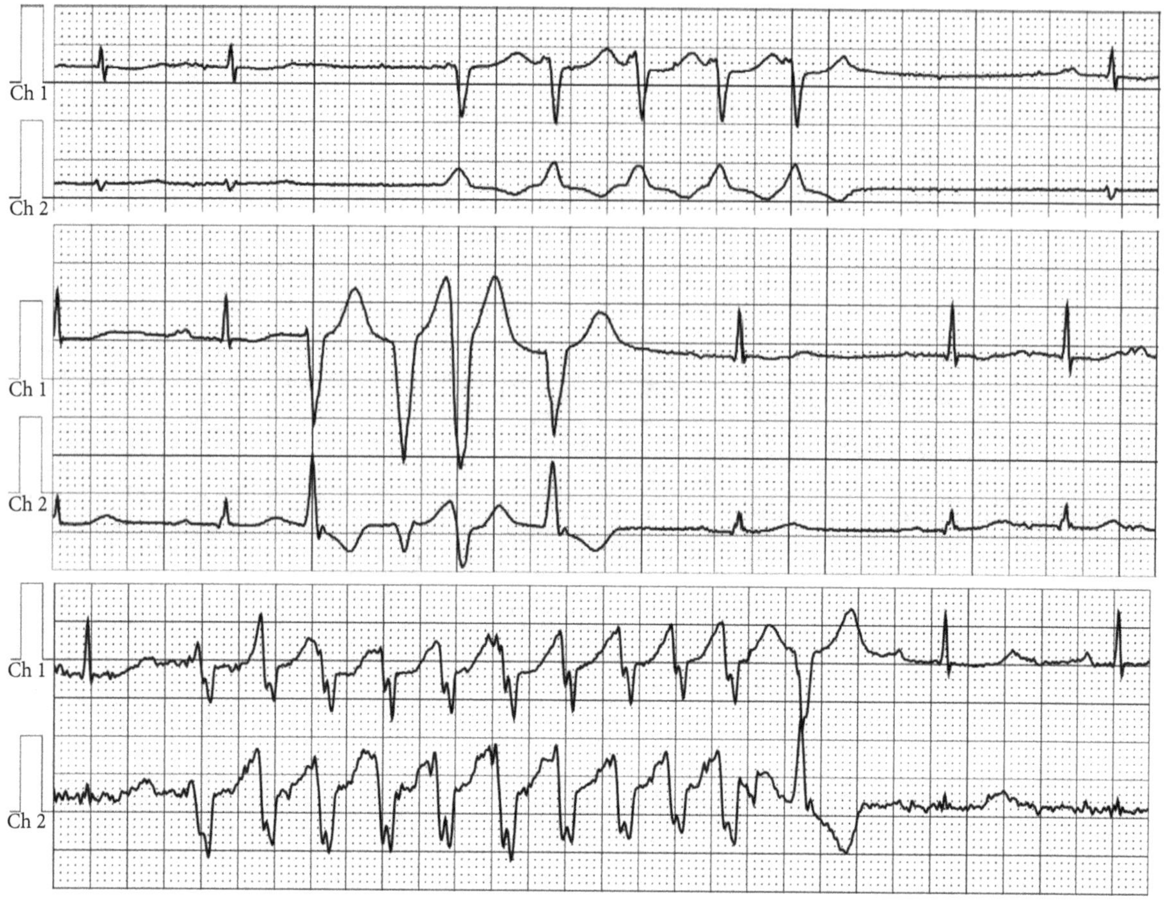

FIGURE 2: Mobile cardiac outpatient telemetry: frequent multifocal ventricular arrhythmias.

was discharged on therapeutic enoxaparin for thromboprophylaxis given limited data on the use of direct oral anticoagulants during breastfeeding.

3. Discussion

The lamin A/C gene (*LMNA*) is located on chromosome 1q21-22 and encodes two main nuclear laminar proteins, lamin A and lamin C, by alternative splicing [1]. These type V intermediate filament proteins are expressed in terminally differentiated somatic cells and are required for normal formation of the cell's nuclear envelope. When these proteins are disrupted, the stability of the nuclear membrane along with DNA replication, transcription, and nuclear organization are threatened [2]. Lamin A/C cardiac disease is inherited in an autosomal dominant pattern; therefore, heterozygotes often manifest disease, although with variable expressivity.

Diseases caused by variants in lamin A/C are collectively termed laminopathies and affect skeletal muscle (e.g., autosomal dominant and recessive Emery-Dreifuss muscular dystrophy, autosomal dominant limb-girdle muscular dystrophy), adipose tissue (e.g., familial partial lipodystrophy), peripheral nervous tissue (e.g., sensory and motor axonal neuropathy), and cardiac muscle [1]. There is wide variability among these phenotypes, with some patients first and only displaying cardiac manifestations characterized by AV conduction abnormalities, arrhythmias, biventricular dysfunction, and advanced heart failure. In addition, the majority of pathogenic *LMNA* variant carriers with muscular dystrophy-predominant symptoms also develop cardiac complications. Natural history studies have shown that conduction disease without other structural heart disease develops in a majority of these patients by the age of 30 with heart failure mostly manifesting around 20 years later [3]. Variants in *LMNA* have been found in 5-8% of familial dilated cardiomyopathy (DCM) cases, making these variants among the most frequently implicated in the development of DCM [1, 2, 4]. Our patient did not exhibit any other laminopathic signs or symptoms, including neuromuscular symptoms, and had stable left ventricular structure and function on her serial third trimester and postpartum transthoracic echocardiograms. She will remain under periodic echocardiographic surveillance.

Conduction disturbances associated with *LMNA* include atrial and ventricular arrhythmias and AV conduction delays and blocks. Typically, sinoatrial disease becomes apparent first and manifests as sinus bradycardia, sick sinus syndrome with sinus arrest and junctional escape rhythms, and first-degree AV delay. Supraventricular arrhythmias include atrial fibrillation, atrial flutter, and atrial tachycardia. In a multicenter international study of *LMNA* pathogenic or likely pathogenic variant carriers, 45% of patients who had atrial

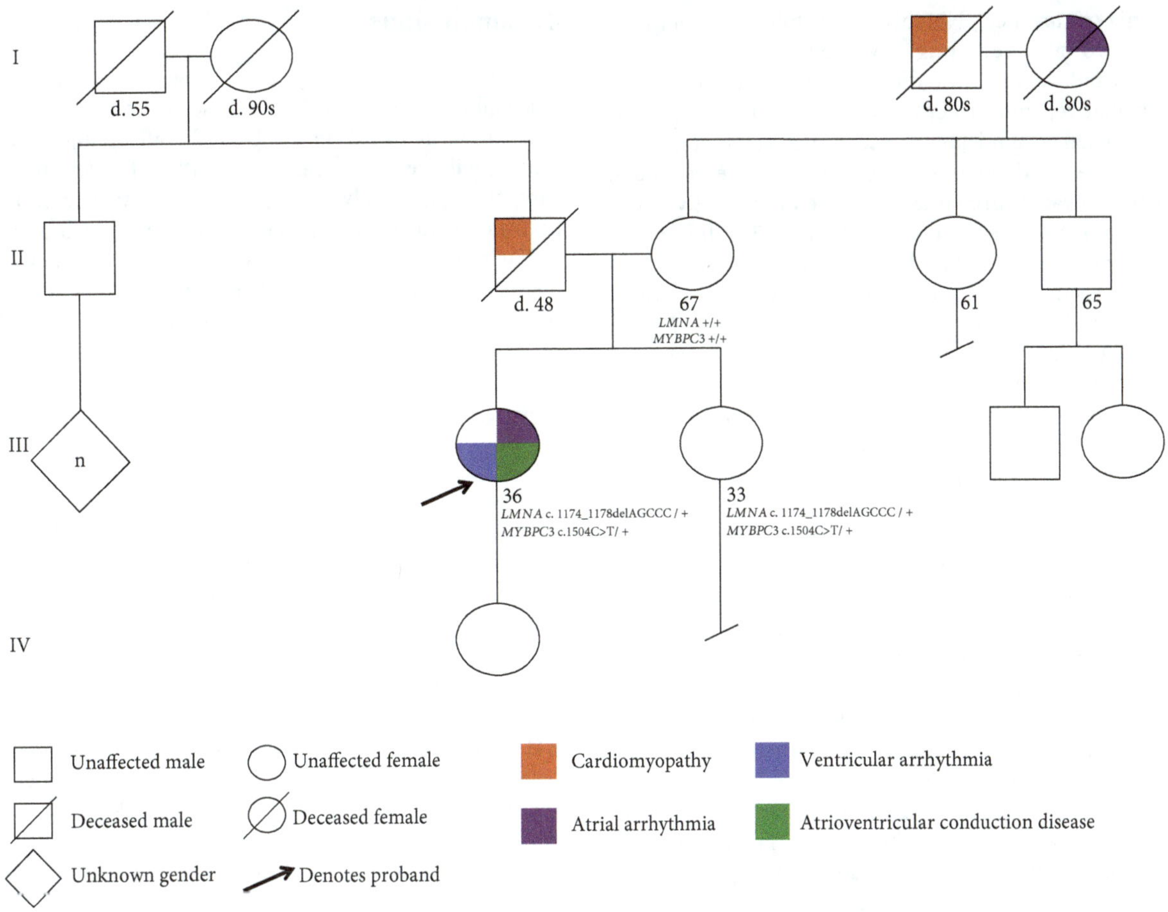

FIGURE 3: Pedigree: numbers below symbols denote current age or age at death. + denotes normal allele.

fibrillation on presentation progressed to persistent or permanent forms within the median follow-up period of 7 years [5]. In comparison to genotype-negative idiopathic DCM patients, *LMNA* variant carriers experienced a significantly higher risk of arterial and venous thromboembolic complications (HR 4.8, 95% CI: 2.2-10.6), raising the possibility of an additional prothrombotic phenotype [6]. Pregnancy is, in itself, a hypercoagulable state, and this combined with our patient's episodes of atrial fibrillation necessitated the consideration of systemic anticoagulation and delivery.

LMNA carriers have significantly worse cardiovascular outcomes compared to other DCM patients with increased mortality due to sudden cardiac death and severe heart failure [1]. In a multicenter European study of 269 *LMNA* variant carriers, independent risk factors for malignant ventricular arrhythmias included nonsustained ventricular tachycardia (VT), left ventricular ejection fraction < 45% at first clinical contact, male sex, and nonmissense (i.e., insertion, deletion, truncations, and splice site) variants [7]. In this same study, there was a high rate of appropriate ICD therapies in patients who had received a primary prevention device (8 per 100 person-years with a median follow-up period of 29 months). Similarly, in another study, 42% of patients with genetically confirmed lamin A/C disease and primary prevention ICDs sustained appropriate shocks [8]. These data are the foundation for the 2015 European Society of Cardiology guideline class IIa recommendation to consider ICD implantation in patients with DCM, a confirmed disease-causing *LMNA* variant, and clinical risk factors [9].

Our patient's known pathogenic variant, positive family history, and documented progressive conduction disease with new and frequent multifocal ventricular arrhythmias were thought to confer a high enough risk of sudden cardiac death to warrant primary prevention ICD implantation, regardless of her pregnant state. The risks of bradycardia and asystole were also important considerations in implanting a pacing system given that these rhythms could be acutely life threatening to the patient and fetus. As the patient was already at 25 weeks gestation at the time of device implantation, the risks of radiation exposure to the fetus were somewhat attenuated. A dual-chamber device can be implanted with very low dose fluoroscopy, as was the case here, with only 2 minutes of low frame rate fluoroscopy used. A significantly higher fluoroscopy dose would have been used to implant a cardiac resynchronization therapy lead; therefore, her device was implanted with appropriate programming to minimize right ventricular pacing.

Data on catheter ablation for management of ventricular arrhythmias in lamin A/C disease are limited. In a recent international multicenter study of 25 *LMNA* patients with drug-refractory VT, catheter ablation was associated with poor procedural success and a very high rate of ventricular arrhythmia recurrence. Notably, at a follow-up, 44% of patients were on or awaiting advanced therapies for end-stage heart failure, and 26% died [10]. Catheter ablation is mostly palliative, and further prospective studies are needed to assess whether guideline-directed medical therapy can delay the onset and progression of advanced heart failure. At this time, heart transplantation is the only curative therapy for lamin A/C cardiac disease. A phase 3, randomized, placebo-controlled clinical trial evaluating the safety and efficacy of a selective oral inhibitor of p32 mitogen-activated protein kinase in treating patients with symptomatic *LMNA* DCM (NCT03439514) is currently enrolling and expected to reach study completion in July 2020 [11].

Arrhythmias are one of the most common cardiac conditions in pregnancy. Contributors to this proarrhythmic state include myocardial stretch due to a 50% increase in blood volume, hormonal changes, and an increase in circulating catecholamines [12]. Supraventricular tachycardias are thought to be the most frequent sustained arrhythmias that women experience during this time [13]. Sustained VT and ventricular fibrillation are quite rare in pregnancy with registry data showing a 1.4% incidence in women with underlying structural heart disease [14].

Data on obstetrical and fetal outcomes in lamin A/C cardiac disease are exceedingly scarce. The only published case series describes 11 pregnancies in 5 *LMNA* variant carriers. Of the 5 women, 4 had palpitations or AV conduction abnormalities prior to or during their pregnancies. No major cardiac events were observed during their pregnancies. Unfortunately, no systematic electrocardiographic data were reported, precluding direct comparison with our patient [15].

The proband and her sister (Figure 3, individual III-3) were both heterozygous for disease-associated variants in *LMNA* and *MYBPC3*. Although the clinical lab interpreted the *MYBPC3* c.1504C>T variant as pathogenic, the variant has conflicting interpretations of pathogenicity in ClinVar [16]. At this time, the proband is only exhibiting a phenotype consistent with the pathogenic *LMNA* variant; her left ventricular wall thickness is normal. Individuals with *LMNA*-related cardiac disease generally exhibit a highly penetrant phenotype, consistent with the proband's presentation and course, while penetrance is reduced for *MYBPC3* variants. The proband and her sister will remain under clinical surveillance for manifestations of *LMNA*-related cardiac disease and of hypertrophic cardiomyopathy. At this time, the proband's sister's clinical phenotyping, consisting of a physical exam, electrocardiogram, and echocardiogram performed at another institution, shows no evidence of disease. She is scheduled to undergo additional phenotyping with cardiac magnetic resonance imaging and ambulatory electrocardiographic monitoring.

To our knowledge, this is the first report of the diagnosis and management of lamin A/C cardiac disease progression during pregnancy. Our patient experienced a typical disease course as described above with progressive sinoatrial and AV abnormalities and ultimately atrial and ventricular tachyarrhythmias necessitating dedicated management, but whether this course was hastened by her pregnancy remains unclear.

4. Conclusions

Progressive conduction system disease in a young individual is a hallmark of lamin A/C disease. With the mean age of mothers at first birth in the United States rising, it is likely that we will see genetic cardiomyopathies like lamin A/C disease, thought usually to present in mid- to late adulthood, become manifest in antepartum and postpartum women [17]. Cardiologists should be aware of *LMNA*-related cardiac disease and the importance of electrocardiographic monitoring in the diagnosis of inherited arrhythmia and cardiomyopathy syndromes.

Acknowledgments

Dr. Reza is supported by the National Institutes of Health National Human Genome Research Institute Ruth L. Kirschstein Institutional National Research Service T32 Award in Genomic Medicine (T32 HG009495). Dr. Owens is supported by the Winkelman Family Fund in Cardiovascular Innovation.

References

[1] M. R. Taylor, P. R. Fain, G. Sinagra et al., "Natural history of dilated cardiomyopathy due to lamin A/C gene mutations," *Journal of the American College of Cardiology*, vol. 41, no. 5, pp. 771–780, 2003.

[2] N. Sylvius and F. Tesson, "Lamin A/C and cardiac diseases," *Current Opinion in Cardiology*, vol. 21, no. 3, pp. 159–165, 2006.

[3] J. H. van Berlo, W. G. de Voogt, A. J. van der Kooi et al., "Meta-analysis of clinical characteristics of 299 carriers of LMNA gene mutations: do lamin A/C mutations portend a high risk of sudden death?," *Journal of Molecular Medicine*, vol. 83, no. 1, pp. 79–83, 2005.

[4] Y. Fu and H. J. Eisen, "Genetics of dilated cardiomyopathy," *Current Cardiology Reports*, vol. 20, no. 11, 2018.

[5] S. Kumar, S. H. Baldinger, E. Gandjbakhch et al., "Long-term arrhythmic and nonarrhythmic outcomes of lamin A/C mutation carriers," *Journal of the American College of Cardiology*, vol. 68, no. 21, pp. 2299–2307, 2016.

[6] I. A. van Rijsingen, A. Bakker, D. Azim et al., "Lamin A/C mutation is independently associated with an increased risk of arterial and venous thromboembolic complications," *International Journal of Cardiology*, vol. 168, no. 1, pp. 472–477, 2013.

[7] I. A. W. van Rijsingen, E. Arbustini, P. M. Elliott et al., "Risk factors for malignant ventricular arrhythmias in lamin A/C mutation carriers: a European cohort study," *Journal of the American College of Cardiology*, vol. 59, no. 5, pp. 493–500, 2012.

[8] C. Meune, J. H. Van Berlo, F. Anselme, G. Bonne, Y. M. Pinto, and D. Duboc, "Primary prevention of sudden death in patients with lamin A/C gene mutations," *New England Journal of Medicine*, vol. 354, no. 2, pp. 209-210, 2006.

[9] S. G. Priori, C. Blomström-Lundqvist, A. Mazzanti et al., "2015 ESC Guidelines for the management of patients with ventricular arrhythmias and the prevention of sudden cardiac death: the Task Force for the Management of Patients with Ventricular Arrhythmias and the Prevention of Sudden Cardiac Death

of the European Society of Cardiology (ESC) Endorsed by: Association for European Paediatric and Congenital Cardiology (AEPC)," *European Heart Journal*, vol. 36, no. 41, pp. 2793–2867, 2015.

[10] S. Kumar, A. F. A. Androulakis, J. M. Sellal et al., "Multicenter experience with catheter ablation for ventricular tachycardia in lamin A/C cardiomyopathy," *Circulation Arrhythmia and Electrophysiology*, vol. 9, no. 8, 2016.

[11] "A study of ARRY-371797 in patients with symptomatic dilated cardiomyopathy due to a lamin A/C gene mutation," https://ClinicalTrials.gov/show/NCT03439514.

[12] C. MacIntyre, C. Iwuala, and R. Parkash, "Cardiac arrhythmias and pregnancy," *Current Treatment Options in Cardiovascular Medicine*, vol. 20, no. 8, p. 63, 2018.

[13] V. R. Vaidya, S. Arora, N. Patel et al., "Burden of arrhythmia in pregnancy," *Circulation*, vol. 135, no. 6, pp. 619–621, 2017.

[14] E. Ertekin, I. M. van Hagen, A. M. Salam et al., "Ventricular tachyarrhythmia during pregnancy in women with heart disease: data from the ROPAC, a registry from the European Society of Cardiology," *International Journal of Cardiology*, vol. 220, pp. 131–136, 2016.

[15] E. Palojoki, M. Kaartinen, R. Kaaja et al., "Pregnancy and childbirth in carriers of the lamin A/C-gene mutation," *European Journal of Heart Failure*, vol. 12, no. 6, pp. 630–633, 2010.

[16] National Center for Biotechnology Information, *ClinVar; [VCV000042540.4]*, United States National Library of Medicine, Bethesda, MD, USA, 2019, September 2019, https://www.ncbi.nlm.nih.gov/clinvar/variation/VCV000042540.4.

[17] T. J. Mathews and B. E. Hamilton, "Mean age of mothers is on the rise: United States 2000–2014," in *NCHS data brief, no 232*, National Center for Health Statistics, Hyattsville, MD, 2016.

41

A Rare Case of Cardiac Recovery after Acute Myocarditis from West Nile Virus Infection

KaChon Lei,[1,2] Wilbur Ji,[1,2] Bhavana Bhaya,[1,2] and Chowdhury Ahsan[1,2]

[1]*Kirk Kerkorian School of Medicine at University of Nevada, Las Vegas, Department of Internal Medicine, USA*
[2]*Kirk Kerkorian School of Medicine at University of Nevada, Las Vegas, Division of Cardiovascular Medicine, USA*

Correspondence should be addressed to KaChon Lei; kachon.lei@unlv.edu

Academic Editor: Yuli Huang

West Nile Virus (WNV) myocarditis is nearly fatal, according to the current medical literature. We report a previously healthy 37-year-old Caucasian male who presented to our facility with two days of progressive lower extremity weakness, fever, edema, and shortness of breath found to have left ventricular global hypokinesis with an ejection fraction of less than 25%, consistent with acute viral myocarditis. He also has concomitant WNV meningoencephalitis due to his altered mentation. He was found to have a positive serum WNV IgM suggestive of a diagnosis of WNV myocarditis. He was intubated and was placed on vasoactive pressors for supportive care due to evidence of mixed cardiogenic and septic shock. After two weeks of hemodynamic support, we discovered a near-complete cardiac recovery, as shown on a repeat transthoracic echocardiography (TTE) and a normalized mean arterial blood pressure. This is a unique case report because near fatality is often associated with WNV myocarditis secondary to tachyarrhythmia, and there are currently no documented cases that are suggestive of cardiac recovery from the current literature.

1. Introduction

West Nile Virus, a mosquito-borne RNA flavivirus, is associated with neuroinvasive disease and systemic illness. Although 80% of infected individuals are asymptomatic, it is the reported etiology of viral encephalitis in the United States (approximately less than 1% of all cases) [1]. The prognosis of WNV infection is controversial, but only approximately 30% of patients will develop systemic symptoms, including fever, headache, ataxia, and weakness [2]. The mortality of WNV infection is 2%, according to the CDC. Young age appears to be the single most significant protective prognostic factor, in addition to immunocompetency. However, the progression of the disease to WNV myocarditis has demonstrated poor clinical outcomes due to rapidly deteriorating cardiorespiratory status and its associated conduction abnormalities [1–3]. Documented cases of WNV myocarditis are common in domesticated animals, with only a few cases reported in humans. WNV myocarditis is not associated with a specific arrhythmia; however, observational studies have suggested that 2nd and 3rd-degree heart blocks are prevalent in WNV infected hosts [4]. Once myocarditis is apparent in the clinical picture, tachyarrhythmias appear inevitable, and the mortality rate approaches 100%. A previous case report showed that patients with WNV myocarditis are at risk of developing idioventricular rhythm and asystole [3]. We herein report a rare case of a 37-year-old male with WNV myocarditis, who presented with shock physiology and had cardiac recovery after receiving supportive care, IVIG, and plasmapheresis.

2. Case Report

A 37-year-old Caucasian man with no past medical history presented to the Emergency Department with a 3-day history of high fevers, diarrhea, and malaise after hiking outdoors. He also visited a nearby hiking trail and swam in a local lake that contained "blue-green algae" and sewage waste. After he went home, his health continued to decline, and Emergency Medical Services was called due to his altered mentation and lethargy. He had no sick contacts, and he did not recall mosquito bites prior to his

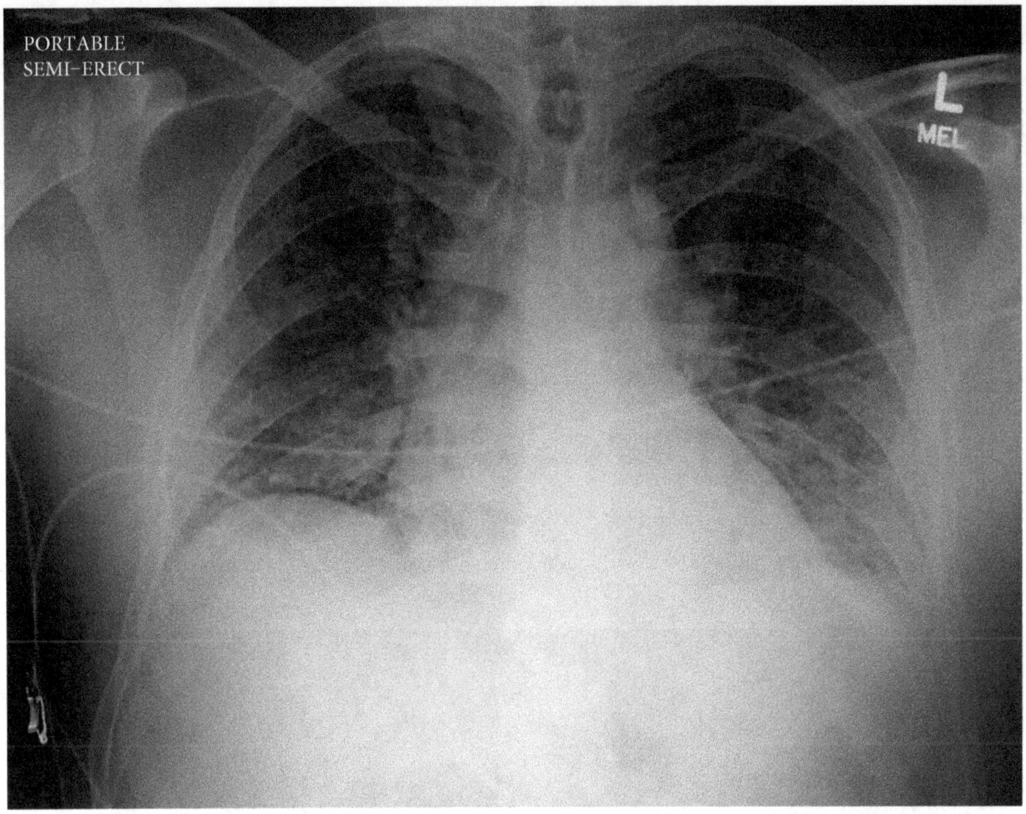

FIGURE 1: Chest X-ray on admission shows bilateral pulmonary infiltrates concerning for pulmonary edema vs. pneumonia.

presentation. He had no significant past medical or surgical history. He did not take any medications and reported no allergies. There is no significant family history of autoimmune and neurological diseases. He denied alcohol, smoking, and recreational drug use. A review of systems showed no other pertinent findings. On admission, he was febrile to 103F, tachycardic to 150 bpm, tachypneic with a respiratory rate of 32 bpm, and hypertensive to 149/115 mmHg. BNP was 1,309 pg/ml. Troponin was elevated at 0.8 μg/dl. Arterial blood gas showed a pH of 7.5 with pCO_2 29.7 mmHg and PO_2 54.3 mmHg, which demonstrated acute hypoxemia with respiratory alkalosis. Physical examination was notable for reduced lower extremity strength bilaterally with diminished deep tendon reflexes. He also had bilateral crackles and 2+ pitting edema at the lower extremities. He was immediately intubated due to rapidly declining oxygen saturation. For the next four days, his Glasgow Coma Scale score dropped from 15 to 5, with no additional sedation given following the 1st day of intubation. He continued to have progressive upper extremity weakness and hearing loss. Laboratory workup on admission showed a complete blood cell count with WBC of 22.6 k/mm^3 with 91% neutrophils. Chest X-ray showed pulmonary edema with bilateral interstitial infiltrates (Figure 1). The complete metabolic panel was grossly unremarkable, except for hypokalemia at 3.0 mEq/dl. EKG demonstrated persistent sinus tachycardia without ST or T wave changes (Figure 2). No AV nodal blocks or other tachyarrhythmias were appreciated. A TTE showed left ventricular global hypokinesis with a reduced ejection fraction of 25-30% without valvular abnormalities (Figure 3). A lumbar puncture was performed, which showed pleocytosis with no evidence of bacterial infection, and the meningitis viral panel was negative (Cytomegalovirus, Enterovirus, Herpes Simplex Virus 1/2, Human Herpesvirus 6, Human Parechovirus, and Varicella Zoster Virus). Lyme, fungal, and Coxsackie viral serology were also negative. The initial WNV IgM using the antibody-capture enzyme-linked immunosorbent assay was negative (Manufacturer: ARUP, ID: 0050228, with clinical sensitivity of 98%, specificity of 92.4%).

At this time, the prevailing working diagnosis was understood to be Guillain-Barré Syndrome, and the patient was treated with IVIG and aggressive diuresis with furosemide. Due to a lack of improvement and worsening respiratory status on mechanical ventilation despite IVIG therapy, he was transitioned to plasmapheresis on hospital day 3. He was placed on norepinephrine and dobutamine due to the concern of mixed cardiogenic and septic shock in this young individual. When his flaccid paralysis and mentation progressively worsened despite plasmapheresis on day 5, we became increasingly concerned about WNV encephalitis. We retested for WNV serology, which ultimately came back IgM positive. Unfortunately, the virus neutralization test was unavailable at our institution. After 14 days of vasopressor/inotropic support, as well as five days of plasmapheresis, empiric antibiotics, and diuresis, the patient's mentation, pulmonary edema, and clinical status improved to the point where he was weaned off of mechanical ventilation.

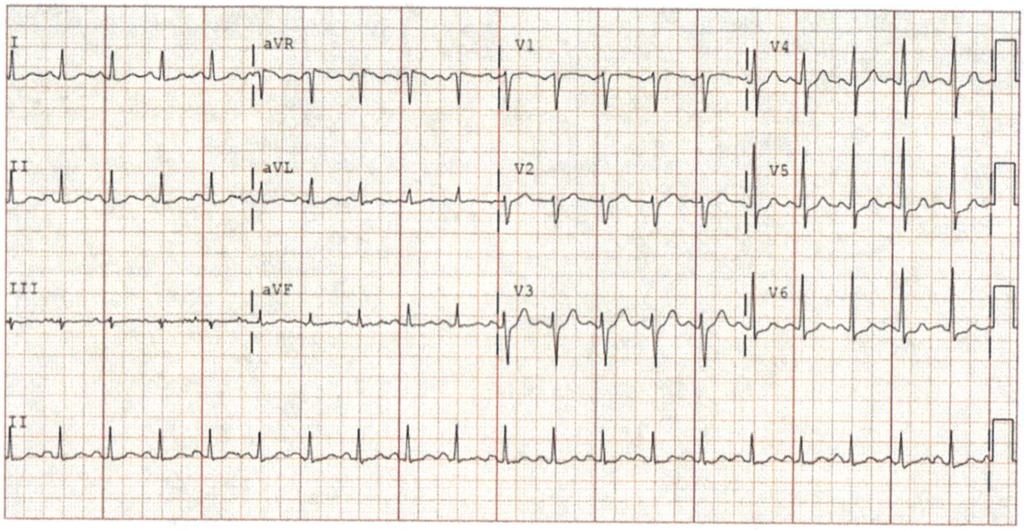

Figure 2: EKG on admission shows sinus tachycardia otherwise normal rhythm with no significant ST changes.

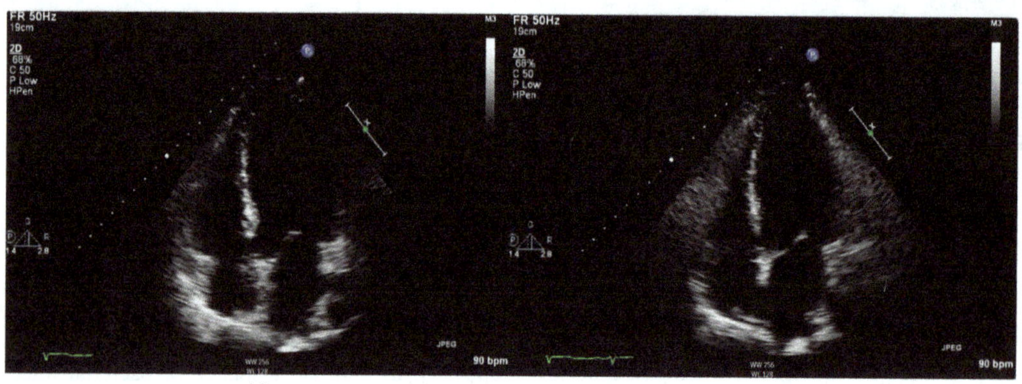

(a) (b)

Figure 3: Four-chamber view of TTE demonstrates global wall motion hypokinesis and reduced LV systolic function on admission in the setting of a structurally normal heart on hospital day 3 after diuresis. (a) Four-chamber view during diastole. (b) Four-chamber view during systole with decreased contractility and minimal changes in LV size.

However, he continued to have significant upper and lower extremity weakness. Repeat TTE now showed EF > 50% with significantly improved global wall motion abnormalities (Figure 4). The patient was transferred to inpatient rehab shortly after extubation. No arrhythmias were detected throughout his hospitalization. He was followed up with his primary care physician, as well as a PM&R physician. Unfortunately, he continues to have residual lower extremity weakness 2 years after his initial hospitalization, and he is currently wheelchair-bound at the time of writing this article. Nevertheless, from a cardiac standpoint, he has complete recovery, and he is not on any medication for congestive heart failure.

3. Discussion

This case highlights a rare presentation of WNV meningoencephalitis complicated by acute viral myocarditis. WNV-associated myocarditis carries a poor prognosis because it can cause fatal arrhythmias, including asystole, ventricular tachycardia, and ventricular fibrillation due to inflammation and scar formation within the heart [4, 5]. However, cardiac involvement due to WNV infection is poorly understood. Based on the current literature, when the patient presents with both WNV meningoencephalitis and myocarditis, survival becomes increasingly unlikely, and mortality approaches near 100% [1–3, 5, 6]. Like most other viral myocarditis, there is no specific treatment for WNV myocarditis except for hemodynamic support, and the possible utility of IVIG and plasmapheresis. The most common causes of acute viral myocarditis are often adenovirus, enterovirus, parvovirus B19, and CMV, with a mortality ranging from 56 to 83 percent [7]. However, this is not the case for WNV myocarditis. In animals, there appears to be a preference for cardiac atrioventricular nodal tissues in WNV infection. In birds, the brain, heart, and lung often carry the highest viral titer. Hemolysin and eosin staining of bird cardiomyocytes infected with WNV also show significant necrosis and neutrophilic infiltration, indicating significant inflammation and scar formation that may lead to life-

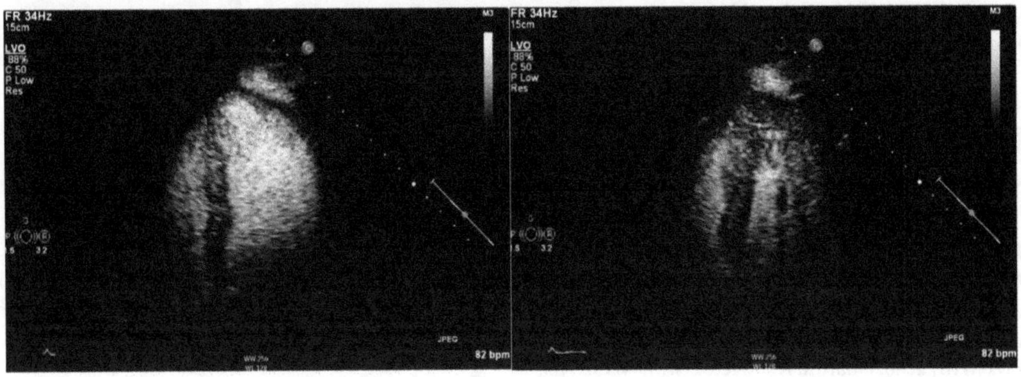

(a) (b)

FIGURE 4: Left ventricular view of TTE with perflutren contrast demonstrates preserved LV ejection fraction with excellent contractility and the absence of thrombus prior to hospital discharge. (a) Left ventricle during diastole. (b) Left ventricle during systole.

threatening arrhythmias [8, 9]. Prolonged sinus pauses have also been described in WNV hosts that eventually required temporary and permanent pacemaker placement [10]. Furthermore, animal studies also show that WNV targets the hyperpolarization-activated cyclic nucleotide-gated potassium channel 4 at the sinoatrial and atrioventricular node in mammals, predisposing them to autonomic dysfunction [11]. This may explain the high mortality rate observed in humans with WNV-associated cardiomyopathy.

The limitation of our case report is that we cannot distinguish our patient's new-onset congestive heart failure from stress-induced cardiomyopathy. In addition, we did not have viral deneutralization testing available at our institution. However, the lack of regional wall motion abnormalities involving the basal segment on TTE is not consistent with stress-induced cardiomyopathy. There were also no significant ST-T changes in the EKG on presentation. We also did not perform coronary angiography and/or left ventriculogram due to the lack of evidence and low pretest probability of coronary artery disease. The clinical presentation of tachycardia, new-onset CHF, and recent viral prodrome makes the diagnosis of WNV myocarditis very likely. The timing of recovery and resolution of left ventricular dysfunction is also more supportive of a viral inflammatory etiology (Figures 3 and 4). Cardiac MRI with late gadolinium enhancement may be helpful in determining the likelihood of life-threatening arrhythmias as it has been shown to have utility in the setting of acute viral myocarditis, as compared to more invasive measures such as endomyocardial biopsy [10].

Fortunately, our patient did not suffer from life-threatening tachyarrhythmias, as demonstrated in the current medical literature. However, patients with WNV myocarditis should remain on continuous cardiac telemetry and avoid clinical volume overload. Early IVIG and plasmapheresis may have helped in his recovery. Perhaps, a combination of unloading strategies such as mechanical circulatory support with ventricular assist devices, pulmonary artery catheter, and diuretic medication to reduce left ventricular end-diastolic pressure can be helpful to prevent tachyarrhythmias in the setting of cardiogenic shock [12]. Further cross-sectional and retrospective studies are required to understand the clinical outcome and prevalence of WNV myocarditis.

Additional Points

Learning Objectives. West Nile Viral myocarditis is a rare complication of WNV infection, and it carries a high mortality rate. Close cardiac monitoring and supportive care should be started promptly on presentation. Early steroid, intravenous immunoglobulin (IVIG), and plasmapheresis, as well as hemodynamic support, are imperative in the treatment of acute WNV myocarditis. Cardiac magnetic resonance imaging (MRI), ventricular assist device, and pulmonary artery catheter are useful tools to help guide diagnoses and treatment plans.

Acknowledgments

We would like to acknowledge Drs. Karen Kang, Kevin Bushey, Haley Roser, and Shadaba Asad for their contribution on images and their clinical expertise provided in this case report.

References

[1] S. Pergam, C. Delong, L. Echevarria, G. Scully, and D. Goade, "Myocarditis in West Nile virus infection," *The American Journal of Tropical Medicine and Hygiene*, vol. 75, no. 6, pp. 1232-1233, 2006.

[2] A. A. Leis and D. S. Stokic, "Neuromuscular manifestations of West Nile virus infection," *Frontiers in Neurology*, vol. 3, p. 37, 2012.

[3] A. Kushawaha, S. Jadonath, and N. Mobarakai, "West Nile virus myocarditis causing a fatal arrhythmia: a case report," *Cases Journal*, vol. 2, no. 1, p. 7147, 2009.

[4] A. V. Bode, J. J. Sejvar, W. J. Pape, G. L. Campbell, and A. A. Marfin, "West Nile virus disease: a descriptive study of 228 patients hospitalized in a 4-county region of Colorado in 2003," *Clinical Infectious Diseases*, vol. 42, no. 9, pp. 1234–1240, 2006.

[5] J. J. Sejvar, "Clinical manifestations and outcomes of West Nile virus infection," *Viruses*, vol. 6, no. 2, pp. 606–623, 2014.

[6] R. L. Debiasi and K. L. Tyler, "West Nile virus meningoencephalitis," *Nature Clinical Practice. Neurology*, vol. 2, no. 5, pp. 264–275, 2006.

[7] R. Dennert, H. J. Crijns, and S. Heymans, "Acute viral myocarditis," *European Heart Journal*, vol. 29, no. 17, pp. 2073–2082, 2008.

[8] S. E. Gibbs, A. E. Ellis, D. G. Mead et al., "West Nile virus detection in the organs of naturally infected blue jays (Cyanocitta cristata)," *Journal of Wildlife Diseases*, vol. 41, no. 2, pp. 354–362, 2005.

[9] A. Wünschmann, J. Shivers, L. Carroll, and J. Bender, "Pathological and immunohistochemical findings in American crows (Corvus brachyrhynchos) naturally infected with West Nile virus," *Journal of Veterinary Diagnostic Investigation*, vol. 16, no. 4, pp. 329–333, 2004.

[10] M. G. Friedrich, U. Sechtem, J. Schulz-Menger et al., "Cardiovascular magnetic resonance in myocarditis: a JACC white paper," *Journal of the American College of Cardiology*, vol. 53, no. 17, pp. 1475–1487, 2009.

[11] H. Wang, V. Siddharthan, J. O. Hall, and J. D. Morrey, "Autonomic nervous dysfunction in hamsters infected with West Nile virus," *PLoS One*, vol. 6, no. 5, article e19575, 2011.

[12] C. Tschöpe, S. Van Linthout, O. Klein et al., "Mechanical unloading by fulminant myocarditis: LV-IMPELLA, ECMELLA, BI-PELLA, and PROPELLA concepts," *Journal of Cardiovascular Translational Research*, vol. 12, no. 2, pp. 116–123, 2019.

42

Takotsubo Syndrome Associated with ST Elevation Myocardial Infarction

Saad Ezad,[1] **Michael McGee**,[1] **and Andrew J. Boyle**[1,2,3]

[1]*John Hunter Hospital, Hunter New England Health, Newcastle, NSW, Australia*
[2]*The University of Newcastle, Newcastle, NSW, Australia*
[3]*Hunter Medical Research Institute, Newcastle, NSW, Australia*

Correspondence should be addressed to Andrew J. Boyle; andrew.boyle@newcastle.edu.au

Academic Editor: Man-Hong Jim

Background. Takotsubo syndrome is a reversible heart failure syndrome which often presents with symptoms and ECG changes that mimic an acute myocardial infarction. Obstructive coronary artery disease has traditionally been seen as exclusion criteria for the diagnosis of takotsubo; however, recent reports have called this into question and suggest that the two conditions may coexist. *Case Summary.* We describe a case of an 83-year-old male presenting with chest pain consistent with acute myocardial infarction. The ECG demonstrated anterior ST elevation with bedside echocardiography showing apical wall motion abnormalities. Cardiac catheterisation found an occluded OM2 branch of the left circumflex artery with ventriculography confirming apical ballooning consistent with takotsubo and not in the vascular territory supplied by the occluded epicardial vessel. Repeat echocardiogram 6 weeks later confirmed resolution of the apical wall motion abnormalities consistent with a diagnosis of takotsubo. *Discussion.* This case demonstrates the finding of takotsubo syndrome in a male patient with acute myocardial infarction. Traditionally, this would preclude a diagnosis of takotsubo; however, following previous reports of takotsubo in association with coronary artery dissection and acute myocardial infarction in female patients, new diagnostic criteria have been proposed which allow the diagnosis of takotsubo in the presence of obstructive coronary artery disease. This case adds to the growing body of literature that suggests takotsubo can coexist with acute myocardial infarction; however, it remains to be elucidated if it is a consequence or cause of myocardial infarction.

1. Introduction

First described in a case series of Japanese patients in 1991 [1], takotsubo syndrome (TTS) is a rapidly reversible heart failure syndrome most commonly seen in postmenopausal women following emotional or physical stress [2]. Various terms have been used to describe this condition including broken heart syndrome [3], takotsubo cardiomyopathy [4], and stress-induced cardiomyopathy [5]. TTS is now the preferred nomenclature as patients with takotsubo do not appear to have primary muscle pathology [6]. Presentation mimics acute myocardial infarction (AMI) with chest pain and dyspnoea often associated with ST segment elevation or T wave inversion. In a contemporary western population, an estimated 0.9% of patients admitted for primary PCI were diagnosed with TTS [7]. However, data from the International Takotsubo Registry has shown coronary artery disease coexists in 15.3% of patients with a diagnosis of TTS [8]. The underlying pathophysiology has yet to be fully understood, although a rapid elevation in circulating catecholamine levels in response to stress has traditionally been believed to be a central feature [9]. More recently, however, it has been demonstrated that plasma catecholamine levels are normal or only mild-moderately elevated in patients with TTS [10] and that local cardiac sympathetic hyperactivation results in myocardial stunning [11].

2. Case Presentation

An 83-year-old gentleman with a past medical history of diet-controlled diabetes mellitus type 2, gout, and hypertension presented to our institution with a 4-hour history of

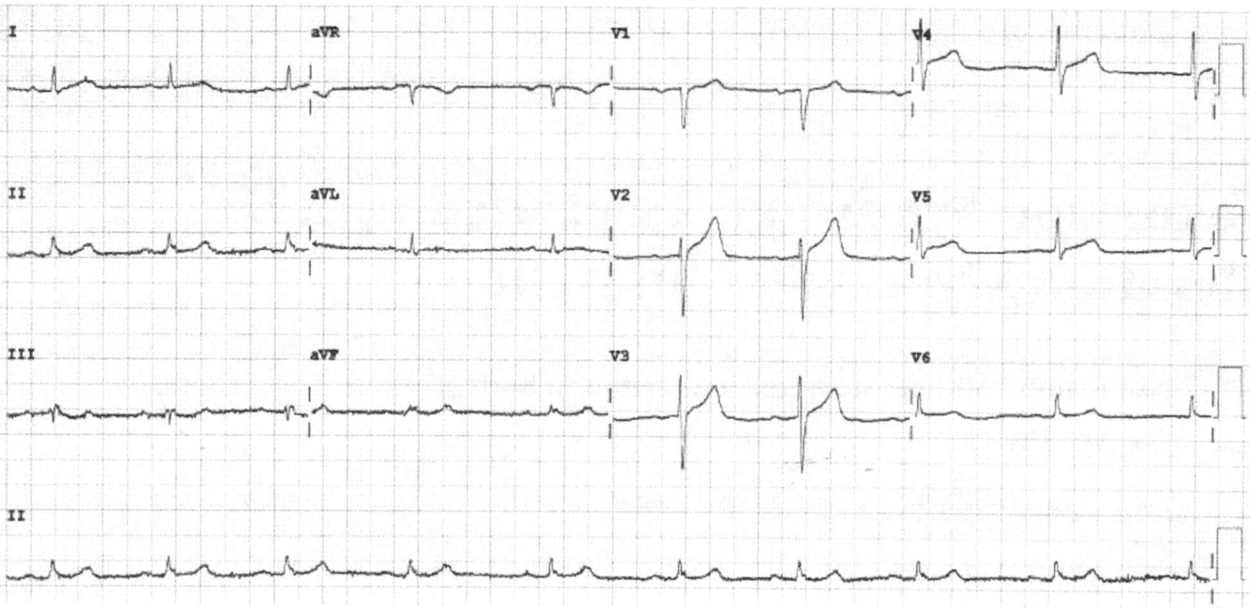

(a)

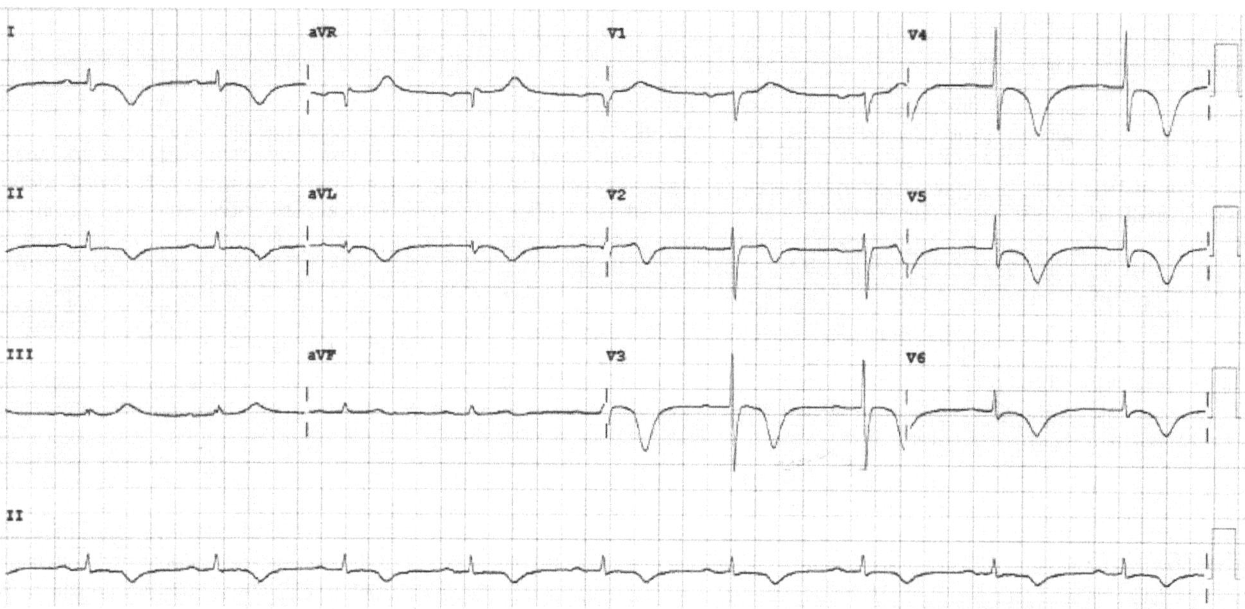

(b)

FIGURE 1: (a) Admission ECG showing minimal anterior ST elevation and concave ST segments in leads II, III, and aVF. (b) ECG 48 hours after presentation demonstrating deep T wave inversion across precordial and limb leads with a prolonged QTc.

upper abdominal pain and lower chest tightness associated with dyspnoea, which was partially relieved by intravenous morphine and sublingual glyceryl trinitrate administered by ambulance paramedics. On arrival in the emergency department, a 12-lead ECG showed minimal anterior ST elevation (Figure 1(a)); therefore, a bedside echocardiogram was performed. This demonstrated hypokinesis of the apical third of the anterior, inferior, and lateral walls. Given the borderline ECG changes and regional wall motion abnormalities on echo, the patient was taken for emergency cardiac catheterisation.

Angiography revealed an occluded obtuse marginal 2 (OM2) branch of the circumflex artery (Figure 2(c)) with minor disease in the other major epicardial arteries (Figures 2(a) and 2(b)). Flow was restored following passage of the guidewire, and thrombus was clearly identifiable in the vessel. The lesion was treated with one 2.5 mm × 15 mm drug-eluting stent resulting in TIMI III flow (Figure 2(d)).

Ventriculogram done in the RAO projection revealed mid and apical hypokinesis and ballooning with preserved basal function (Figures 2(e) and 2(f)). Ventriculogram from the LAO projection showed posterior wall hypokinesis more

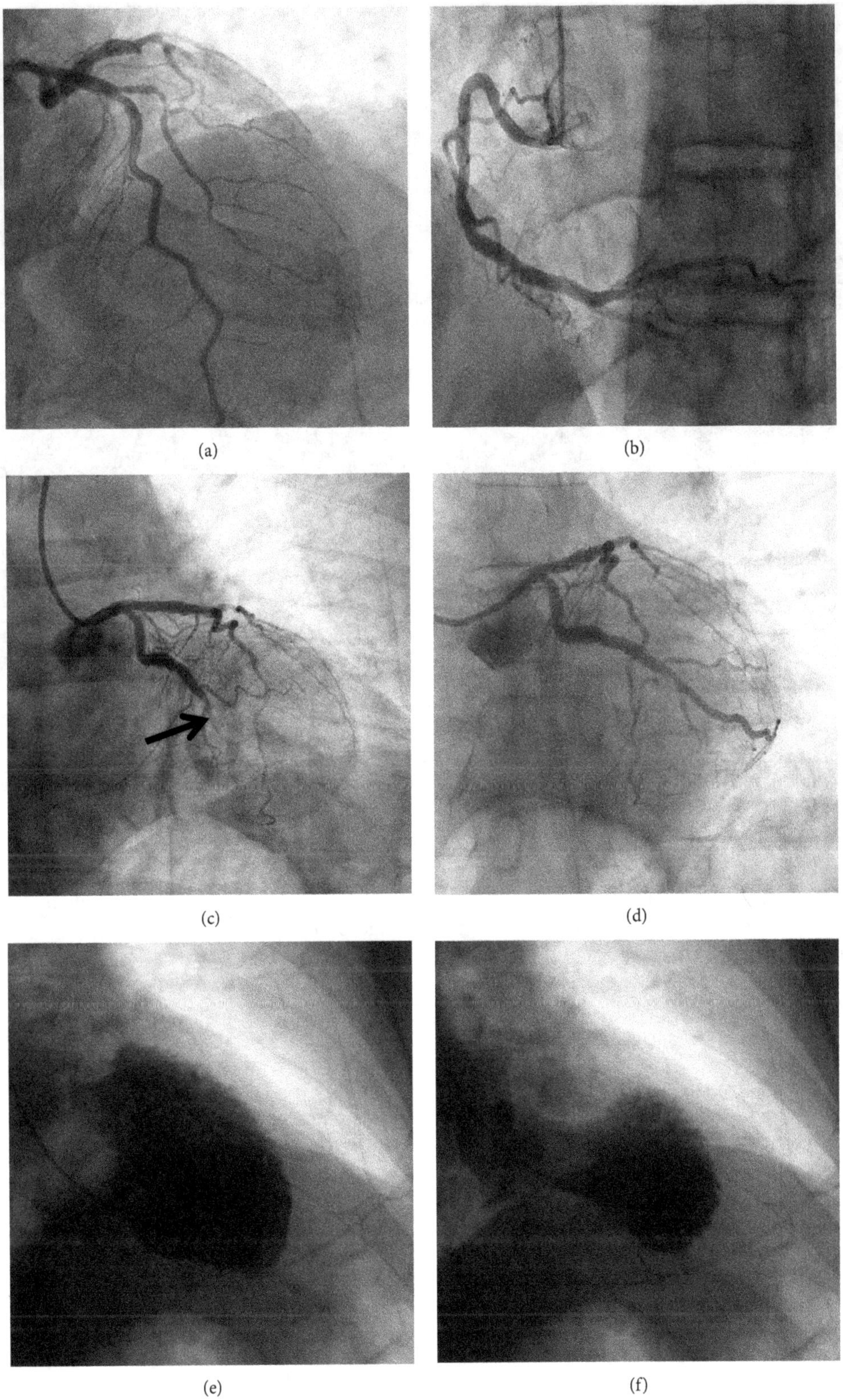

Figure 2: Coronary angiography on admission. (a) Minor disease in the left anterior descending artery. (b) Mild-moderate disease in the right coronary artery. (c) Occluded OM2 branch (arrow) of the left circumflex artery. (d) TIMI III flow post percutaneous coronary intervention (PCI) with drug-eluting stent (DES). Left ventriculogram in the right anterior oblique (RAO) projection during diastole (e) and systole (f) showing mid apical pattern of takotsubo syndrome with sparing of the apical tip.

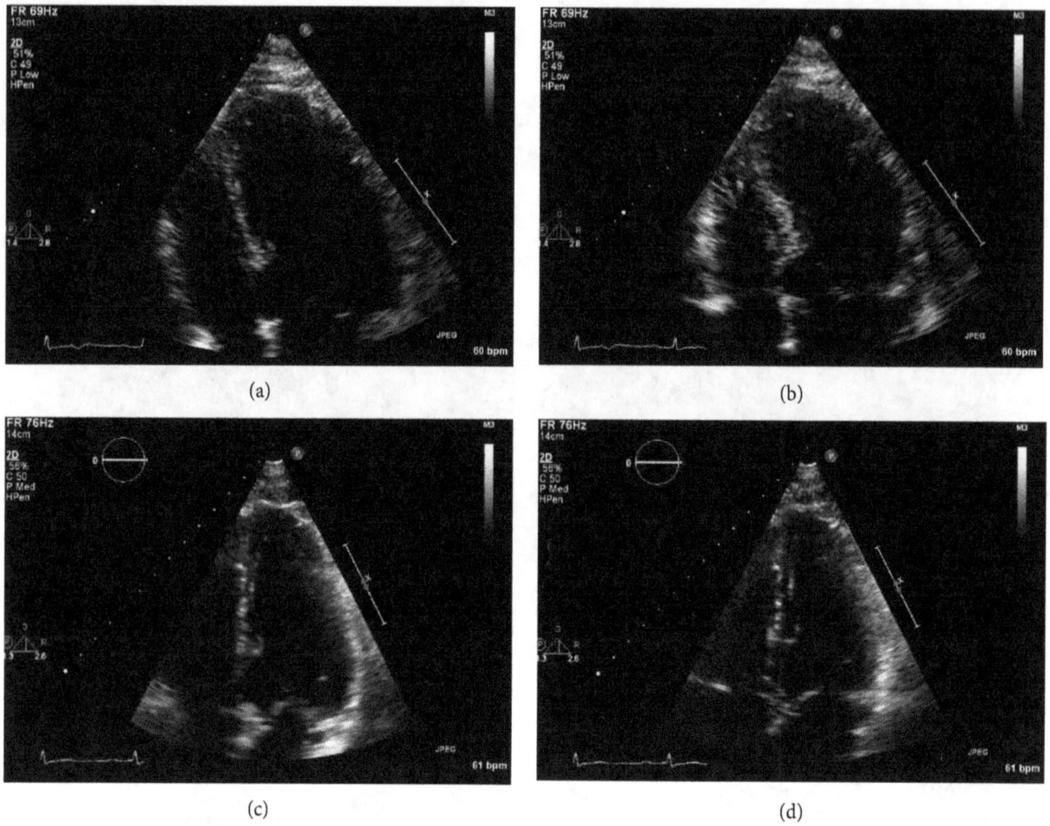

FIGURE 3: Transthoracic echocardiogram on admission and 6-week follow-up. Apical 4 chamber window at end-diastole (a) and at end-systole (b) showing apical dilatation during acute presentation. (c) Apical 4 chamber window at end-diastole at 6-week follow-up. (d) Apical 4 chamber window at end-systole at 6-week follow-up revealing resolution of apical ballooning.

in keeping with the ischaemic territory affected by acute plaque rupture.

A venous blood gas revealed haemoglobin of 145 g/L (ref 120-170 g/L), normal electrolytes, and blood glucose of 8.7 mmol/L (ref 3.5-7.7 mmol/L). The patient's initial troponin I was 365 ng/L (ref <26 ng/L) and peaked at 17,180 ng/L the following day. His ECG evolved to show deep symmetrical T wave inversion across the anterolateral and limb leads, clearly more extensive than the distribution of the infarct artery (Figure 1(b)) associated with the prolongation of the QT interval. Formal echocardiogram performed 6 hours following percutaneous coronary intervention (PCI) showed severe apical ballooning and hypokinesis extending to mid cavity with preservation of basal function, consistent with TTS. The posterolateral wall was also noted to be akinetic in keeping with a region of infarction. There was mild LV systolic dysfunction (EF 45%).

The patient was commenced on perindopril and atorvastatin in addition to dual antiplatelet therapy with aspirin and clopidogrel. On further questioning, no acute emotional triggers in the patient's life could be identified. On day 3 of the patient's admission, troponin was down trending at 8907 ng/L. He was discharged 4 days after presentation, following an uncomplicated inpatient stay. Follow-up echocardiography performed 6 weeks after discharge demonstrated restoration of normal LV systolic function and resolution of the previously seen regional wall motion abnormalities (Figure 3).

3. Discussion

The current Mayo diagnostic criteria [12] require the presence of a transient regional wall motional abnormality, which extends beyond a single epicardial vascular distribution, and the absence of obstructive coronary artery disease or evidence of acute plaque rupture. However, several recent reports of TTS in association with coronary artery dissection [13] and acute myocardial infarction [14, 15] have led to newly proposed diagnostic criteria which state that TTS may exist as a comorbidity with a variety of illnesses including acute coronary syndromes [16].

To our knowledge, this is a unique case describing the association of acute myocardial infarction (AMI) caused by acute plaque rupture and TTS in a male patient. The lack of an emotional trigger in this case suggests a possible causal relationship between the two conditions. The stress associated with AMI could conceivably have resulted in sympathetic activation causing TTS in a distribution not perfused by the occluded OM2 artery. Alternatively, postischaemic myocardial stunning has been proposed as a possible trigger factor [17]. Conversely, AMI may be triggered by TTS [18]. A recent report described a case of thromboembolism from a left ventricular thrombus as a result of TTS causing AMI [19]. Alternatively, pain has been described as a trigger for TTS [20], and the chest pain from AMI could potentially have triggered sympathetic activation.

Frangieh et al. found that T wave inversion on presentation was twice as common in TTS (45%) compared with AMI (22%) [21]. The lack of T wave inversion on presentation in this case followed by the development of deep T wave inversion across the precordial leads could suggest that AMI was the initial pathology followed by TTS. Furthermore, the QTc interval increased from 390 msec on the presentation to 527 msec when the T wave inversion evolved. A prolonged QT interval has also been associated with TTS rather than AMI [21, 22]. A shorter time to peak troponin (<6 hours) and smaller troponin rise have been found to be predictive of TTS [22], in contrast to our case where a large troponin rise was seen which peaked 24 hours after admission.

This case adds to the growing body of literature suggesting TTS and coronary artery disease may not be mutually exclusive as once thought; however, more work is required to identify the nature of the link and whether TTS is the cause or consequence of AMI in those patients in whom it coexists.

Consent

The authors confirm that written consent for submission and publication of this case report including images and associated text has been obtained from the patient.

References

[1] K. Dote, H. Sato, H. Tateishi, T. Uchida, and M. Ishihara, "Myocardial stunning due to simultaneous multivessel coronary spasms: a review of 5 cases," *Journal of Cardiology*, vol. 21, no. 2, pp. 203–214, 1991.

[2] E. Bossone, G. Savarese, F. Ferrara et al., "Takotsubo cardiomyopathy: overview," *Heart Failure Clinics*, vol. 9, no. 2, pp. 249–266, 2013.

[3] A. Mukherjee, B. Sunkel-Laing, and N. Dewhurst, "'Broken heart' syndrome in Scotland: a case of Takotsubo cardiomyopathy in a recently widowed lady," *Scottish Medical Journal*, vol. 58, no. 1, pp. e15–e19, 2013.

[4] S. W. Sharkey, J. R. Lesser, M. S. Maron, and B. J. Maron, "Why not just call it tako-tsubo cardiomyopathy: a discussion of nomenclature," *Journal of the American College of Cardiology*, vol. 57, no. 13, pp. 1496-1497, 2011.

[5] B. J. Maron, J. A. Towbin, G. Thiene et al., "Contemporary definitions and classification of the cardiomyopathies: an American Heart Association Scientific Statement from the Council on Clinical Cardiology, Heart Failure and Transplantation Committee; Quality of Care and Outcomes Research and Functional Genomics and Translational Biology Interdisciplinary Working Groups; and Council on Epidemiology and Prevention," *Circulation*, vol. 113, no. 14, pp. 1807–1816, 2006.

[6] A. R. Lyon, E. Bossone, B. Schneider et al., "Current state of knowledge on takotsubo syndrome: a position statement from the taskforce on takotsubo syndrome of the Heart Failure Association of the European Society of Cardiology," *European Journal of Heart Failure*, vol. 18, no. 1, pp. 8–27, 2016.

[7] R. Showkathali, H. Patel, A. Ramoutar et al., "Typical takotsubo cardiomyopathy in suspected ST elevation myocardial infarction patients admitted for primary percutaneous coronary intervention," *European Journal of Internal Medicine*, vol. 25, no. 2, pp. 132–136, 2014.

[8] C. Templin, J. R. Ghadri, J. Diekmann et al., "Clinical features and outcomes of takotsubo (stress) cardiomyopathy," *The New England Journal of Medicine*, vol. 373, no. 10, pp. 929–938, 2015.

[9] I. S. Wittstein, D. R. Thiemann, J. A. C. Lima et al., "Neurohumoral features of myocardial stunning due to sudden emotional stress," *The New England Journal of Medicine*, vol. 352, no. 6, pp. 539–548, 2005.

[10] S. Y-Hassan, "Plasma epinephrine levels and its causal link to takotsubo syndrome revisited: critical review with a diverse conclusion," *Cardiovascular Revascularization Medicine*, 2018.

[11] S. Y-Hassan and R. De Palma, "Contemporary review on the pathogenesis of takotsubo syndrome: the heart shedding tears. Norepinephrine churn and foam at the cardiac sympathetic nerve terminals," *International Journal of Cardiology*, vol. 228, pp. 528–536, 2017.

[12] A. Prasad, A. Lerman, and C. S. Rihal, "Apical ballooning syndrome (Tako-Tsubo or stress cardiomyopathy): a mimic of acute myocardial infarction," *American Heart Journal*, vol. 155, no. 3, pp. 408–417, 2008.

[13] S. Y-Hassan and L. Henareh, "Spontaneous coronary artery dissection triggered post-ischemic myocardial stunning and takotsubo syndrome: two different names for the same condition," *Cardiovascular Revascularization Medicine*, vol. 14, no. 2, pp. 109–112, 2013.

[14] I. S. Hurtado Rendón, D. Alcivar, J. P. Rodriguez-Escudero, and K. Silver, "Acute myocardial infarction and stress cardiomyopathy are not mutually exclusive," *The American Journal of Medicine*, vol. 131, no. 2, pp. 202–205, 2018.

[15] G. Abreu, S. Rocha, N. Bettencourt et al., "An unusual trigger causing takotsubo syndrome," *International Journal of Cardiology*, vol. 223, pp. 118–120, 2016.

[16] J. E. Madias, "Why the current diagnostic criteria of takotsubo syndrome are outmoded: a proposal for new criteria," *International Journal of Cardiology*, vol. 174, no. 3, pp. 468–470, 2014.

[17] S. Y-Hassan, R. Themudo, and E. Maret, "Spontaneous coronary artery dissection and takotsubo syndrome: the chicken or the egg causality dilemma," *Catheterization and Cardiovascular Interventions*, vol. 89, no. 7, pp. 1215–1218, 2017.

[18] J. E. Madias, "On a plausible association of spontaneous coronary artery dissection and takotsubo syndrome," *Canadian Journal of Cardiology*, vol. 31, no. 11, article 1410.e1, 2015.

[19] S. Y-Hassan, S. Holmin, G. Abdula, and F. Böhm, "Thromboembolic complications in takotsubo syndrome: review and demonstration of an illustrative case," *Clinical Cardiology*, vol. 42, no. 2, pp. 312–319, 2019.

[20] M. J. Daly and L. J. Dixon, "Takotsubo cardiomyopathy in two preoperative patients with pain," *Anesthesia & Analgesia*, vol. 110, no. 3, pp. 708–711, 2010.

[21] A. H. Frangieh, S. Obeid, J. R. Ghadri et al., "ECG criteria to differentiate between takotsubo (stress) cardiomyopathy and myocardial infarction," *Journal of the American Heart Association*, vol. 5, no. 6, article e003418, 2016.

[22] G. Vaidya, A. J. Jaiswal, and B. Madhira, "'GET QT': clinical criteria to differentiate takotsubo cardiomyopathy from STEMI," *International Cardiovascular Forum Journal*, vol. 5, pp. 53–57, 2016.

43

Noncompaction and Takotsubo Syndrome in a Neuromuscular Disorder

Josef Finsterer,[1] **Claudia Stöllberger**,[2] **and Walter Benedikt Winkler**[2]

[1]*Krankenanstalt Rudolfstiftung, Vienna, Austria*
[2]*2nd Medical Department with Cardiology and Intensive Care Medicine, Krankenanstalt Rudolfstiftung, Vienna, Austria*

Correspondence should be addressed to Josef Finsterer; fifigs1@yahoo.de

Academic Editor: Nurten Sayar

Background. Takotsubo syndrome (TTS) in patients with left ventricular hypertrabeculation/noncompaction (LVHT) has been reported in four patients, and a TTS plus LVHT plus a neuromuscular disorder (NMD) was only reported once so far. Here, we present the fifth patient with LVHT and TTS and the second patient with LVHT, TTS, and a NMD. *Methods and Results.* The patient is a 68 yo female hobby choir singer with a history of skin dermatofibroma, skin fibrokeratoma, arterial hypertension, hyperlipidemia, hypothyroidism, anemia, hyponatremia, diverticulosis, LVHT detected at age 60 y, five syncopes, a liver cyst, and carotid endarterectomy 2 months prior to admission because of sudden-onset chest pain. Workup revealed ST elevation, troponin elevation, and mild coronary artery sclerosis. Ventriculography and transthoracic echocardiography (TTE) showed the apical type of a TTS. ECG normalised within 10 w and TTE within 6 w under beta-blockers and ATII-blockers. The TTS was triggered by being offended of being unable to sing anymore after endarterectomy. Neurological workup suggested the presence of a NMD. *Conclusions.* This case shows that LVHT occurs in NMD patients and that patients with LVHT and a NMD may develop a TTS. Whether patients with LVHT and a NMD are particularly prone to develop a TTS requires further confirmation. NMD patients with LVHT should avoid stress not to trigger a TTS.

1. Introduction

Only few patients with left ventricular hypertrabeculation (LVHT), also known as noncompaction, have been reported who also developed a Takotsubo syndrome (TTS) [1–4]. This unusual combination has been reported in a patient with a Beals-Hecht syndrome [1], a female with myotonic dystrophy type 1 [2], a 76 yo female without other concomitant diseases [3], and in a 12 yo female with low-grade glioma of the cerebellar vermis [4]. Here, we report a fifth patient with LVHT who developed a TTS shortly after carotid endarterectomy.

2. Methods and Results

The patient is a 68 yo Caucasian female, height 170 cm, weight 68 kg, with a previous history of smoking (20 pack-years) until age 50 y, arterial hypertension since age 40 y, and resection of a dermatofibroma on the right upper arm and a fibrokeratoma of the 3rd digit of the left foot at age 50 y. The individual history was further positive for struma nodosa and Hashimoto thyroiditis since age 58 y, hyperlipidemia since at least age 58 y, a liver cyst in segments 6/7, diverticulosis of the colon, first detected at age 58 y, and myoma resection. Also, since age 58 y, she temporarily experienced a few panic attacks for which she was hospitalised once at age 60 y. Since age 59 y, she reported a mild sleep disorder. Mild anemia of unknown cause was recognised since age 59 y. Since at least age 59 y, recurrent hyponatremia in the absence of taking diuretics or serotonin reuptake inhibitors was noted. LVHT was first diagnosed at age 60 y and confirmed at age 68 y (Figure 1). Since age 63 y, she experienced recurrent nausea and abdominal pain with a tendency for constipation and flatulence. Gastroscopy and colonoscopy only revealed the known diverticulosis. Workup for secondary arterial hypertension at age 67 y was negative. Parathyroid hormone, renin, aldosterone, and ACTH levels were all in the normal range. There was recurrent transient

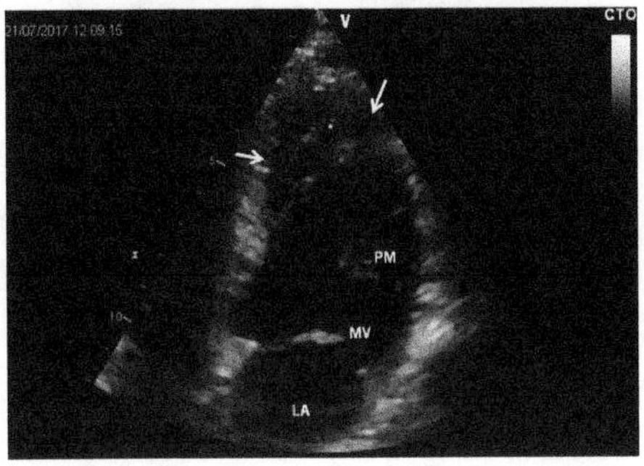

FIGURE 1: Echocardiographic apical five chamber view from 2017 showing hypertrabeculation/noncompaction in the apex (arrows). LA: left atrium; MV: mitral valve; PM: anterolateral papillary muscle.

lymphocytosis, but workup for malignancy was negative. The family history was positive for epilepsy (2nd brother), dementia (2nd brother), migraine (daughter), arterial hypertension (father, mother, and 1st sister), arrhythmias (2nd sister), diabetes (father), tuberculosis with osteomyelitis (1st sister), Graves' disease (daughter), and coronary heart disease (father and 1st brother). She was a passionate hobby choir singer since years.

Workup for two syncopes at age 67 y (the second with secessus urinae) and three syncopes before revealed normal systolic function and confirmed previously diagnosed LVHT on transthoracic echocardiography (TTE). Long-term electrocardiogram (ECG) had not been carried out so far. Concerning the neurological history, she reported muscle cramps under simvastatin, exercise intolerance, and easy fatigability. Upon the neurological exam, an exaggerated masseter reflex, generally reduced tendon reflexes, and fasciculations of the right adductor pollicis muscle were found. Electroencephalography (EEG), cerebral computed tomography (CCT), and cerebral magnetic resonance imaging (MRI) were normal, but carotid ultrasound and MR angiography (MRA) revealed a high-grade stenosis of the left internal carotid artery. This is why she underwent carotid endarterectomy of the left internal and common carotid artery. Postoperatively, she experienced recurrent collapses, hypertensive crises, and uncertainty and fear but no further syncope.

Two months after surgery, she developed sudden onset thoracic pain. Since ECG showed ST elevation and troponin was elevated, myocardial infarction was suspected. However, acute coronary angiography revealed only mild coronary sclerosis but ventriculography showed the apical type of a TTS (Figure 2), which was confirmed by TTE. Already 6 d after the onset of symptoms, TTE showed almost normal systolic function, mild myocardial thickening, diastolic dysfunction grade 2, and regional apical akinesia/hypokinesia. TTE normalised completely within 6 w and the ECG within 10 w. The presumed trigger of the TTS was being offended of being unable to sing again. The cause of hyponatremia remained speculative. A syndrome of inadequate ADH secretion (SIADH) was excluded, and the patient was asked to salt the food more extensively. She is currently taking acetyl-salicylic acid, bisoprolol, candesartan, rilmenidine, and simvastatin.

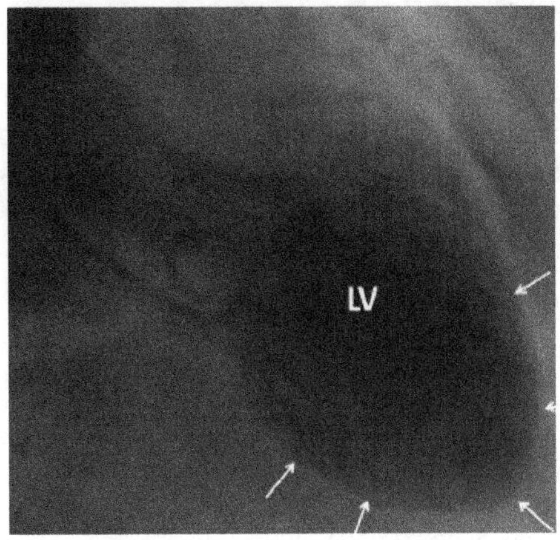

FIGURE 2: Ventriculography showing apical ballooning (arrows) of the left ventricle (LV).

3. Discussion

The patient is interesting for the coincidence of LVHT and a TTS and the presence of a NMD. A coincidence of LVHT and a TTS has been reported only in four patients before [1–4], suggesting that LVHT does not promote the development of a TTS. However, systematic investigations on the question if cardiomyopathy is generally a predisposing factor for the development of a TTS are not available. Thus, it is still conceivable that cardiomyopathy is less resistant to a catecholamine storm than the normal myocardium and that LVHT is nonetheless a risk factor for the development of a TTS.

Concerning the notion that LVHT occurs in up to 80% of the patients with a NMD [5], the present case confirms such a relation. The neurological history revealed muscle cramps under simvastatin, exercise intolerance, and easy fatigability, and the neurological exam revealed generally reduced tendon reflexes and fasciculation in the right adductor pollicis muscle, suggesting the presence of a NMD. The type of NMD, however, remained speculative since further workup for a NMD was not feasible. Anyhow, a metabolic NMD is more likely than a structural NMD.

LVHT is frequently complicated by ventricular arrhythmias, heart failure, or embolism [6]. None of these conditions had been recognised yet in the present patient, but it cannot be excluded that TTS is another, hitherto, not recognised complication of LVHT. In this respect, it is conceivable that already little distress, less than in cardiologically healthy patients, triggers the development of a TTS. Whether the five syncopes were rather due to ventricular arrhythmias, due to transient heart failure, or due to cardiovascular embolism than due to the carotid artery stenosis remains speculative. Seizures were excluded as a cause of the syncopes.

In conclusion, this case shows that LVHT occurs in NMD patients and that patients with LVHT and a NMD may experience a TTS. Whether patients with LVHT and a NMD are particularly prone to develop a TTS requires further investigations. NMD patients with LVHT should avoid extreme stress not to trigger a TTS.

Authors' Contributions

JF was assigned in patient care, design, literature search, discussion, and the first draft of the manuscript. CS and W-BW contributed to the patient care, literature search, discussion, and critical comments of the manuscript. All three authors contributed equally in this study.

References

[1] T. Matsumoto, A. Watanabe, M. Migita et al., "Transient cardiomyopathy in a patient with congenital contractural arachnodactyly (Beals syndrome)," *Journal of Nippon Medical School*, vol. 73, no. 5, pp. 285–288, 2006.

[2] J. Finsterer, C. Stöllberger, A. Hornykewycz, and M. Gencik, "Noncompaction predisposing for recurrent Takotsubo syndrome in myotonic dystrophy 1," *International Journal of Cardiology*, vol. 168, no. 2, pp. e38–e39, 2013.

[3] T. D. Karamitsos, S. Bull, N. Spyrou, S. Neubauer, and J. B. Selvanayagam, "Tako-tsubo cardiomyopathy presenting with features of left ventricular non-compaction," *International Journal of Cardiology*, vol. 128, no. 1, pp. e34–e36, 2008.

[4] G. De Rosa, M. Pardeo, C. Di Rocco et al., "Neurogenic stunned myocardium presenting as left ventricular hypertrabeculation in childhood: a variant of Takotsubo cardiomyopathy?," *Pediatric Critical Care Medicine*, vol. 12, no. 6, pp. e420–e423, 2011.

[5] C. Stöllberger, J. Finsterer, and G. Blazek, "Left ventricular hypertrabeculation/noncompaction and association with additional cardiac abnormalities and neuromuscular disorders," *The American Journal of Cardiology*, vol. 90, no. 8, pp. 899–902, 2002.

[6] J. Finsterer, C. Stöllberger, and J. A. Towbin, "Left ventricular noncompaction cardiomyopathy: cardiac, neuromuscular, and genetic factors," *Nature Reviews Cardiology*, vol. 14, no. 4, pp. 224–237, 2017.

Permissions

All chapters in this book were first published by Hindawi Publishing Corporation; hereby published with permission under the Creative Commons Attribution License or equivalent. Every chapter published in this book has been scrutinized by our experts. Their significance has been extensively debated. The topics covered herein carry significant findings which will fuel the growth of the discipline. They may even be implemented as practical applications or may be referred to as a beginning point for another development.

The contributors of this book come from diverse backgrounds, making this book a truly international effort. This book will bring forth new frontiers with its revolutionizing research information and detailed analysis of the nascent developments around the world.

We would like to thank all the contributing authors for lending their expertise to make the book truly unique. They have played a crucial role in the development of this book. Without their invaluable contributions this book wouldn't have been possible. They have made vital efforts to compile up to date information on the varied aspects of this subject to make this book a valuable addition to the collection of many professionals and students.

This book was conceptualized with the vision of imparting up-to-date information and advanced data in this field. To ensure the same, a matchless editorial board was set up. Every individual on the board went through rigorous rounds of assessment to prove their worth. After which they invested a large part of their time researching and compiling the most relevant data for our readers.

The editorial board has been involved in producing this book since its inception. They have spent rigorous hours researching and exploring the diverse topics which have resulted in the successful publishing of this book. They have passed on their knowledge of decades through this book. To expedite this challenging task, the publisher supported the team at every step. A small team of assistant editors was also appointed to further simplify the editing procedure and attain best results for the readers.

Apart from the editorial board, the designing team has also invested a significant amount of their time in understanding the subject and creating the most relevant covers. They scrutinized every image to scout for the most suitable representation of the subject and create an appropriate cover for the book.

The publishing team has been an ardent support to the editorial, designing and production team. Their endless efforts to recruit the best for this project, has resulted in the accomplishment of this book. They are a veteran in the field of academics and their pool of knowledge is as vast as their experience in printing. Their expertise and guidance has proved useful at every step. Their uncompromising quality standards have made this book an exceptional effort. Their encouragement from time to time has been an inspiration for everyone.

The publisher and the editorial board hope that this book will prove to be a valuable piece of knowledge for researchers, students, practitioners and scholars across the globe.

List of Contributors

Irushna Perera and Sanjeewa Rajapakse
Colombo North Teaching Hospital, Ragama, Sri Lanka

Shamila T. De Silva
Colombo North Teaching Hospital, Ragama, Sri Lanka
Faculty of Medicine, University of Kelaniya, Sri Lanka

Fadi Kandah, Tanya Deol, Pooja Dhruva and Zachary Chandler
Internal Medicine, UF Health Jacksonville, Dept. of Medicine, 655 W 8th Street, Jacksonville, FL 32209 -6595, USA

Thaer Musa and Gladys Velarde
Cardiology, UF Health Jacksonville, Dept. of Cardiology, 655 W 8th Street, Jacksonville, FL 32209-6595, USA

Tarun Dalia
Internal Medicine, University of Kansas Medical Center, Kansas City, KS 66160, USA

Bashar S. Amr and Jared Kvapil
Department of Cardiovascular Medicine, University of Kansas Medical Center, Kansas City, KS 66160, USA

Ankit Agrawal
Internal Medicine Residency Program, Rutgers Robert Wood Johnson Medical School-Saint Peter's University Hospital, New Brunswick, NJ 08901, USA

Archana Gautam
Montgomery Internal Medicine Residency Program, University of Alabama, Montgomery, Alabama 36116, USA

Venkata Rakesh Sethapati
Department of Pathology & Laboratory Medicine, University of Kansas Medical Center, Kansas City, KS 66160, USA

Huihui Ma, Jing Zhang, Yongmei Zhou, Tao He, Jianhong Tao and Xiaoping Li
Department of Cardiology, Sichuan Provincial People's Hospital, University of Electronic Science and Technology of China, Chengdu, Sichuan 610072, China
Chinese Academy of Sciences Sichuan Translational Medicine Research Hospital, Chengdu 610072, China

Xin Cao
Chengdu University of Traditional Chinese Medicine, Chengdu, Sichuan 610075, China

Rong Luo
Institute of Geriatric Cardiovascular Disease, Chengdu Medical College, Chengdu, Sichuan 610500, China

Ian Garrahy, Peter Nicholas III and Oreoluwa Oladiran
Department of Internal Medicine, Reading Hospital and Medical Center, Tower Health, West Reading, PA, USA

Salik Nazir
Department of Cardiology, University of Toledo Medical Center, Toledo, Ohio, USA

Michael J. McGee
School of Medicine and Public Health, University of Newcastle, Newcastle, NSW, Australia
Cardiovascular Department, John Hunter Hospital, Newcastle, NSW, Australia
Hunter Medical Research Institute, Newcastle, NSW, Australia

William Yu, Joshua McCarthy, Malcolm Barlow and Rosemary Hackworthy
Cardiovascular Department, John Hunter Hospital, Newcastle, NSW, Australia

Nicholas Mencer and Larry Todd Justice
Department of Interventional Cardiology Methodist Medical Center, Oak Ridge, Tennessee 37748, USA

William Black and Kayleigh Litton
Department of Interventional Cardiology, The University of Tennessee Knoxville, Knoxville, Tennessee 37996, USA

Fusako Sera, Shunsuke Nishimura, Kei Nakamoto, Yasumasa Tsukamoto, Isamu Mizote, Tomohito Ohtani, Shungo Hikoso and Yasushi Sakata
Department of Cardiovascular Medicine, Osaka University Graduate School of Medicine, Osaka, Japan

Tomoko Inoue
Department of Cardiovascular Medicine, Osaka University Graduate School of Medicine, Osaka, Japan
Department of Cardiorenal and Cerebrovascular Medicine, Faculty of Medicine, Kagawa University, Kagawa, Japan

Tetsuo Minamino
Department of Cardiorenal and Cerebrovascular Medicine, Faculty of Medicine, Kagawa University, Kagawa, Japan

Yoshihiko Ikeda and Hatsue Ishibashi-Ueda
Department of Pathology, National Cardiovascular Center, Osaka, Japan

Yumiko Hori and Eiichi Morii
Department of Pathology, Osaka University Graduate School of Medicine, Osaka, Japan

Gift Echefu and Daniel Hammett
Baton Rouge General Medical Center Internal Medicine Residency Program, Baton Rouge, LA, USA

Amir Ausef
Hospital Medicine Group, Baton Rouge General Medical Center, Baton Rouge, LA, USA

Lance LaMotte
Baton Rouge Cardiology Center, Baton Rouge, LA, USA
Martin Chaumont, Rachid Briki, Philippe Unger and Nadia Debbas
Cardiology Department, CHU Saint-Pierre, 322 rue Haute, B-1000 Brussels, Belgium

Marc Blaimont
Cardiology Department, Hôpital de Jolimont, 7100 La Louvière, Belgium

Laura Onderko, Benjamin Starobin, Amy E. Riviere, Patrick K. Hohl, Colin T. Phillips, Roisin B. Morgan, Aimee Welsh, Sanjeev A. Francis and Maxwell Eyram Afari
Cardiovascular Disease Service Line, Maine Medical Center, Portland, Maine, USA

Abdulbaril Olagunju
Department of Medicine, Creighton University, Phoenix, AZ, USA

Chandana Shekar, Anantharam Kalya, Farouk Mookadam and Samuel Unzek
Heart Center, Banner University Medical Center, University of Arizona College of Medicine-Phoenix, Phoenix, AZ, USA

Michael Morris
Department of Diagnostic Radiology, Banner University Medical Center, University of Arizona College of Medicine-Phoenix, Phoenix, AZ, USA

Malik Shehadeh
Medstar Washington Hospital Center, Washington, D. C, USA

Ana Barac
Medstar Washington Hospital Center, Washington, D. C, USA
Medstar Heart and Vascular Institute, Washington, D. C, USA

Rachel Marcus
Medstar Union Memorial Hospital and Latin American Society of Chagas (LASOCHA), USA

Mohammed Abdullahi Talle and Faruk Buba
Department of Medicine, College of Medical Sciences, University of Maiduguri, Nigeria
Cardiology Unit, Department of Medicine, University of Maiduguri Teaching Hospital, Maiduguri, Nigeria

Aimé Bonny
University of Douala, Cameroon

Musa Mohammed Baba
Department of Medicine, College of Medical Sciences, University of Maiduguri, Nigeria
Cardiology Unit, Department of Medicine, College of Medical Sciences, Gombe State University, Gombe, Nigeria

Vishal I. Patel
St. Mary Medical Center, Department of Internal Medicine, USA
UCLA David Geffen School of Medicine, USA

Serap Sobnosky
St. Mary Medical Center, Department of Internal Medicine, USA
UCLA David Geffen School of Medicine, USA
St. Mary Medical Center, Department of Cardiology, USA

Elyssa Cohen, Conor P. O'Halloran, Philip T. Thrush and Paul Tannous
Ann & Robert H. Lurie Children's Hospital of Chicago, Chicago, IL, USA
Northwestern University Feinberg School of Medicine, Chicago, IL, USA

T. Marsha Ma
Loyola University Medical Center, Chicago, IL, USA

Robert Lembo, Paul Wesley and Joe B. Calkins
Department of Cardiovascular Medicine, Medical College of Georgia, 1120 15th Street, Augusta, GA 30912, USA

Fariba Alaei
Pediatric Cardiology Department, Mofid Children's Hospital, Faculty of Medicine, Shahid Beheshti University of Medical Sciences, Tehran, Iran

Marjan Shakiba and Hedyeh Saneifard
Pediatric Endocrinology and Metabolism Department, Mofid Children's Hospital, Faculty of Medicine, Shahid Beheshti University of Medical Sciences, Tehran, Iran

Kourosh Vahidshahi
Pediatric Cardiology, Shahid Modarres Hospital, Faculty of Medicine, Shahid Beheshti University of Medical Sciences, Tehran, Iran

Mastaneh Alaei
Blood Transfusion Research Center, High Institute for Research and Education in Transfusion Medicine, Tehran, Iran

Julia Tian and Asif Uddin
Department of Medicine, Northwell Health at Staten Island University Hospital, Staten Island, NY 10305, USA

Philippe Akhrass
Department of Electrophysiology, Northwell Health at Staten Island University Hospital, Staten Island, NY 10305, USA

Tomoyuki Watanabe
Division of Internal Medicine, Health Co-op, Watari Hospital, Fukushima, Japan

Toshihiro Terui
Division of Internal Medicine, Health Co-op, Watari Hospital, Fukushima, Japan
International Community Health, Graduate School of Medicine, Fukushima Medical University, Fukushima, Japan
Department of Neuropsychiatry, Fukushima Medical University, Fukushima, Japan

Masumi Iwai-Takano
Department of Epidemiology, Fukushima Medical University, Fukushima, Japan
Division of Cardiovascular Surgery, Fukushima Medical University, Fukushima, Japan
Fukushima Prefectural General Hygiene Institute, Fukushima, Japan

Juan Vaz
Department of Medicine, Halmstad Hospital, Halmstad, Sweden

Rikard Berggren
Department of Cardiology, Halmstad Hospital, Halmstad, Sweden

Berne Eriksson
Department of Medicine, Halmstad Hospital, Halmstad, Sweden
Krefting Research Centre, Institute of Medicine, University of Gothenburg, Gothenburg, Sweden

Kolade M. Agboola, Barry A. Boilson, Naveen L. Pereira and Jacob C. Jentzer
Department of Cardiovascular Medicine, Mayo Clinic College of Medicine, Rochester, MN 55905, USA

Trevon McGill
Department of General Internal Medicine, Mayo Clinic College of Medicine, Rochester, MN 55905, USA

Hugo R. Martinez
Cincinnati Children's Hospital Medical Center, Heart Institute, Cincinnati, OH, USA

Adrienne M. Hammill
Department of Pediatrics, University of Cincinnati College of Medicine, Cincinnati, OH, USA
Cincinnati Children's Hospital Medical Center, Division of Hematology, Cincinnati, OH, USA

Chet Villa, Matthew Bacon, Samuel G. Wittekind and Angela Lorts
Cincinnati Children's Hospital Medical Center, Heart Institute, Cincinnati, OH, USA
Department of Pediatrics, University of Cincinnati College of Medicine, Cincinnati, OH, USA

Christian Georgi, Michael Neuß, Viviane Möller, Martin Seifert, and Christian Butter
Heart Center Brandenburg-Department of Cardiology and Medical School Brandenburg Theodor Fontane, Bernau bei Berlin, Germany

Nathan Zaher, Rashid Al Hussain and Diane Levine
Department of Internal Medicine, Wayne State University/Detroit Medical Center, Michigan, USA

Hammam Shereef
Department of Internal Medicine, Beaumont Hospital-Dearborn, Michigan, USA

John Dawdy and M. Chadi Alraies
Division of Cardiology, Wayne State University/ Detroit Medical Center, Michigan, USA

A. Ganes and L. Segan
Department of Cardiology, Barwon Health, Bellerine Street, Geelong, VIC 3220, Australia

Daniel Costa
Department of Cardiology, Kettering General Hospital NS Foundation Trust, Rothwell Road, Kettering, NN16 8UZ, UK

Azhar Farooqui
Department of Cardiology, Kettering General Hospital NS Foundation Trust, Rothwell Road, Kettering, NN16 8UZ, UK
University Hospitals of Leicester NHS Trust, Leicester, UK

Tin Lwin
Department of Cardiology, Kettering General Hospital NS Foundation Trust, Rothwell Road, Kettering, NN16 8UZ, UK
Department of Cardiology, Castle Hill Hospital, UK

Simon Hetherington and Raj Mattu
Department of Cardiology, Kettering General Hospital NS Foundation Trust, Rothwell Road, Kettering, NN16 8UZ, UK
University of Leicester, Leicester, UK

Christopher Nnaoma, Christoph Sossou, Tobi Ogundare and Ogechukwu Chika-Nwosuh
Internal Medicine Resident, Newark Beth Israel Medical Center, Newark, NJ, USA

Amee Sodha
Teaching Attending Physician, Newark Beth Israel Medical Center, Newark, NJ, USA

Cynthia McKinney
Medical Student, St. George's University School of Medicine, Grenada

Jose Bustillo
Associate Program Director, Internal Medicine, Newark Beth Israel Medical Center, Newark, NJ, USA

Kalaimani Elango
Department of Cardiology-University of Nevada, Las Vegas-Kirk Kirkorian School of Medicine, USA

Sadaf Fakhra
Department of Internal Medicine-University of Nevada, Las Vegas-Kirk Kirkorian School of Medicine, USA

Shabada Asad
Department of Infectious Disease-University of Nevada, Las Vegas-Kirk Kirkorian School of Medicine, USA

Sunny Patel
Department of Medicine, Long Island Jewish Forest Hills, Northwell Health, New York, USA

Sepideh Nabatian and Michael Goyfman
Department of Cardiology, Long Island Jewish Forest Hills, Northwell Health, New York, USA

Michael H. Chiu, Cvetan Trpkov, Saman Rezazedeh and Derek S. Chew
Libin Cardiovascular Institute of Alberta, Cummings School of Medicine, University of Calgary, Alberta, Canada

Mohammad Dlewati, Kyeeun Park and Saumya Rawat
Division of Internal Medicine, Memorial Healthcare System, Hollywood, Florida, USA

Jorge Conte and Kashmira Bhadha
Division of Internal Medicine, Memorial Healthcare System, Hollywood, Florida, USA
Division of Cardiology, Memorial Healthcare System, Hollywood, Florida, USA

Ian Lancaster, Jeffrey Steinhoff, Jose Mosco-Guzman, and Deep Patel
HCA Healthcare/USF Morsani College of Medicine GME/Largo Medical Center, USA

N. F. N. Sakul and Nikhita Balabbigari
Department of Internal Medicine, Overlook Medical Center, Summit, NJ 07901, USA

Srijan Shrestha and Sapan Talati
Department of Cardiology, Morristown Medical Center, Morristown, NJ 07960, USA

Rebecca A. Ocher
Department of Medicine, University of California, Los Angeles, Los Angeles, California, USA

Erika Padilla, Jonathan C. Hsu and Pam R. Taub
Division of Cardiovascular Medicine, Department of Medicine, University of California, San Diego, California, USA

Ariyon Schreiber
University of Nevada Las Vegas School of Medicine, Department of Medicine, USA

Michael Gardner, Chris Sossou and Natasha Greene
Department of Cardiology, University of Nevada, Las Vegas, Las Vegas, USA

Young Min Cho, Abdullah Asreb, Riaz Mahmood and Ahmad Moaz
Internal Medicine Residency Program, Northeast Georgia Medical Center, Gainesville, Georgia, USA

Ugochukwu Egolum
Georgia Heart Institute, Northeast Georgia Medical Center, Gainesville, Georgia, USA

Aneesh Bapat, Abhishek Maan and E. Kevin Heist
Cardiac Arrhythmia Service, Massachusetts General Hospital, Boston, MA 02114, USA

Evan Harmon, Sebastian Estrada, Sula Mazimba and Younghoon Kwon
University of Virginia Health System, Charlottesville, VA, USA

Ryan J. Koene
Cleveland Clinic Foundation, Cleveland, OH, USA

Nosheen Reza, Jessica L. Chowns, Amy Marzolf, Jessica Kim and Anjali Tiku Owens
Center for Inherited Cardiovascular Disease, Division of Cardiovascular Medicine, Perelman School of Medicine, University of Pennsylvania, Philadelphia, PA, USA

Lisa D. Levine
Maternal and Child Health Research Center, Department of Obstetrics and Gynecology, Perelman School of Medicine, University of Pennsylvania, Philadelphia, PA, USA

Gregory Supple
Cardiac Electrophysiology Section, Division of Cardiovascular Medicine, Perelman School of Medicine, University of Pennsylvania, Philadelphia, PA, USA

KaChon Lei, Wilbur Ji, Bhavana Bhaya and Chowdhury Ahsan
Kirk Kerkorian School of Medicine at University of Nevada, Las Vegas, Department of Internal Medicine, USA
Kirk Kerkorian School of Medicine at University of Nevada, Las Vegas, Division of Cardiovascular Medicine, USA

Saad Ezad and Michael McGee
John Hunter Hospital, Hunter New England Health, Newcastle, NSW, Australia

Andrew J. Boyle
John Hunter Hospital, Hunter New England Health, Newcastle, NSW, Australia
The University of Newcastle, Newcastle, NSW, Australia
Hunter Medical Research Institute, Newcastle, NSW, Australia

Josef Finsterer
Krankenanstalt Rudolfstiftung, Vienna, Austria

Claudia Stöllberger and Walter Benedikt Winkler
Krankenanstalt Rudolfstiftung, Vienna, Austria
2nd Medical Department with Cardiology and Intensive Care Medicine, Krankenanstalt Rudolfstiftung, Vienna, Austria

Index